IARC MONOGRAPHS
ON THE
EVALUATION OF THE CARCINOGENIC RISK
OF CHEMICALS TO HUMANS:

Some *N*-Nitroso Compounds

Volume 17

This publication represents the views and expert opinions
of an IARC Working Group on the
Evaluation of the Carcinogenic Risk of Chemicals to Humans
which met in Lyon,
10-15 October 1977

May, 1978

IARC MONOGRAPHS

In 1971, the International Agency for Research on Cancer (IARC) initiated a programme on the evaluation of the carcinogenic risk of chemicals to humans involving the production of critically evaluated monographs on individual chemicals.

The role of the monograph programme is to collect all available relevant experimental and epidemiological data about groups of chemicals to which humans are known to be exposed, to evaluate these data in terms of human risk with the help of international working groups of acknowledged experts in chemical carcinogenesis and related fields, and to publish and disseminate the conclusions of those working groups as a series of IARC Monographs.

ISBN 92 832 12177

PRINTED IN SWITZERLAND

IARC WORKING GROUP ON THE EVALUATION OF THE CARCINOGENIC
RISK OF CHEMICALS TO HUMANS:

SOME *N*-NITROSO COMPOUNDS

Lyon, 10-15 October 1977

Members[1]

Dr J.R. Allen, Professor of Pathology, University of Wisconsin, The Medical School Department of Pathology, 470 North Charter Street, Madison, Wisconsin 53706, USA

Dr B.K. Armstrong, University of Western Australia, Department of Medicine, Medical School Building, Queen Elizabeth II Medical Centre, Nedlands, Western Australia 6009, Australia

Professor P. Bannasch, Abteilung für Cytopathologie, Institut für Experimentelle Pathologie, Deutsches Krebsforschungszentrum, Postfach, 6900 Heidelberg 1, FRG

Dr G. Bochert, Institut für Toxikologie und Embryonal-Pharmakologie der Freien Universität Berlin, Garystrasse 9, 1000 Berlin 33, FRG

Dr J. Cooper[2], Division of Cancer Cause and Prevention, National Cancer Institute, Bethesda, Maryland, USA

Dr D.H. Fine, Senior Scientist, Thermo Electron Research Center, 101 First Avenue, Waltham, Massachusetts 02154, USA

Dr W. Lijinsky, Director, Chemical Carcinogenesis Program, Frederick Cancer Research Center, PO Box B, Frederick, Maryland 21701, USA

Dr P.N. Magee, Director, Fels Research Institute, Temple University, School of Medicine, Philadelphia, Pennsylvania 19140, USA (*Chairman*)

Professor U. Mohr, Director, Abteilung für Experimentelle Pathologie, Medizinische Hochschule Hannover, Karl-Wiechert-Allee 9, 3000 Hannover 61, FRG

---

[1]Unable to attend: Dr G. Eisenbrand, Institut für Toxikologie und Chemotherapie, Deutsches Krebsforschungszentrum, Im Neuenheimer Feld 280, 6900 Heidelberg 1, FRG

[2]Present address: Unit of Epidemiology and Biostatistics, International Agency for Research on Cancer, 150 Cours Albert Thomas, 69372 Lyon Cédex 2, France

Dr A.E. Pegg, Professor, Department of Physiology, The Milton S. Hershey Medical Center, The Pennsylvania State University, Hershey, Pennsylvania 17033, USA

Professor R. Preussmann, Institut für Toxikologie und Chemotherapie, Deutsches Krebsforschungszentrum, Im Neuenheimer Feld 280, 6900 Heidelberg 1, FRG (*Vice-Chairman*)

Professor C. Rappe, Department of Organic Chemistry, Umeå University, S-901 87 Umeå, Sweden

Dr B.W. Stewart, School of Pathology, University of New South Wales, PO Box 1, Kensington, New South Wales 2033, Australia

Professor S.R. Tannenbaum, Professor of Food Chemistry, Department of Nutrition and Food Science, Massachusetts Institute of Technology, Cambridge, Massachusetts 02139, USA

Dr E. Vogel, Department of Radiation Genetics and Chemical Mutagenesis of the State University of Leiden, Wassenaarseweg 72, Leiden, The Netherlands

Observers

Dr H.E. Christensen, Chief, Information Processing Unit, Room 31, International Register of Potentially Toxic Chemicals, United Nations Environment Programme, World Health Organization, 1211 Geneva 27, Switzerland

Dr K.E. McCaleb, Director, Chemical-Environmental Program, Chemical Industries Center, SRI International, Menlo Park, California 94025, USA (*Rapporteur sections 2.1 and 2.2*)

Mrs M.-T. van der Venne, Commission of the European Communities, Health and Safety Directorate, Bâtiment Jean Monnet, Plateau du Kirchberg, Boîte Postale 1907, Luxembourg, Great Duchy of Luxembourg

Representative from the National Cancer Institute

Dr S. Siegel, Coordinator, Technical Information Activities, Technical Information Resources Branch, Room 3A-06, Landow Building, Carcinogenesis Bioassay Testing Program, Division of Cancer Cause and Prevention, National Cancer Institute, Bethesda, Maryland 20014, USA

Secretariat

Dr H. Bartsch, Unit of Chemical Carcinogenesis (*Rapporteur section 3.2*)

Dr L. Griciute, Chief, Unit of Environmental Carcinogens

Dr J.E. Huff, Unit of Chemical Carcinogenesis (*Secretary*)

Mrs D. Mietton, Unit of Chemical Carcinogenesis (*Library assistant*)

Dr R. Montesano, Unit of Chemical Carcinogenesis
(*Rapporteur section 3.1*)

Mrs C. Partensky, Unit of Chemical Carcinogenesis (*Technical editor*)

Mrs I. Peterschmitt, Unit of Chemical Carcinogenesis, WHO, Geneva
(*Bibliographic researcher*)

Dr V. Ponomarkov, Unit of Chemical Carcinogenesis

Dr R. Saracci, Unit of Epidemiology and Biostatistics
(*Rapporteur section 3.3*)

Dr L. Tomatis, Chief, Unit of Chemical Carcinogenesis
(*Head of the Programme*)

Mr E.A. Walker, Unit of Environmental Carcinogens
(*Rapporteur sections 1 and 2.3*)

Mrs E. Ward, Montignac, France (*Editor*)

Mr J.D. Wilbourn, Unit of Chemical Carcinogenesis (*Co-secretary*)

Secretarial assistance

Miss A.V. Anderson

Mrs M.-J. Ghess

Miss R.B. Johnson

NOTE TO THE READER

The term 'carcinogenic risk' in the IARC Monograph series is taken to mean the probability that exposure to the chemical will lead to cancer in humans.

Inclusion of a chemical in the monographs does not imply that it is a carcinogen, only that the published data have been examined. Equally, the fact that a chemical has not yet been evaluated in a monograph does not mean that it is not carcinogenic.

Anyone who is aware of published data that may alter the evaluation of the carcinogenic risk of a chemical for humans is encouraged to make this information available to the Unit of Chemical Carcinogenesis, International Agency for Research on Cancer, Lyon, France, in order that the chemical may be considered for reevaluation by a future Working Group.

Although every effort is made to prepare the monographs as accurately as possible, mistakes may occur. Readers are requested to communicate any errors to the Unit of Chemical Carcinogenesis, so that corrections can be reported in future volumes.

CONTENTS

IARC MONOGRAPH PROGRAMME ON THE EVALUATION OF THE CARCINOGENIC RISK OF CHEMICALS TO HUMANS

PREAMBLE

BACKGROUND

In 1971, the International Agency for Research on Cancer (IARC) initiated a programme on the evaluation of the carcinogenic risk of chemicals to humans centred on the production of critically evaluated monographs on individual chemicals. Since 1972, the programme has undergone considerable expansion, primarily with the scientific collaboration and financial support of the US National Cancer Institute.

The criteria established in 1971 to evaluate the carcinogenic risk of chemicals to humans were adopted in essence by all the working groups whose deliberations resulted in the first 16 volumes of the *IARC Monograph* series. In October 1977, a joint IARC/WHO *ad hoc* Working Group met to reevaluate these guiding criteria; this preamble reflects the results of their deliberations[1].

OBJECTIVE AND SCOPE

The objective of the monograph programme is to collect all available relevant experimental and epidemiological data about groups of chemicals to which humans are known to be exposed, to evaluate these data in terms of human risk with the help of international working groups of experts in chemical carcinogenesis and related fields, and to publish and disseminate the conclusions of those working groups as a series of monographs.

The critical evaluations of experimental data given in these monographs are intended to assist national and international authorities in formulating decisions concerning preventive measures. The WHO publications on food additives[2], drugs[3], pesticides and contaminants[4] and occupational carcinogens[5] are particularly informative.

Since the programme began in 1971, 17 volumes have been published[6-22] in the *IARC Monograph* series, and 380 separate chemicals have been evaluated (see cumulative index to the monographs, p. 353). Each volume is printed in 4000 copies and distributed *via* the World Health Organization (WHO) publications service (see inside covers for a listing of IARC publications and back outside cover for distribution and sales services).

The *IARC Monographs* are recognized as an authoritative source of information on the carcinogenicity of environmental chemicals. The first users' survey, made in 1976, indicates that the monographs are consulted routinely by various agencies in 24 countries.

SELECTION OF CHEMICALS FOR MONOGRAPHS

The chemicals (natural and synthetic, mixtures and manufacturing processes) are selected for evaluation on the basis of two main criteria: (1) there is evidence of human exposure, and (2) there is some experimental evidence of carcinogenicity and/or there is some evidence or suspicion of a risk to humans. *Inclusion of a chemical in a volume does not imply that the chemical is carcinogenic, only that the published data have been examined. The evaluations must be consulted to ascertain the conclusions of the Working Group. Equally, the fact that a chemical has not appeared in a monograph does not mean that the chemical is not carcinogenic.*

The scientific literature is monitored for published data relevant to the monograph programme. Additionally, the IARC Survey of Chemicals Being Tested for Carcinogenicity[23-29] often indicates those chemicals that are to be scheduled for future meetings. The major aims of the survey are to prevent unnecessary duplication of research, to increase communication among scientists, and to make a census of chemicals that are being tested and of available research facilities.

When new, relevant information becomes available concerning a chemical(s) which has already been evaluated, or when new principles for evaluating carcinogenic risk receive acceptance, reevaluations may be made at subsequent meetings, and a monograph(s) may be revised and published.

WORKING PROCEDURES

Approximately one year in advance of a working group meeting, a list of the substances to be considered is prepared by IARC in consultation with other experts. Subsequently, all relevant biological data are collected by IARC; in this context, US Public Health Service Publication No. 149[30-35] has been particularly valuable and has been used in conjunction with other recognized sources of information on chemical carcinogenesis. The major effort in the collection of data and the preparation of first drafts for the sections on chemical and physical properties, on production, use and occurrence and on analysis is made by SRI International under a separate contract with the US National Cancer Institute. Most of the data they provide on production, use and occurrence concern the United States and Japan; SRI and IARC try to supplement this information with that from other sources in Europe. Important bibliographical sources for mutagenicity and teratogenicity data are the Environmental Mutagen Informational Center and the Environmental Teratology Information Center, both located at the Oak Ridge National Laboratory, USA.

Six to nine months before the meeting, reprints of articles containing relevant biological data are sent to an expert(s), or are used by the IARC staff, for the preparation of first drafts of the monographs. These drafts are edited by IARC staff and are sent prior to the meeting to all participants of the Working Group for their comments. The Working Group then meets in Lyon for seven to eight days to discuss and finalize the texts of the monographs and to formulate the evaluations. After the meeting, the master copy of each monograph is verified by consulting the original literature, then edited and prepared for reproduction. The monographs appear in print within six months after adjournment of the Working Group meeting.

DATA FOR EVALUATIONS

With regard to biological data, generally only reports that have been published or accepted for publication are reviewed by the working groups. The monographs do not cite all of the literature on a particular chemical:

only those data considered by the Working Group to be relevant to the evaluation of the carcinogenic risk of the chemical to humans are included.

Anyone who is aware of data that have been published or are in press which are relevant to the evaluations of the carcinogenic risk to humans of chemicals for which monographs have appeared is urged to make them available to the Unit of Chemical Carcinogenesis, International Agency for Research on Cancer, Lyon, France.

THE WORKING GROUP

During a meeting the tasks of the Working Group are generally fivefold: (1) to confirm that all relevant published data are included; (2) to ensure that the summaries of data enable the reader to follow the reasoning of the committee; (3) to judge the significance of the experimental and epidemiological results; (4) to select and summarize the data on which to base an evaluation; and (5) to formulate an evaluation of the carcinogenic risk of the chemical.

Working Group participants who contributed to the consideration and evaluation of chemicals within a particular volume are listed, with their addresses, at the beginning of each publication (see p. 3). Each member serves as an individual scientist and not as a representative of any organization or government. In addition, observers are often invited from national and international agencies, organizations and industries.

GENERAL PRINCIPLES FOR EVALUATING THE CARCINOGENIC RISK OF CHEMICALS

The widely accepted meaning of the term 'chemical carcinogenesis', and that used in these monographs, is the induction by chemicals of neoplasms that are not usually observed, the earlier induction by chemicals of neoplasms that are usually observed, and/or the induction by chemicals of more neoplasms than are usually found, although fundamentally different mechanisms may be involved in these three phenomena. Etymologically, the term 'carcinogenesis' means the induction of cancer, that is, of malignant neoplasms; however, the commonly accepted meaning is the induction of various types of neoplasms or of a combination of malignant and benign tumours.

Within the monographs, the words 'tumour' and neoplasm' are used interchangeably (In scientific literature the terms 'tumourigen', 'oncogen' and 'blastomogen' have all been used synonymously with 'carcinogen', although occasionally 'tumourigen' has been used specifically to denote the induction of benign tumours).

The term 'carcinogenic risk' in this *IARC Monograph* series is taken to mean the probability that exposure to the chemical will lead to cancer in humans.

Experimental Evidence

Qualitative aspects

Both the interpretation and evaluation of a particular study as well as the overall assessment of the carcinogenic activity of a chemical involve several qualitatively important considerations, including:
(1) the experimental conditions under which the chemical was tested, including route of administration and exposure, species, strain, sex, age, etc.; (2) the consistency with which the chemical has been shown to be carcinogenic, e.g., in how many species and at which tumour sites(s); (3) the spectrum of neoplastic response, from benign neoplasia to multiple malignant tumours (this consideration warrants special attention); (4) the stage of tumour formation in which a chemical may be involved: some chemicals act as complete carcinogens and have initiating and promoting activity, while others are promoters only; and 5) the possible role of modifying agents.

Many chemicals induce both benign and malignant tumours; few instances are recorded in which only benign neoplasms are induced by chemicals that have been studied extensively. Benign tumours may represent a stage in the evolution of a malignant neoplasm or they may be 'end-points' which do not readily undergo transition to malignant neoplasms. If a substance is found to induce only benign neoplasms in experimental animals, the chemical should be suspected of being a carcinogen and requires further investigation.

Hormonal carcinogenesis

Hormonal carcinogenesis presents certain distinctive features: the chemicals involved occur both naturally and exogenously; in most instances, long exposure is required; tumours occur in the target issue in association with a stimulation of non-neoplastic growth, but in some cases, hormones promote the proliferation of tumour cells in a target organ. Hormones that occur in excessive amounts, hormone-mimetic agents and agents that cause hyperactivity or imbalance in the endocrine system may require evaluative methods comparable with those used to identify chemical carcinogens; particular emphasis must be laid on quantitative aspects and duration of exposure. Some chemical carcinogens have significant side effects on the endocrine system, which may also result in hormonal carcinogenesis. Synthetic hormones and anti-hormones can be expected to possess other pharmacological and toxicological actions in addition to those on the endocrine system, and in this respect they must be treated like any other chemical with regard to intrinsic carcinogenic potential.

Quantitative aspects

Dose-response studies are important in the evaluation of carcinogenesis: the confidence with which a carcinogenic effect can be established is strengthened by the observation of an increasing incidence of neoplasms with increasing exposure.

The assessment of carcinogenicity in animals is frequently complicated by recognized differences among the test animals (species, strain, sex, age), in route(s) of administration and in dose/duration of exposure; often, target organs at which a cancer occurs and its histological type may vary with these conditions. Nevertheless, indices of carcinogenic potency in particular experimental systems (for instance, the dose-rate required under continuous exposure to halve the probability of the animals remaining tumourless[36]) have been formulated in the hope that, at least among categories of fairly similar agents, such indices may be of some predictive value in other systems, including humans.

Chemical carcinogens differ widely in the dose required to produce a given level of tumour induction, although many of them share common biological properties which include metabolism to reactive (electrophilic[37-39]) intermediates capable of interacting with DNA. The reason for this variation in dose-response is not understood but may be due either to differences within a common metabolic process or to the operation of qualitatively distinct mechanisms.

Statistical analysis of animal studies

Tumours which would have arisen had an animal lived longer may not be observed because of the death of the animal from unrelated causes, and proper allowance must be made for this possibility. Various analytical techniques have been developed which use the assumption of independence of competing risks to allow for the effects of intercurrent mortality on the final numbers of tumour-bearing animals in particular treatment groups.

For externally visible tumours and for neoplasms that cause death, methods such as Kaplan-Meier (i.e., 'life-table', 'product-limit' or 'actuarial') estimates[36], with associated significance tests[40,41], are recommended.

For internal neoplasms which are discovered 'incidentally'[40] at autopsy but which did not cause the death of the host, different estimates[42] and significance tests[40,41] may be necessary for the unbiased study of the numbers of tumour-bearing animals.

All of these methods[36,40,41,42] can be used to analyse the numbers of animals bearing particular tumour types, but they do not distinguish between animals with one or many such tumours. In experiments which end at a particular fixed time with the simultaneous sacrifice of many animals, analysis of the total numbers of internal neoplasms per animal found at autopsy at the end of the experiment is straightforward. However, there are no adequate statistical methods for analysing the numbers of particular neoplasms that kill an animal host.

There are problems not only of differential survival but of differential toxicity, which may be manifested by unequal growth and weight gain in treated and control animals. These complexities should also be considered in the interpretation of data, or, better, in the experimental design.

Evidence of Carcinogenicity in Humans

Evidence of carcinogenicity in humans can be derived from three types of study, the first two of which usually provide only suggestive evidence: (1) reports concerning individual cancer patients (case reports), including a history of exposure to the supposed carcinogenic agent; (2) descriptive epidemiological studies in which the incidence of cancer in human populations is found to vary (spatially or temporally) with exposure to the agent); and (3) analytical epidemiological studies (e.g., case-control or cohort studies) in which individual exposure to the agent is found to be associated with an increased risk of cancer.

An analytical study that shows a positive association between an agent and a cancer may be interpreted as implying causality to a greater or lesser extent, if the following criteria are met: (1) There is no identifiable positive bias (By 'positive bias' is meant the operation of factors in study design or execution which lead erroneously to a more strongly positive association between an agent and disease than in fact exists. Examples of positive bias include, in case-control studies, more nearly complete ascertainment of exposure to the agent in cases than in controls and, in cohort studies, more nearly complete detection of cancer in individuals exposed to the agent than in individuals not exposed). (2) The possibility of positive confounding has been considered (By 'positive confounding' is meant a situation in which the relationship between an agent and a disease is rendered more strongly positive than it truly is as a result of an association between that agent and another agent which either causes or prevents the disease. An example of positive confounding is the association between coffee consumption and lung cancer, which results from their joint association with cigarette smoking). (3) The association is unlikely to be due to chance alone. (4) The association is strong. (5) There is a dose-response relationship.

In some instances, a single epidemiological study may be strongly indicative of a cause-effect relationship, however, the most convincing evidence of causality comes when several independent studies done under different circumstances result in 'positive' findings.

Analytical epidemiological studies that show no association between an agent and a cancer ('negative' studies) should be interpreted according to criteria analogous to those listed above: (1) There is no identifiable negative bias. (2) The possibility of negative confounding has been considered. (3) The possible effects of misclassification of exposure or outcome have been considered.

In addition, it must be recognized that in any study there are confidence limits around the estimate of association or relative risk. In a study regarded as 'negative', the upper confidence limit may indicate a relative risk substantially greater than unity; in that case, the study excludes only relative risks that are above this upper limit. This usually means that a 'negative' study must be large to be convincing. Confidence in a 'negative' result is increased when several independent studies carried out under different circumstances are in agreement.

Finally, a 'negative' study may be considered to be relevant only to dose levels within or below the range of those observed in the study and is pertinent only if sufficient time has elapsed since first human exposure to the agent. Experience with human cancers of known etiology suggests that the period from first exposure to a chemical carcinogen to development of clinically observed cancer is usually measured in decades and may be in excess of 30 years.

Experimental Data Relevant to the Evaluation of Carcinogenic Risk to Humans

No adequate criteria are presently available to interpret experimental carcinogenicity data directly in terms of carcinogenic potential for humans. Nonetheless, utilizing data collected from appropriate tests in animals, positive extrapolations to possible human risk can reasonably be approximated.

Information compiled from the first 17 volumes of the *Monographs*[43-45] shows that of about 26 chemicals or manufacturing processes now generally accepted to cause cancer in humans, all but possibly two (arsenic and benzene) of those which have been tested appropriately produce cancer in at least one animal species. For several (aflatoxins, 4-aminobiphenyl, diethylstilboestrol, melphalan, mustard gas and vinyl chloride), evidence of carcinogenicity in experimental animals preceded evidence obtained from epidemiological studies or case reports.

In general, the evidence that a chemical produces tumours in experimental animals is of two degrees: (1) *sufficient evidence* of carcinogenicity is indicated by the production of malignant tumours; and (2) *limited evidence* of carcinogenicity reflects the qualitative and/or quantitative limitations of the experimental results.

For many of the chemicals evaluated in the first 17 volumes of the *IARC Monographs* for which there is *sufficient evidence* of carcinogenicity in animals, data relating to carcinogenicity for humans are either insufficient or nonexistent. In the absence of adequate data on humans, it is reasonable to regard for practical purposes such chemicals as if they were carcinogenic to humans.

Sufficient evidence of carcinogenicity is provided by experimental studies that show an increased incidence of malignant tumours: (a) in multiple species or strains, and/or (b) in multiple experiments (routes and/or doses), and/or (c) to an unusual degree (with regard to incidence, site, type and/or precocity of onset). Additional evidence may be provided by data concerning dose-response, mutagenicity or structure.

In the present state of knowledge, it would be difficult to define a predictable relationship between the dose (mg/kg bw/day) of a particular chemical required to produce cancer in test animals and the dose which would produce a similar incidence of cancer in humans. The available data suggest, however, that such a relationship may exist[46], at least for certain classes of carcinogenic chemicals. Data that provide *sufficient evidence* of carcinogenicity in test animals may therefore be used in an approximate quantitative evaluation of the human risk at some given exposure level, provided that the nature of the chemical concerned and the physiological, pharmacological and toxicological differences between the test animals and humans are taken into account. However, no acceptable methods are currently available for quantifying the possible errors in such a procedure, whether it is used to generalize between species or to extrapolate from high to low doses. The methodology for such quantitative extrapolation to humans requires further development.

Evidence for the carcinogenicity of some chemicals in experimental animals may be limited for two reasons. Firstly, experimental data may be restricted to such a point that it is not possible to determine a causal relationship between administration of a chemical and the development of a particular lesion in the animals. Secondly, there are certain neoplasms, including lung tumours and hepatomas in mice, which have been considered of lesser significance than neoplasms occurring at other sites for the purpose of evaluating the carcinogenic risk of chemicals to humans. Such tumours occur spontaneously in high incidence in these animals, and their malignancy is often difficult to establish. An evaluation of the significance of these tumours following administration of a chemical is the responsibility of the particular Working Group preparing the individual monograph, and it has not been possible to set down rigid guidelines; the relevance of these tumours must be determined by considerations which include experimental design and completeness of reporting.

Some chemicals for which there is *limited evidence* of carcinogenicity in animals have also been studied in humans with, in general, inconclusive results. While such chemicals may indeed be carcinogenic to humans, more experimental and epidemiological investigation is required.

Hence, '*sufficient evidence*' of carcinogenicity and '*limited evidence*' of carcinogenicity do not indicate categories of chemicals: the inherent definitions of those terms indicate varying degrees of experimental evidence, which may change if and when new data on the chemicals become available. The main drawback to any rigid classification of chemicals with regard to their carcinogenic capacity is the as yet incomplete knowledge of the mechanism(s) of carcinogenesis.

In recent years, several short-term tests for the detection of potential carcinogens have been developed. When only inadequate experimental data are available, positive results in validated short-term tests (see p. 25) are an indication that the compound is a potential carcinogen and that it should be tested in animals for an assessment of its carcinogenicity. Negative results from short-term tests cannot be considered sufficient evidence to rule out carcinogenicity. Whether short-term tests will eventually attain a stature similar to that of long-term tests in predicting carcinogenicity in humans will depend on further demonstrations of consistency with long-term experiments and with data from humans.

EXPLANATORY NOTES ON THE MONOGRAPH CONTENTS

Chemical and Physical Data (Section 1)

The Chemical Abstracts Service Registry Number and the latest Chemical Abstracts Primary Name (9th Collective Index) are recorded in section 1. Other synonyms and trade names are given, but this list is often not comprehensive. Further, some of the trade names are those of mixtures in which the compound being evaluated is only one of the ingredients.

The structural and molecular formulae, molecular weight and chemical and physical properties are given. The properties listed refer to the pure substance, unless otherwise specified, and include, in particular, data that might be relevant to carcinogenicity (for example, lipid solubility) and those that concern identification. A separate description of the composition of technical products includes available information on impurities and formulated products.

Production, Use, Occurrence and Analysis (Section 2)

The purpose of section 2 is to provide indications of the extent of past and present human exposure to this chemical.

Synthesis

Since cancer is a delayed toxic effect, the dates of first synthesis and of first commercial production of the chemical are provided. In addition, methods of synthesis used in past and present commercial production are described. This information allows a reasonable estimate to be made of the time before which no human exposure could have occurred.

Production

Since Europe, Japan and the United States are reasonably representative industrialized areas of the world, most data on production, foreign trade and uses are obtained from those countries. It should not, however, be inferred that those nations are the sole or even the major sources of users of any individual chemical.

Production and foreign trade data are obtained from both governmental and trade publications by chemical economists in the three geographical areas. In some cases, separate production data on organic chemicals manufactured in the United States are not available because their publication could disclose confidential information. In such cases, an indication of the minimum quantity produced can be obtained from the number of companies reporting commercial production. Each company is required to report on individual chemicals if the sales value or the weight of the annual production of a chemical exceeds a specified minimum level. These levels vary for chemicals classified for different uses, e.g., medicinals, plastics; however, the minimal annual sales value is between $1000 and $50,000 and the minimal annual weight of production is between 450 and 22,700 kg. Data on production in some European countries are obtained by means of general questionnaires sent to companies thought to produce the compounds being evaluated. Information from the completed questionnaires is compiled by country, and the resulting estimates of production are included in the individual monographs.

Use

Information on uses is meant to serve as a guide only and is not complete. It is usually obtained from published data but is often complemented by direct contact with manufacturers of the chemical. In the case of drugs, mention of their therapeutic uses does not necessarily represent current practice nor does it imply judgement as to their clinical efficacy.

Statements concerning regulations and standards (e.g., pesticide registrations, maximum levels permitted in foods, occupational standards and allowable limits) in specific countries are mentioned as examples only. They may not reflect the most recent situation, since such legislation is in a constant state of change; nor should it be taken to imply that other countries do not have similar regulations.

Occurrence

Information on the occurrence of a chemical in the environment is obtained from published data, including that derived from the monitoring and surveillance of levels of the chemical in occupation environments, air, water, soil, foods and tissues of animals and humans. When available, data on the generation, persistence and bioaccumulation of a chemical are also included.

Analysis

The purpose of the section on analysis is to give the reader an indication, rather than a complete review, of methods cited in the literature. No attempt is made to evaluate critically or to recommend any of the methods.

Biological Data Relevant to the Evaluation of Carcinogenic Risk to Humans (Section 3)

In general, the data recorded in section 3 are summarized as given by the author; however, certain shortcomings of reporting, of statistical analysis or of experimental design are commented upon by the Working Group in square brackets. The nature and extent of impurities/contaminants in the chemicals being tested are given when available.

Carcinogenicity and related studies in animals

The monographs are not intended to cover all reported studies. Some studies are purposely omitted (1) because they are inadequate, as judged from previously described criteria[47-50] (e.g., too short a duration, too few animals, poor survival); (2) because they only confirm findings that have already been fully described; or (3) because they are judged irrelevant for the purpose of the evaluation. In certain cases, however, such studies are mentioned briefly, particularly when the information is considered to be a useful supplement to other reports or when it is the only data available. Their inclusion does not, however, imply acceptance of the adequacy of their experimental design and/or of the analysis and interpretation of their results.

Mention is made of all routes of administration by which the compound has been adequately tested and of all species in which relevant tests have been done[4,50]. In most cases, animal strains are given (general characteristics of mouse strains have been reviewed[51]). Quantitative data are given to indicate the order of magnitude of the effective carcinogenic doses. In general, the doses and schedules are indicated as they appear in the original paper; sometimes units have been converted for easier comparison. Experiments on the carcinogenicity of known metabolites, chemical precursors, analogues and derivatives, and experiments on factors that modify the carcinogenic effect are also reported.

Other relevant biological data

Lethality data are given when available, and other data on toxicity are included when considered relevant. The metabolic data are restricted to studies that show the metabolic fate of the chemical in animals and man, and comparisons of data from animals and humans are made when possible. Information is also given on absorption, distribution, excretion and placental transfer.

Embryotoxicity and teratogenicity

Data on teratogenicity from studies in experimental animals and observations in humans are also included. There appears to be no necessary causal relationship between teratogenicity[52] and carcinogenicity, but chemicals often have both properties. Evidence of teratogenicity suggests transplacental transfer, which is a prerequisite for transplacental carcinogenesis.

Mutagenicity and other short-term tests

Data from indirect tests are also included. Since most of these tests have the advantage of taking less time and being less expensive than mammalian carcinogenicity studies, they are generally known as 'short-term' tests. They comprise assay procedures which rely on the induction of biological and biochemical effects in *in vivo* and/or *in vitro* systems. The end-point of the majority of these tests is not the production of neoplasms in animals but changes at the molecular, cellular or multicellular level: these include the induction of DNA damage and repair, mutagenesis in bacteria and other organisms, transformation of mammalian cells in culture, and other systems.

The short-term tests are proposed for use (1) in predicting potential carcinogenicity in the absence of carcinogenicity data in animals, (2) as a contribution in deciding which chemicals should be tested in animals, (3) in identifying active fractions of complex mixtures containing carcinogens, (4) for recognizing active metabolites of known carcinogens in human and/or animal body fluids and (5) to help elucidate mechanisms of carcinogenesis.

Although the theory that cancer is induced as a result of somatic mutation suggests that agents which damage DNA *in vivo* may be carcinogens, the precise relevance of short-term tests to the mechanism by which cancer is induced is not known. Predictions of potential carcinogenicity are currently based on correlations between responses in short-term tests and data from animal carcinogenicity and/or human epidemiological studies. This approach is limited because the number of chemicals known to be carcinogenic in humans is insufficient to provide a basis for validation, and most validation studies involve chemicals that have been evaluated for carcinogenicity only in animals. The selection of chemicals is in turn limited to those classes for which data on carcinogenicity are available. The results of validation studies could be strongly influenced by such selection of chemicals and by the proportion of carcinogens in the series of chemicals tested; this should be kept in mind when evaluating the predictivity of a particular test. The usefulness of any test is reflected by its ability to classify carcinogens and noncarcinogens, using the animal data as a standard; however, animal tests may not always provide a perfect standard. The attainable level of correlation between short-term tests and animal bioassays is still under investigation.

Since many chemicals require metabolism to an active form, test systems that do not take this into account may fail to detect certain potential carcinogens. The metabolic activation systems used in short-term tests (for example, the cell-free systems used in bacterial tests) are meant to simulate the intact human. Each has its advantages and limitations; thus, more confidence can be placed in the conclusions when negative or positive results for a chemical are confirmed in several such test systems. Deficiencies in metabolic competence may lead to misclassification of chemicals, which means that not all tests are suitable for assessing the potential carcinogenicity of all classes of compounds.

The present state of knowledge does not permit the selection of a specific test(s) as the most appropriate for identifying potential carcinogenicity. Before the results of a particular test can be considered to be fully acceptable for predicting potential carcinogenicity, certain criteria should be met: (1) the test should have been validated with respect to known animal carcinogens and found to have a high capacity for discriminating between carcinogens and noncarcinogens, and (2) when possible, a structurally related carcinogen(s) and noncarcinogen(s) should have been tested simultaneously with the chemical in question. The results should have been reproduced in different laboratories, and a prediction of carcinogenicity should have been confirmed in additional test systems. Confidence in positive results is increased if a mechanism of action can be deduced and if appropriate dose-response data are available. For optimum usefulness, data on purity must be given.

The short-term tests in current use that have been the most extensively validated are the *Salmonella typhimurium* plate-incorporation assay[53-57], the X-linked recessive lethal test in *Drosophila melanogaster*[58], unscheduled DNA synthesis[59] and *in vitro* transformation[57,60]. Each is compatible with current concepts of the possible mechanism(s) of carcinogenesis.

An adequate assessment of the genetic activity of a chemical depends on data from a wide range of test systems. The monographs include, therefore, data not only from those already mentioned, but also on the induction of point mutations in other systems[61-66], of structural[67] and numerical chromosome aberrations, including dominant lethal effects[68], of mitotic recombination in fungi[61] and of sister chromatid exchanges[69,70].

The existence of a correlation between quantitative aspects of mutagenic and carcinogenic activity has been suggested[4,68-74], but it is not sufficiently well established to allow general use.

Further information about mutagenicity and other short-term tests is given in references 71-77.

Case reports and epidemiological studies

Observations in humans are summarized in this section.

Summary of Data Reported and Evaluation (Section 4)

Section 4 summarizes the relevant data from animals and humans and gives the critical views of the Working Group on those data.

Experimental data

Data relevant to the evaluation of the carcinogenicity of a chemical in animals are summarized in this section. Results from validated mutagenicity and other short-term tests are reported if the Working Group considered the data to be relevant. Dose-response data are given when available. An assessment of the carcinogenicity of the chemical in animals is made on the basis of all of the available data.

The animal species mentioned are those in which the carcinogenicity of the substance was clearly demonstrated. The route of administration used in experimental animals that is similar to the possible human exposure is given particular mention. Tumour sites are also indicated. If the substance has produced tumours after prenatal exposure or in single-dose experiments, this is indicated.

Human data

Human exposure to the chemical is summarized, and the significance of data on production, use and occurrence and other relevant biological data is discussed. Case reports and epidemiological studies that are considered to be pertinent to an assessment of human carcinogenicity are described. Adequate dose-response data are given when available. An assessment of the carcinogenicity of the chemical in humans is made on the basis of all of the available evidence.

Evaluation

This section comprises the overall evaluation by the Working Group of the carcinogenic risk of the chemical to humans. All of the data in the monograph, and particularly the summarized information on experimental and human data, are considered in order to make an evaluation. In addition, recommendations are made regarding areas in which further investigation is considered to be necessary.

References

1. IARC (1977) Technical Report 77/002, Preamble, International Agency for Research on Cancer, Lyon

2. WHO (1961) Fifth Report of the Joint FAO/WHO Expert Committee on Food Additives. Evaluation of carcinogenic hazard of food additives. Wld Hlth Org. techn. Rep. Ser., No. 220, pp. 5, 18, 19

3. WHO (1969) Report of a WHO Scientific Group. Principles for the testing and evaluation of drugs for carcinogenicity. Wld Hlth Org. techn. Rep. Ser., No. 426, pp. 19, 21, 22

4. WHO (1974) Report of a WHO Scientific Group. Assessment of the carcinogenicity and mutagenicity of chemicals. Wld Hlth Org. techn. Rep. Ser., No. 546

5. WHO (1964) Report of a WHO Expert Committee. Prevention of cancer. Wld Hlth Org. techn. Rep. Ser., No. 276, pp. 29, 30

6. IARC (1972) IARC Monographs on the Evaluation of the Carcinogenic Risk of Chemicals to Man, 1, Some Inorganic Substances, Chlorinated Hydrocarbons, Aromatic Amines, *N*-Nitroso Compounds and Natural Products, Lyon, 184 pages

7. IARC (1973) IARC Monographs on the Evaluation of the Carcinogenic Risk of Chemicals to Man, 2, Some Inorganic and Organometallic Compounds, Lyon, 181 pages

8. IARC (1973) IARC Monographs on the Evaluation of the Carcinogenic Risk of Chemicals to Man, 3, Certain Polycyclic Aromatic Hydrocarbons and Heterocyclic Compounds, Lyon, 271 pages

9. IARC (1974) IARC Monographs on the Evaluation of the Carcinogenic Risk of Chemicals to Man, 4, Some Aromatic Amines, Hydrazine and Related Substances, *N*-Nitroso Compounds and Miscellaneous Alkylating Agents, Lyon, 286 pages

10. IARC (1974) IARC Monographs on the Evaluation of the Carcinogenic Risk of Chemicals to Man, 5, Some Organochlorine Pesticides, Lyon, 241 pages

11. IARC (1974) IARC Monographs on the Evaluation of the Carcinogenic Risk of Chemicals to Man, 6, Sex Hormones, Lyon, 243 pages

12. IARC (1974) IARC Monographs on the Evaluation of the Carcinogenic Risk of Chemicals to Man, 7, Some Anti-thyroid and Related Substances, Nitrofurans and Industrial Chemicals, Lyon, 326 pages

13. IARC (1975) IARC Monographs on the Evaluation of the Carcinogenic Risk of Chemicals to Man, 8, Some Aromatic Azo Compounds, Lyon, 357 pages

14. IARC (1975) IARC Monographs on the Evaluation of the Carcinogenic Risk of Chemicals to Man, 9, Some Aziridines, *N*-, *S*- and *O*-Mustards and Selenium, Lyon, 268 pages

15. IARC (1976) IARC Monographs on the Evaluation of the Carcinogenic Risk of Chemicals to Man, 10, Some Naturally Occurring Substances, Lyon, 353 pages

16. IARC (1976) IARC Monographs on the Evaluation of the Carcinogenic Risk of Chemicals to Man, 11, Cadmium, Nickel, Some Epoxides, Miscellaneous Industrial Chemicals and General Considerations on Volatile Anaesthetics, Lyon, 306 pages

17. IARC (1976) IARC Monographs on the Evaluation of the Carcinogenic Risk of Chemicals to Man, 12, Some Carbamates, Thiocarbamates and Carbazides, Lyon, 282 pages

18. IARC (1977) IARC Monographs on the Evaluation of the Carcinogenic Risk of Chemicals to Man, 13, Some Miscellaneous Pharmaceutical Substances, Lyon, 255 pages

19. IARC (1977) IARC Monographs on the Evaluation of the Carcinogenic Risk of Chemicals to Man, 14, Asbestos, Lyon, 106 pages

20. IARC (1977) IARC Monographs on the Evaluation of the Carcinogenic Risk of Chemicals to Man, 15, Some Fumigants, the Herbicides 2,4-D and 2,4,5-T, Chlorinated Dibenzodioxins and Miscellaneous Industrial Chemicals, Lyon, 354 pages

21. IARC (1977) IARC Monographs on the Evaluation of the Carcinogenic Risk of Chemicals to Man, 16, Some Aromatic Amines and Related Nitro Compounds - Hair Dyes, Colouring Agents and Miscellaneous Industrial Chemicals, Lyon, 400 pages

22. IARC (1978) IARC Monographs on the Evaluation of the Carcinogenic Risk of Chemicals to Humans, 17, Some *N*-Nitroso Compounds, Lyon, 365 pages

23. IARC (1973) IARC Information Bulletin on the Survey of Chemicals Being Tested for Carcinogenicity, No. 1, Lyon, 52 pages

24. IARC (1973) IARC Information Bulletin on the Survey of Chemicals Being Tested for Carcinogenicity, No. 2, Lyon, 77 pages

25. IARC (1974) IARC Information Bulletin on the Survey of Chemicals Being Tested for Carcinogenicity, No. 3, Lyon, 67 pages

26. IARC (1974) IARC Information Bulletin on the Survey of Chemicals Being Tested for Carcinogenicity, No. 4, Lyon, 97 pages

27. IARC (1975) IARC Information Bulletin on the Survey of Chemicals Being Tested for Carcinogenicity, No. 5, Lyon, 88 pages

28. IARC (1976) IARC Information Bulletin on the Survey of Chemicals Being Tested for Carcinogenicity, No. 6, Lyon, 360 pages

29. IARC (1978) IARC Information Bulletin on the Survey of Chemicals Being Tested for Carcinogenicity, No. 7, Lyon, 460 pages

30. Hartwell, J.L. (1951) Survey of Compounds which have been Tested for Carcinogenic Activity, Washington DC, US Government Printing Office (Public Health Service Publication No. 149)

31. Shubik, P. & Hartwell, J.L. (1957) Survey of Compounds which have been Tested for Carcinogenic Activity, Washington DC, US Government Printing Office (Public Health Service Publication No. 149: Supplement 1)

32. Shubik, P. & Hartwell, J.L. (1969) Survey of Compounds which have been Tested for Carcinogenic Activity, Washington DC, US Government Printing Office (Public Health Service Publication No. 149: Supplement 2)

33. Carcinogenesis Program National Cancer Institute (1971) Survey of Compounds which have been Tested for Carcinogenic Activity, Washington DC, US Government Printing Office (Public Health Service Publication No. 149: 1968-1969)

34. Carcinogenesis Program National Cancer Institute (1973) Survey of Compounds which have been Tested for Carcinogenic Activity, Washington DC, US Government Printing Office (Public Health Service Publication No. 149: 1961-1967)

35. Carcinogenesis Program National Cancer Institute (1974) Survey of Compounds which have been Tested for Carcinogenic Activity, Washington DC, US Government Printing Office (Public Health Service Publication No. 149: 1970-1971)

36. Pike, M.C. & Roe, F.J.C. (1963) An actuarial method of analysis of an experiment in two-stage carcinogenesis. Brit. J. Cancer, 17, 605-610

37. Miller, E.C. & Miller, J.A. (1966) Mechanisms of chemical carcinogenesis: nature of proximate carcinogens and interactions with macromolecules. Pharmacol. Rev., 18, 805-838

38. Miller, J.A. (1970) Carcinogenesis by chemicals: an overview - G.H.A. Clowes Memorial Lecture. Cancer Res., 30, 559-576

39. Miller, J.A. & Miller, E.C. (1976) The metabolic activation of chemical carcinogens to reactive electrophiles. In: Yuhas, J.M., Tennant, R.W. & Reagon, J.D., eds, Biology of Radiation Carcinogenesis, New York, Raven Press

40. Peto, R. (1974) Guidelines on the analysis of tumours rates and death rates in experimental animals. Brit. J. Cancer, 29, 101-105

41. Peto, R. (1975) Letter to the editor. Brit. J. Cancer, 31, 697-699

42. Hoel, D.G. & Walburg, H.E. (1972) Statistical analysis of survival experiments. J. nat. Cancer Inst., 49, 361-372

43. Tomatis, L. (1977) The value of long-term testing for the implementation of primary prevention. In: Hiatt, H.H., Watson, J.D. & Winsten, J.A., eds, Origins of Human Cancer, Book C, Cold Spring Harbor, N.Y., Cold Spring Harbor Laboratory, pp. 1339-1357

44. IARC (1977) Annual Report 1977, Lyon, International Agency for Research on Cancer, pp. 89-93

45. Tomatis, L., Agthe, C., Bartsch, H., Huff, J., Montesano, R., Saracci, R., Walker, E. & Wilbourn, J. (1978) Evaluation of the carcinogenicity of chemicals: a review of the IARC Monograph Programme, 1971-1977. Cancer Res., 38, 877-885

46. Rall, D.P. (1977) Species differences in carcinogenesis testing. In: Hiatt, H.H., Watson, J.D. & Winsten, J.A., eds, Origins of Human Cancer, Book C, Cold Spring Harbor, N.Y., Cold Spring Harbor Laboratory, pp. 1383-1390

47. WHO (1958) Second Report of the Joint FAO/WHO Expert Committee on Food Additives. Procedures for the testing of intentional food additives to establish their safety for use. Wld Hlth Org. techn. Rep. Ser., No. 144

48. WHO (1967) Scientific Group. Procedures for investigating intentional and unintentional food additives. Wld Hlth Org. techn. Rep. Ser., No. 348

49. Berenblum, I., ed. (1969) Carcinogenicity testing. UICC techn. Rep. Ser., 2

50. Sontag, J.M., Page, N.P. & Saffiotti, U. (1976) Guidelines for carcinogen bioassay in small rodents. National Cancer Institute Carcinogenesis techn. Rep. Ser., No. 1

51. Committee on Standardized Genetic Nomenclature for Mice (1972) Standardized nomenclature for inbred strains of mice. Fifth listing. Cancer Res., 32, 1609-1646

52. Wilson, J.G. & Fraser, F.C. (1977) Handbook of Teratology, New York, Plenum Press

53. Ames, B.N., Durston, W.E., Yamasaki, E. & Lee, F.D. (1973) Carcinogens are mutagens: a simple test system combining liver homogenates for activation and bacteria for detection. Proc. nat. Acad. Sci. (Wash.), 70, 2281-2285

54. McCann, J., Choi, E., Yamasaki, E. & Ames, B.N. (1975) Detection of carcinogens as mutagens in the *Salmonella*/microsome test: assay of 300 chemicals. Proc. nat. Acad. Sci. (Wash.), 72, 5135-5139

55. McCann, J. & Ames, B.N. (1976) Detection of carcinogens as mutagens in the *Salmonella*/microsome test: assay of 300 chemicals: discussion. Proc. nat. Acad. Sci. (Wash.), 73, 950-954

56. Sugimura, T., Sato, S., Nagao, M., Yahagi, T., Matsushima, T., Seino, Y., Takeuchi, M. & Kawachi, T. (1977) Overlapping of carcinogens and mutagens. In: Magee, P.N., Takayama, S., Sugimura, T. & Matsushima, T., eds, Fundamentals in Cancer Prevention, Baltimore, University Park Press, pp. 191-215

57. Purchase, I.F.M., Longstaff, E., Ashby, J., Styles, J.A., Anderson, D., Lefevre, P.A. & Westwood, F.R. (1976) Evaluation of six short term tests for detecting organic chemical carcinogens and recommendations for their use. Nature (Lond.), 264, 624-627

58. Vogel, E. & Sobels, F.H. (1976) The function of *Drosophila* in genetic toxicology testing. In: Hollaender, A., ed., Chemical Mutagens: Principles and Methods for Their Detection, Vol. 4, New York, Plenum Press, pp. 93-142

59. San, R.H.C. & Stich, H.F. (1975) DNA repair synthesis of cultured human cells as a rapid bioassay for chemical carcinogens. Int. J. Cancer, 16, 284-291

60. Pienta, R.J., Poiley, J.A. & Lebherz, W.B. (1977) Morphological transformation of early passage golden Syrian hamster embryo cells derived from cryopreserved primary cultures as a reliable *in vitro* bioassay for identifying diverse carcinogens. Int. J. Cancer, 19, 642-655

61. Zimmermann, F.K. (1975) Procedures used in the induction of mitotic recombination and mutation in the yeast *Saccharomyces cerevisiae*. Mutation Res., 31, 71-86

62. Ong, T.-M. & de Serres, F.J. (1972) Mutagenicity of chemical carcinogens in *Neurospora crassa*. Cancer Res., 32, 1890-1893

63. Huberman, E. & Sachs, L. (1976) Mutability of different genetic loci in mammalian cells by metabolically activated carcinogenic polycyclic hydrocarbons. Proc. nat. Acad. Sci. (Wash.), 73, 188-192

64. Krahn, D.F. & Heidelburger, C. (1977) Liver homogenate-mediated mutagenesis in Chinese hamster V79 cells by polycyclic aromatic hydrocarbons and aflatoxins. Mutation Res., 46, 27-44

65. Kuroki, T., Drevon, C. & Montesano, R. (1977) Microsome-mediated mutagenesis in V79 Chinese hamster cells by various nitrosamines. Cancer Res., 37, 1044-1050

66. Searle, A.G. (1975) The specific locus test in the mouse. Mutation Res., 31, 277-290

67. Evans, H.J. & O'Riordan, M.L. (1975) Human peripheral blood lymphocytes for the analysis of chromosome aberrations in mutagen tests. Mutation Res., 31, 135-148

68. Epstein, S.S., Arnold, E., Andrea, J., Bass, W. & Bishop, Y. (1972) Detection of chemical mutagens by the dominant lethal assay in the mouse. Toxicol. appl. Pharmacol., 23, 288-325

69. Perry, P. & Evans, H.J. (1975) Cytological detection of mutagen-carcinogen exposure by sister chromatid exchanges. Nature (Lond.), 258, 121-125

70. Stetka, D.G. & Wolff, S. (1976) Sister chromatid exchange as an assay for genetic damage induced by mutagen-carcinogens. I. *In vivo* test for compounds requiring metabolic activation. Mutation Res., 41, 333-342

71. Bartsch, H. & Grover, P.L. (1976) Chemical carcinogenesis and mutagenesis. In: Symington, T. & Carter, R.L., eds, Scientific Foundations of Oncology, Vol. IX, Chemical Carcinogenesis, London, Heinemann Medical Books Ltd, pp. 334-342

72. Hollaender, A., ed. (1971a,b, 1973, 1976) Chemical Mutagens: Principles and Methods for Their Detection, Vols 1-4, New York, Plenum Press

73. Montesano, R. & Tomatis, L., eds (1974) Chemical Carcinogenesis Essays, Lyon (IARC Scientific Publications No. 10)

74. Ramel, C., ed. (1973) Evaluation of genetic risk of environmental chemicals: report of a symposium held at Skokloster, Sweden, 1972. Ambio Special Report, No. 3

75. Stoltz, D.R., Poirier, L.A., Irving, C.C., Stich, H.F., Weisburger, J.H. & Grice, H.C. (1974) Evaluation of short-term tests for carcinogenicity. Toxicol. appl. Pharmacol., 29, 157-180

76. Montesano, R., Bartsch, H. & Tomatis, L., eds (1976) Screening Tests in Chemical Carcinogenesis, Lyon (IARC Scientific Publications No. 12)

77. Committee 17 (1975) Environmental mutagenic hazards. Science, 187, 503-514

GENERAL REMARKS ON THE SUBSTANCES CONSIDERED

In this seventeenth volume of the *IARC Monograph* series, certain *N*-nitroso compounds are evaluated. Among these are a number of *N*-nitrosamines that have been tested for carcinogenicity and that have been shown to occur in the environment; the nitrosamides, *N*-nitroso-*N*-ethylurea and *N*-nitroso-*N*-methylurea; and the anticancer drug, streptozotocin, which is related structurally to the latter nitrosamide. Monographs on *N*-nitrosodiethylamine, *N*-nitrosodimethylamine, *N*-nitroso-*N*-ethylurea and *N*-nitroso-*N*-methylurea appeared in volume 1 of the *IARC Monographs*, and monographs on *N*-nitrosodi-*n*-butylamine and streptozotocin were published in volume 4; new data on these compounds have been included in the present volume.

In addition, a monograph on polychlorinated biphenyls, published in volume 7 of the *IARC Monographs*, was re-examined and updated to include recent observations on the effects of this class of chemicals on humans. The resulting monograph will be combined with a future one on polybrominated biphenyls, and these are to be published as a separate volume.

Following the observation in animals of the toxic (Barnes & Magee, 1954) and carcinogenic effects of *N*-nitrosodimethylamine (Magee & Barnes, 1956), studies were made of the biological activities of a variety of *N*-nitroso compounds. The hepatotoxic effect of *N*-nitrosodimethylamine in humans was reported in 1937 by Freund (1937), who described clinical and autopsy findings in two chemists accidentally poisoned with this compound. The carcinogenicity of several *N*-nitroso compounds was extensively investigated and reported by Druckrey *et al.* (1967) and was reviewed by Magee & Barnes (1967). More recently, reviews on their toxicity (Magee & Swann, 1969), carcinogenicity and metabolism (Magee *et al.*, 1975, 1976), teratogenicity (Druckrey, 1973a,b) and mutagenicity (Montesano & Bartsch, 1976; Neale, 1976) have also appeared. The carcinogenicity studies have demonstrated that these *N*-nitroso compounds have a high degree of specificity in inducing tumours in various species and among target organs within the same species. This group of carcinogens has provided a unique research tool for elucidating the possible mechanism(s) of cancer induction by chemical substances at cellular and molecular levels (Magee *et al.*, 1976; Pegg, 1977).

The observation of severe liver disease in sheep fed a diet containing fishmeal preserved with nitrite (Koppang *et al.*, 1964) and the identification of *N*-nitrosodimethylamine as the toxic principle in such products (Ender *et al.*, 1964; Sakshaug *et al.*, 1965) led to widespread efforts to evaluate levels of *N*-nitroso compounds in food destined for human and animal consumption.

Humans may be exposed to *N*-nitroso compounds in several ways: formation in the environment and subsequent absorption from food, water, air or industrial and consumer products; formation in the human body from precursors ingested separately in food, water or air; from the consumption or smoking of tobacco; and from naturally occurring compounds.

It has been known since 1865 that the reaction of dimethylamine hydrochloride with sodium nitrite at an acidic pH yields *N*-nitrosodimethylamine (Fridman *et al.*, 1971). It has been suggested (Druckrey *et al.*, 1963; Lijinsky & Epstein, 1970; Sander, 1967) that this reaction could occur in the acid conditions of the mammalian stomach between ingested nitrite and amines, and there is now substantial evidence that *N*-nitrosamines can be formed in this way. The phenomenon was first demonstrated by Sander *et al.* (1968).

Nitrite and nitrate are added to some foods, particularly meats and fish, as processing aids and as agents to prevent formation of botulinum toxin. White (1975) estimated that about 80% of the total nitrate ingested daily (106 mg) originates from vegetables, and about 70% of nitrite that enters the stomach (12.8 mg) comes from the saliva. Regulations exist in many countries to control the addition of nitrate and nitrite to food products. In order to prevent the possible formation of *N*-nitrosamines from, for example, mixtures of spices with nitrites and/or nitrates used in commercial meat and poultry curing (known as curing premixes), the US Food and Drug Administration has made a regulation that allows the use of these premixes only if the nitrites and/or nitrates are packaged separately from the spices with instructions on the label that they are not to be combined until just prior to use (US Food and Drug Administration, 1973). Nitrate reduction by bacteria could also lead to the formation of *N*-nitrosamines either *in vivo* (Hawksworth & Hill, 1971) or in the environment (Ayanaba *et al.*, 1973).

Little is known about the metabolism of nitrate in man. Nitrite is formed in the oral cavity by bacterial reduction of nitrate, and the normal concentration range in individuals who do not consume large amounts of nitrate is 6-10 mg/l of saliva (Tannenbaum *et al.*, 1974). When foods that contain nitrate, such as certain root and leafy vegetables, are consumed, salivary nitrate and nitrite levels are elevated to hundreds of mg/l (Spiegelhalder *et al.*, 1976; Tannenbaum *et al.*, 1976). Under normal conditions, nitrite arises in the stomach from the swallowing of saliva (Klein *et al.*, 1978), but bacterial reduction of nitrate may continue in the stomachs of individuals who have low gastric acidity or anacidity; low gastric acidity has been related to the etiology of gastric cancer (Cuello *et al.*, 1976).

Nitrosatable substances that occur in the environment include secondary and tertiary amines, quaternary ammonium compounds, ureas, carbamates and guanidines. Some of these compounds are found ubiquitously in nature; nitrosation of a number of agricultural chemicals has been shown to occur (Eisenbrand *et al.*, 1974; Elespuru & Lijinsky, 1973; Preussmann, 1975; Sen *et al.*, 1974), and various drugs carry nitrosatable alkyl amino or amido groups (Lijinksy, 1974; Lijinsky & Greenblatt, 1972). The chemical kinetics of nitrosation have been reviewed recently by Mirvish (1975).

The drug amidopyrine can react rapidly with traces of nitrosating agents (even gaseous nitrogen oxides), resulting in the formation of *N*-nitrosodimethylamine; a wide variety of commercial drugs containing amidopyrine have been found to have traces of this carcinogen (Eisenbrand *et al.*, 1978).

Evidence that *N*-nitroso compounds are formed in the body from amine precursors is based on: (a) their detection in gastric juices *in vitro* and in the mammalian or human stomach *in vivo*; and (b) the observation of acute toxic and carcinogenic effects as well as damage to cellular macromolecules after simultaneous administration of nitrite and various amines and amides (Magee *et al.*, 1976; Preussmann, 1975). Recently,

N-nitrosodiethyl- and -dimethylamines have been detected in human blood after the consumption of a meal consisting of normal dietary items (Fine *et al.*, 1977a).

The amount of *N*-nitroso compounds formed by nitrosation is affected by many factors, such as basicity of the amine, pH and substrate concentration. Nucleophilic ions such as thiocyanate increase the rate of *N*-nitrosamine formation (Boyland *et al.*, 1971; Fan & Tannenbaum, 1973). *C*-Nitrosophenols, the product of the nitrosation of phenols, catalyse *N*-nitrosamine formation (Davies *et al.*, 1978); other naturally occurring phenols may either inhibit or promote formation under different conditions (Walker *et al.*, 1975). Nitrosation may be promoted in certain environments by the presence of bacteria (Archer *et al.*, 1978; Klubes *et al.*, 1972). Ascorbic acid (Mirvish *et al.*, 1972) and α-tocopherol (Mergens *et al.*, 1978) inhibit the formation of *N*-nitroso compounds.

Other, as yet unexplored possibilities for the formation of *N*-nitroso compounds are: transnitrosation reactions (Singer *et al.*, 1978); nitrosation in organic solutions of strongly basic amines even by inorganic nitrite (Angeles *et al.*, 1978); and nitrosation even under strongly alkaline conditions with nitrogen oxides (Challis *et al.*, 1978).

Human exposure to *N*-nitroso compounds can also occur from contact with exogenously formed *N*-nitroso compounds. The occurrence of nitrosamines in foodstuffs has been reviewed recently (Crosby, 1976; Crosby & Sawyer, 1976). Significant levels of *N*-nitrosamines have also been found in cosmetics (Fan *et al.*, 1977a).

The possible formation of *N*-nitrosamines in cigarette smoke was originally suggested by Druckrey & Preussmann (1962), since tobacco contains several nitrosatable amines and nitrosating agents. Subsequently, nitrosamines were found in tobacco and tobacco smoke (Brunnemann & Hoffmann, 1978; Hoffmann *et al.*, 1974, 1976) and in indoor atmospheres under conditions of excessive tobacco smoking (Brunnemann & Hoffmann, 1978).

The occupational hazards associated with the use of *N*-nitroso compounds in industry have been outlined by Magee (1972). Some are used as organic accelerators and antioxidants in the production of rubber (Boyland *et al.*,

1968). *N*-Nitrosodimethylamine was detected as a pollutant in the air of a factory producing dimethylamine; its concentration correlated with the concentrations of nitrogen dioxide and secondary amine in the air (Bretschneider & Matz, 1974, 1976). *N*-Nitrosodimethylamine and three unidentified *N*-nitroso compounds were also detected in samples of air in the vicinity of a plant manufacturing 1,1-dimethylhydrazine, a rocket propellant of which *N*-nitrosodimethylamine is a precursor, and in the vicinity of a factory manufacturing amines (Fine *et al.*, 1976a,b,c). Another source of human exposure to *N*-nitroso compounds may be the nitrite salts used as corrosion inhibitors in packaging materials (Archer & Wishnok, 1976), in synthetic cutting fluids (Fan *et al.*, 1977b; Rappe & Zingmark, 1978; Zingmark & Rappe, 1977) and in some widely used herbicides (Fine *et al.*, 1977b) (see also monographs on *N*-nitrosodi-*n*-butylamine, *N*-nitrosodimethylamine and *N*-nitrosodiethanolamine).

There is considerable evidence that nitrosation reactions can occur in soils, organic waste or water in areas where industrial or other waste discharges contain large amounts of amines (Ayanaba *et al.*, 1973; Tate & Alexander, 1975).

The relevance of these traces of *N*-nitroso compounds to a possible risk to humans has yet to be established. However, a large variety of animal species and organs are susceptible to their carcinogenic action, and samples of human liver and lung are capable of forming alkylating (Harris *et al.*, 1977; Montesano & Magee, 1970) and mutagenic (Bartsch *et al.*, 1976; Czygan *et al.*, 1973) metabolites. The exceedingly difficult question of whether a proportion of human cancer or transmissible genetic damage could be attributed to these groups of carcinogens has not so far been answered, although some studies have indirectly examined the possible role of *N*-nitrosamines in the etiology of a number of human cancers (Correa *et al.*, 1975; Cuello *et al.*, 1976; Hill *et al.*, 1973; Joint Iran-IARC Study Group, 1977; Zaldívar & Wetterstrand, 1975).

At present, however, it may be difficult, if not impossible, to demonstrate in the general population a cause-effect relationship between exposure to low levels of *N*-nitrosamines and the incidence of certain human cancers, although the existence of such a correlation remains a working hypothesis.

Most of the chemical and physical properties of the nitrosamines described in these monographs were taken from Druckrey *et al.* (1967). The principal techniques employed for the analysis of volatile *N*-nitrosamines have been described in a recent publication (Preussmann *et al.*, 1978). The relative merits of high- and low-resolution mass spectrometry are discussed, since use of mass spectrometry as a confirmatory technique is particularly important. In this respect, those data reported in the section on occurrence which have not been confirmed by this technique have been marked with a footnote. This does not necessarily imply that the data are unreliable, but, in assessing the significance of such data, emphasis should be placed on those that have been confirmed by mass spectrometry. In certain instances, *N*-nitroso compounds may be formed as artefacts during an analytical procedure; in these cases mass spectrometry adds little to the value of the data (Fine *et al.*, 1977b).

References

Angeles, R.M., Keefer, L.K., Roller, P.P. & Uhm, S.J. (1978) Chemical models for possible artifactual nitrosamine formation in environmental analysis. In: Walker, E.A., Castegnaro, M., Griciute, L. & Lyle, R.E., eds, Environmental Aspects of *N*-Nitroso Compounds, Lyon (IARC Scientific Publications No. 19) (in press)

Archer, M.C. & Wishnok, J.S. (1976) Nitrosamine formation in corrosion-inhibiting compositions containing nitrite salts of secondary amines. J. environm. Sci. Hlth, A11, 583-590

Archer, M.C., Yang, H.S. & Okun, J.D. (1978) Acceleration of nitrosamine formation at pH 3.5 by microorganisms. In: Walker, E.A., Castegnaro, M., Griciute, L. & Lyle, R.E., eds, Environmental Aspects of *N*-Nitroso Compounds, Lyon (IARC Scientific Publications No. 19) (in press)

Ayanaba, A., Verstraete, W. & Alexander, M. (1973) Possible microbial contribution to nitrosamine formation in sewage and soil. J. nat. Cancer Inst., 50, 811-813

Barnes, J.M. & Magee, P.N. (1954) Some toxic properties of dimethylnitrosamine. Brit. J. industr. Med., 11, 167-174

Bartsch, H., Camus, A. & Malaveille, C. (1976) Comparative mutagenicity of *N*-nitrosamines in a semi-solid and in a liquid incubation system in the presence of rat or human tissue fractions. Mutation Res., 37, 149-162

Boyland, E., Carter, R.L., Gorrod, J.W. & Roe, F.J.C. (1968) Carcinogenic properties of certain rubber additives. Europ. J. Cancer, 4, 233-239

Boyland, E., Nice, E. & Williams, K. (1971) The catalysis of nitrosation by thiocyanate from saliva. Fd Cosmet. Toxicol., 9, 639-643

Bretschneider, K. & Matz, J. (1974) Nitrosamine (NA) in der atmosphärischen [Luft] und in der Luft am Arbeitsplatz. Arch. Geschwulstforch., 43, 36-41

Bretschneider, K. & Matz, J. (1976) Occurrence and analysis of nitrosamines in air. In: Walker, E.A., Bogovski, P. & Griciute, L., eds, Environmental *N*-Nitroso Compounds Analysis and Formation, Lyon (IARC Scientific Publications No. 14), pp. 395-399

Brunnemann, K.D. & Hoffmann, D. (1978) Chemical studies on tobacco smoke. LIX. Analysis of volatile nitrosamines in tobacco smoke and polluted indoor environments. In: Walker, E.A., Castegnaro, M., Griciute, L. & Lyle, R.E., eds, Environmental Aspects of *N*-Nitroso Compounds, Lyon (IARC Scientific Publications No. 19) (in press)

Challis, B.C., Edwards, A., Hunma, R.R., Kyrptopoulos, S.A. & Outram, J.R. (1978) Rapid formation of *N*-nitrosamines from nitrogen oxides under neutral and alkaline conditions. In: Walker, E.A., Castegnaro, M., Griciute, L. & Lyle, R.E., eds, Environmental Aspects of *N*-Nitroso Compounds, Lyon (IARC Scientific Publications No. 19) (in press)

Correa, P., Haenszel, W., Cuello, C., Tannenbaum, S. & Archer, M. (1975) A model for gastric cancer epidemiology. Lancet, ii, 58-60

Crosby, N.T. (1976) Nitrosamines in foodstuffs. Residue Rev., 64, 77-135

Crosby, N.T. & Sawyer, R. (1976) *N*-Nitrosamines: a review of chemical and biological properties and their estimation in foodstuffs. Adv. Fd Res., 22, 1-71

Cuello, C., Correa, P., Haenszel, W., Gordillo, G., Brown, C., Archer, M.C. & Tannenbaum, S. (1976) Gastric cancer in Colombia. I. Cancer risk and suspect environmental agents. J. nat. Cancer Inst., 57, 1015-1020

Czygan, P., Greim, H., Garro, A.J., Hutterer, F., Rudick, J., Schaffner, F. & Popper, H. (1973) Cytochrome P-450 content and the ability of liver microsomes from patients undergoing abdominal surgery to alter the mutagenicity of a primary and a secondary carcinogen. J. nat. Cancer Inst., 51, 1761-1764

Davies, R., Dennis, M.J., Massey, R.C. & McWeeny, D.J. (1978) Some effects of phenol- and thiol-nitrosation reactions on *N*-nitrosamine formation. In: Walker, E.A., Castegnaro, M., Griciute, L. & Lyle, R.E., eds, Environmental Aspects of *N*-Nitroso Compounds, Lyon (IARC Scientific Publications No. 19) (in press)

Druckrey, H. (1973a) Chemical structure and action in transplacental carcinogenesis and teratogenesis. In: Tomatis, L. & Mohr, U., eds, Transplacental Carcinogenesis, Lyon (IARC Scientific Publications No. 4), pp. 45-58

Druckrey, H. (1973b) Specific carcinogenic and teratogenic effects of 'indirect' alkylating methyl and ethyl compounds, and their dependency on stages of ontogenic developments. Xenobiotica, 3, 271-303

Druckrey, H. & Preussmann, R. (1962) Zur Entstehung carcinogener Nitrosamine am Beispiel des Tabakrauchs. Naturwissenschaften, 49, 498-499

Druckrey, H., Steinhoff, D., Beuthner, H., Schneider, H. & Klärner, P. (1963) Prüfung von Nitrit auf chronisch toxische Wirkung an Ratten. Arzenimittel-Forsch., 13, 320-323

Druckrey, H., Preussmann, R., Ivankovic, S. & Schmähl, D. (1967) Organotrope carcinogene Wirkungen bei 65 verschiedenen *N*-Nitroso-Verbindungen an BD-Ratten. Z. Krebsforsch., 69, 103-201

Eisenbrand, G., Ungerer, O. & Preussmann, R. (1974) Formation of *N*-nitroso compounds from agricultural chemicals and nitrite. In: Bogovski, P. & Walker, E.A., eds, *N*-Nitroso Compounds in the Environment, Lyon (IARC Scientific Publications No. 9), pp. 71-74

Eisenbrand, G., Spiegelhalder, B., Janzowski, C., Kann, J. & Preussmann, R. (1978) Volatile and non-volatile *N*-nitroso compounds in foods and other environmental media. In: Walker, E.A., Castegnaro, M., Griciute, L. & Lyle, R.E., eds, Environmental Aspects of *N*-Nitroso Compounds, Lyon (IARC Scientific Publications No. 19) (in press)

Elespuru, R.K. & Lijinsky, W. (1973) The formation of carcinogenic nitroso compounds from nitrite and some types of agricultural chemicals. Fd Cosmet. Toxicol., 11, 807-817

Ender, F., Havre, G., Helgebostad, A., Koppang, N., Madsen, R., Ceh, L. & Bjӧrnson, O. (1964) Isolation and identification of a hepatotoxic factor in herring meal produced from sodium nitrite preserved herring. Naturwissenschaften, 51, 637-638

Fan, T.-Y. & Tannenbaum, S.R. (1973) Factors influencing the rate of formation of nitrosomorpholine from morpholine and nitrite: acceleration by thiocyanate and other anions. J. agric. Fd. Chem., 21, 237-240

Fan, T.-Y., Goff, U., Song, L., Fine, D.H., Arsenault, G.P. & Biemann, K. (1977a) *N*-Nitrosodiethanolamine in cosmetics, lotions and shampoos. Fd Cosmet. Toxicol., 15, 423-430

Fan, T.-Y., Morrison, J., Rounbehler, D.P., Ross, R., Fine, D.H., Miles, W. & Sen, N.P. (1977b) *N*-Nitrosodiethanolamine in synthetic cutting fluids: a part-per-hundred impurity. Science, 196, 70-71

Fine, D.H., Rounbehler, D.P., Belcher, N.M. & Epstein, S.S. (1976a) *N*-Nitroso compounds: detection in ambient air. Science, 192, 1328-1330

Fine, D.H., Rounbehler, D.P., Pellizzari, E.D., Bunch, J.E., Berkley, R.W., McCrae, J., Bursey, J.T., Sawicki, E., Krost, K. & DeMarrais, G.A. (1976b) *N*-Nitrosodimethylamine in air. Bull. environm. Contam. Toxicol., 15, 739-746

Fine, D., Rounbehler, D.P., Sawicki, E., Krost, K. & DeMarrais, G.A. (1976c) *N*-Nitroso compounds in the ambient community air of Baltimore, Maryland. Analyt. Lett., 9, 595-604

Fine, D.H., Ross, R., Rounbehler, D.P., Silvergleid, A. & Song, L. (1977a) Formation *in vivo* of volatile *N*-nitrosamines in man after ingestion of cooked bacon and spinach. Nature (Lond.), 265, 753-755

Fine, D.H., Rounbehler, D.P., Fan, T. & Ross, R. (1977b) Human exposure to *N*-nitroso compounds in the environment. In: Hiatt, H.H., Watson, J.D. & Winsten, J.A., eds., Origins of Human Cancer, Book A, Cold Spring Harbor, N.Y., Cold Spring Harbor Laboratory, pp. 293-307

Freund, H.A. (1937) Clinical manifestations and studies in parenchymatous hepatitis. Ann. intern. Med., 10, 1144-1155

Fridman, A.L., Mukhametshin, F.M. & Novikov, S.S. (1971) Advances in the chemistry of aliphatic *N*-nitrosamines. Russ. chem. Rev., 40, 34-50

Harris, C.C., Autrup, H., Stoner, G.D., McDowell, E.M., Trump, B.F. & Schafer, P. (1977) Metabolism of dimethylnitrosamine and 1,2-dimethylhydrazine in cultured human bronchi. Cancer Res., 37, 2309-2311

Hawksworth, G.M. & Hill, M.J. (1971) Bacteria and the *N*-nitrosation of secondary amines. Brit. J. Cancer, 25, 520-526

Hill, M.J., Hawksworth, G. & Tattersall, G. (1973) Bacteria, nitrosamines and cancer of the stomach. Brit. J. Cancer, 28, 562-567

Hoffmann, D., Rathkamp, G. & Liu, Y.Y. (1974) Chemical studies on tobacco smoke. XXVI. On the isolation and identification of volatile and non-volatile *N*-nitrosamines and hydrazines in cigarette smoke. In: Bogovski, P. & Walker, E.A., eds, *N*-Nitroso Compounds in the Environment, Lyon (IARC Scientific Publications No. 9), pp. 159-165

Hoffmann, D., Hecht, S.S., Ornaf, R.M., Wynder, E.L. & Tso, T.C. (1976) Chemical studies on tobacco smoke. XLII. Nitrosonornicotine: presence in tobacco, formation and carcinogenicity. In: Walker, E.A., Bogovski, P. & Griciute, L., eds, Environmental *N*-Nitroso Compounds Analysis and Formation, Lyon (IARC Scientific Publications No. 14), pp. 307-320

Joint Iran-International Agency for Research on Cancer Study Group (1977) Esophageal cancer studies in the Caspian littoral of Iran: results of population studies - a prodrome. J. nat. Cancer Inst., 59, 1127-1138

Klein, D., Gaconnet, N., Poullain, B. & Debry, G. (1978) Possibility of nitrosation during human digestion. I. Evaluation of precursors and affecting factors *in vivo*. II. Effect of meal on the reaction. In: Walker, E.A., Castegnaro, M., Griciute, L. & Lyle, R.E., eds, Environmental Aspects of *N*-Nitroso Compounds, Lyon (IARC Scientific Publications No. 19) (in press)

Klubes, P., Cerna, I., Rabinowitz, A.D. & Jondorf, W.R. (1972) Factors affecting dimethylnitrosamine formation from simple precursors by rat intestinal bacteria. Fd Cosmet. Toxicol., 10, 757-767

Koppang, N., Slagsvold, P., Hansen, M.A., Sögnen, E. & Svenkerud, R. (1964) Feeding experiments with meal produced from herring preserved with sodium nitrite and formalin. Nord. Vet.-Med., 16, 343-362

Lijinsky, W. (1974) Reaction of drugs with nitrous acid as a source of carcinogenic nitrosamines. Cancer Res., 34, 255-258

Lijinsky, W. & Epstein, S.S. (1970) Nitrosamines as environmental carcinogens. Nature (Lond.), 225, 21-23

Lijinsky, W. & Greenblatt, M. (1972) Carcinogen dimethylnitrosamine produced *in vivo* from nitrite and aminopyrine. Nature New Biol., 236, 177-178

Magee, P.N. (1972) Possibilities of hazard from nitrosamines in industry. Ann. occup. Hyg., 15, 19-22

Magee, P.N. & Barnes, J.M. (1956) The production of malignant primary hepatic tumours in the rat by feeding dimethylnitrosamine. Brit. J. Cancer, 10, 114-122

Magee, P.N. & Barnes, J.M. (1967) Carcinogenic nitroso compounds. Adv. Cancer Res., 10, 163-246

Magee, P.N. & Swann, P.F. (1969) Nitroso compounds. Brit. med. Bull., 25, 240-244

Magee, P.N., Pegg, A.E. & Swann, P.F. (1975) Molecular mechanisms of chemical carcinogenesis. In: Altmann, H.-W. *et al.*, eds, Handbuch der Allgemeinen Pathologie, Vol. 6, Berlin, Springer, pp. 329-419

Magee, P.N., Montesano, R. & Preussmann, R. (1976) *N*-Nitroso compounds and related carcinogens. In: Searle, C.E., ed., Chemical Carcinogens (ACS Monograph 173), Washington DC, American Chemical Society, pp. 491-625

Mergens, W.J., Kamm, J.J., Newmark, H.L., Fiddler, W. & Pensabene, J. (1978) *Alpha*-tocopherol: uses in preventing nitrosamine formation. In: Walker, E.A., Castegnaro, M., Griciute, L. & Lyle, R.E., eds, Environmental Aspects of *N*-Nitroso Compounds, Lyon (IARC Scientific Publications No. 19) (in press)

Mirvish, S.S. (1975) Formation of *N*-nitroso compounds: chemistry, kinetics, and *in vivo* occurrence. Toxicol. appl. Pharmacol., 31, 325-351

Mirvish, S.S., Wallcave, L., Eagen, M. & Shubik, P. (1972) Ascorbate-nitrite reaction: possible means of blocking the formation of carcinogenic *N*-nitroso compounds. Science, 177, 65-68

Montesano, R. & Bartsch, H. (1976) Mutagenic and carcinogenic *N*-nitroso compounds: possible environmental hazards. Mutation Res., 32, 179-228

Montesano, R. & Magee, P.N. (1970) Metabolism of dimethylnitrosamine by human liver slices *in vitro*. Nature (Lond.), 228, 173-174

Neale, S. (1976) Mutagenicity of nitrosamides and nitrosamidines in microorganisms and plants. Mutation Res., 32, 229-266

Pegg, A.E. (1977) Formation and metabolism of alkylated nucleosides: possible role in carcinogenesis by nitroso compounds and alkylating agents. Adv. Cancer Res., 25, 195-269

Preussmann, R. (1975) Chemische Carcinogene in der menschlichen Umwelt. In: Altmann, H.-W. *et al.*, eds, Handbuch der Allgemeinen Pathologie, Vol. 6, Berlin, Springer, pp. 421-594

Preussmann, R., Walker, E.A., Wasserman, A.E. & Castegnaro, M., eds (1978) Environmental Carcinogens - Selected Methods of Analysis, Vol. 1, Nitrosamines, Lyon (IARC Scientific Publications No. 18) (in press)

Rappe, C. & Zingmark, P.-A. (1978) Formation of *N*-nitrosamines in cutting fluids. In: Walker, E.A., Castegnaro, M., Griciute, L. & Lyle, R.E., eds, Environmental Aspects of *N*-Nitroso Compounds, Lyon (IARC Scientific Publications No. 19) (in press)

Sakshaug, J., Sögnen, E., Hansen, M.A. & Koppang, N. (1965) Dimethylnitrosamine: its hepatotoxic effect in sheep and its occurrence in toxic batches of herring meal. Nature (Lond.), 206, 1261-1262

Sander, J. (1967) Kann Nitrit in der menschlichen Nahrung Ursache einer Krebsentstehung durch Nitrosaminbildung sein? Arch. Hyg. (Berl.), 151, 22-28

Sander, J., Schweinsberg, F. & Menz, H.-P. (1968) Untersuchungen über die Entstehung cancerogener Nitrosamine im Magen. Hoppe-Seyler's Z. physiol. Chem., 349, 1691-1697

Sen, N.P., Donaldson, B.A. & Charbonneau, C. (1974) Formation of nitrosodimethylamine from the interaction of certain pesticides and nitrite. In: Bogovski, P. & Walker, E.A., eds, *N*-Nitroso Compounds in the Environment, Lyon (IARC Scientific Publications No. 9), pp. 75-79

Singer, S.S., Lijinsky, W. & Singer, G.M. (1978) Transnitrosation: an important aspect of the chemistry of aliphatic nitrosamines. In: Walker, E.A., Castegnaro, M., Griciute, L. & Lyle, R.E., eds, Environmental Aspects of *N*-Nitroso Compounds, Lyon (IARC Scientific Publications No. 19) (in press)

Spiegelhalder, B., Eisenbrand, G. & Preussmann, R. (1976) Influence of dietary nitrate on nitrite content of human saliva: possible relevance to *in vivo* formation of *N*-nitroso compounds. Fd Cosmet. Toxicol., 14, 545-548

Tannenbaum, S.R., Sinskey, A.J., Weisman, M. & Bishop, W. (1974) Nitrite in human saliva: its possible relationship to nitrosamine formation. J. nat. Cancer Inst., 53, 79-84

Tannenbaum, S.R., Weisman, M. & Fett, D. (1976) The effect of nitrate intake on nitrite formation in human saliva. Fd Cosmet. Toxicol., 14, 549-552

Tate, R.L., III & Alexander, M. (1975) Stability of nitrosamines in samples of lake water, soil, and sewage. J. nat. Cancer Inst., 54, 327-330

US Food and Drug Administration (1973) Nitrites and/or nitrates combined with spices in curing premixes. Fed. Regist., 38, 31679-31680

Walker, E.A., Pignatelli, B. & Castegnaro, M. (1975) Effects of gallic acid on nitrosamine formation. Nature (Lond.), 258, 176

White, J.W., Jr (1975) Relative significance of dietary sources of nitrate and nitrite. J. agric. Fd Chem., 23, 886-891

Zaldívar, R. & Wetterstrand, W.H. (1975) Further evidence of a positive correlation between exposure to nitrate fertilizers ($NaNO_3$ and KNO_3) and gastric cancer death rates: nitrites and nitrosamines. Experientia, 31, 1354-1355

Zingmark, P.-A. & Rappe, C. (1977) On the formation of *N*-nitrosodiethanolamine in a grinding fluid concentrate after storage. Ambio, 6, 237-238

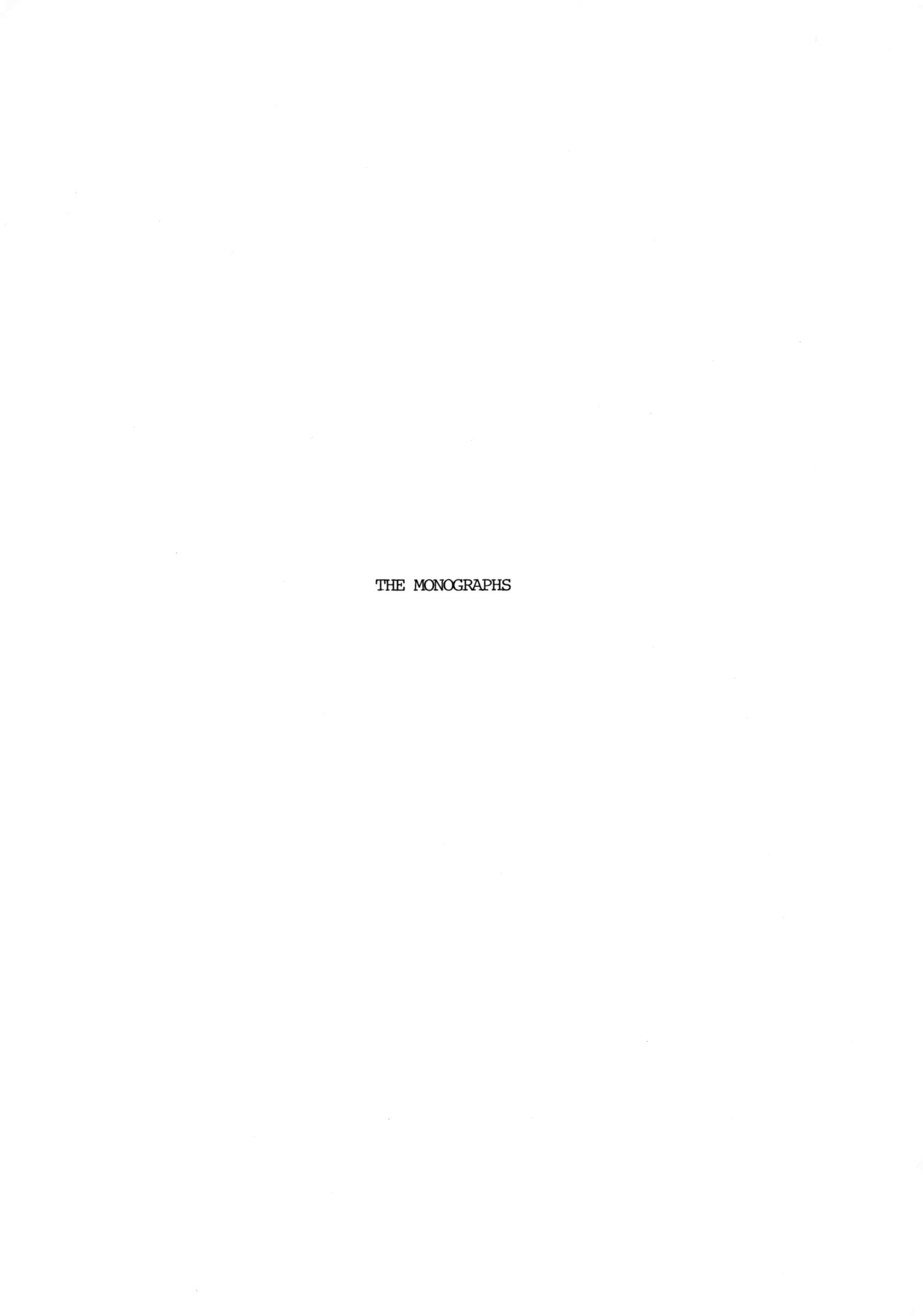

THE MONOGRAPHS

N-NITROSODI-*n*-BUTYLAMINE

This substance was considered previously by an IARC Working Group, in June 1973 (IARC, 1974). Since that time new data have become available, and these have been incorporated into the monograph and taken into account in the present evaluation.

1. Chemical and Physical Data

1.1 Synonyms and trade names

Chem. Abstr. Services Reg. No.: 924-16-3

Chem. Abstr. Name: *N*-Butyl-*N*-nitroso-1-butamine

DBNA; DBN; *N,N*-di-*n*-butylnitrosamine; di-*n*-butylnitrosamine; NDBA

1.2 Structural and molecular formulae and weight

$$O{=}N{-}N\begin{matrix} \diagup CH_2{-}CH_2{-}CH_2{-}CH_3 \\ \diagdown CH_2{-}CH_2{-}CH_2{-}CH_3 \end{matrix}$$

$C_8H_{18}N_2O$ Mol. wt: 158.2

1.3 Chemical and physical properties of the pure substance

(a) Description: Yellow oil

(b) Boiling-point: 116°C (14 mm) (Druckrey *et al.*, 1967)

(c) Density: d_4^{20} 0.9009

(d) Refractive index: n_D^{20} 1.4475

(e) Spectroscopy data: λ_{max} 233 and 347 nm (E_1^1 = 441.7 and 5.6) in water (Druckrey *et al.*, 1967); mass spectroscopy data are given by Pensabene *et al.* (1972) and Rainey *et al.* (1978).

(f) Solubility: Soluble in water, 0.12% (Druckrey *et al.*, 1967), organic solvents and vegetable oils

(g) Volatility: Can be steam-distilled quantitatively (Eisenbrand *et al.*, 1970)

(h) Stability: Stable at room temperature for more than 14 days in neutral or alkaline aqueous solutions in the dark (Druckrey *et al.*, 1967); slightly less stable in acidic solutions; light-sensitive, especially to ultra-violet light

(i) Reactivity: Strong oxidants (peracids) oxidize it to the corresponding nitramine; can be reduced to the corresponding hydrazine and/or amine; relatively resistant to hydrolysis, but can easily be split by hydrogen bromide in acetic acid (Eisenbrand & Preussmann, 1970). Photochemically reactive (Fridman *et al.*, 1971). The preparation of various derivatives has been discussed (Preussmann *et al.*, 1978).

1.4 Technical products and impurities

No data were available to the Working Group.

2. Production, Use, Occurrence and Analysis

2.1 Production and use

For background information on this section, see preamble, p. 22.

(a) Production

N-Nitrosodi-*n*-butylamine (NDBA) was first prepared by Linnemann in 1872 (Prager *et al.*, 1922). It can be made by the reaction of dibutylamine with nitrous acid (Druckrey *et al.*, 1967).

Although NDBA is available in small quantities for research purposes, no evidence was found that it has been manufactured commercially.

(b) Use

NDBA has been used in the synthesis of di-*n*-butylhydrazine (Derr, 1960; Joffe, 1958), although there is no indication that it has been used commercially in this way.

2.2 Occurrence

(a) Tobacco smoke

Analysis of the smoke from 11 different kinds of cigarettes from 2 countries revealed 3 ng/cigarette NDBA in the smoke condensate (McCormick *et al.*, 1973).

(b) Water

Cohen & Bachman (1978) reported 0.82 μg/l[1] in the effluent from 1/18 chemical factories (a coke plant).

(c) Food and feed

NDBA has been found at a level of 290 μg/kg[1] in soya bean oil (Hedler *et al.*, 1972); and 20-30 μg/kg[1] have been found in cheese (Cerutti *et al.*, 1975), although Alliston *et al.* (1972), Eisenbrand *et al.* (1978) and Sen *et al.* (1978), among others, did not detect NDBA in cheese.

Less than 1 μg/kg[1] was found in pork luncheon meat (Alliston *et al.*, 1972). Stephany *et al.* (1976) found 0.4-3.9 μg/kg in salami-like sausages, 0.2-0.7 μg/kg in cooked and smoked ham, 0.4-0.6 μg/kg in bacon-like products, 0.0-0.09 μg/kg in smoked ham and beef meat, 0.0-1.1 μg/kg in fried minced meat and 0.0-2.1 μg/kg in luncheon meat.

Gough (1978) found 0.2 and 0.5 μg/kg[1] NDBA in 2/30 tinned and powdered soups and 0.04 and 0.3 μg/kg[1] in 2/6 tinned meals, but none in a further 228 food samples. Havery *et al.* (1978) did not find NDBA in 106 food samples, and Eisenbrand *et al.* (1978) found none in 34 cured meat products.

Levels of 0.-4.1 μg/kg have been found in experimental animal feed (IARC, 1977).

(d) Vapour-phase corrosion inhibitors

Archer & Wishnok (1976) found 100 mg/kg NDBA in a commercial corrosion-resistant film of unknown source and composition.

---

[1]These results were not confirmed by mass spectroscopy (see also 'General Remarks on the Substances Considered', p. 40).

2.3 Analysis

An IARC Manual gives selected methods for the analysis of volatile *N*-nitrosamines, including NDBA (Preussmann *et al.*, 1978).

3. Biological Data Relevant to the Evaluation of Carcinogenic Risk to Man

3.1 Carcinogenicity and related studies in animals

(a) Oral administration

Mouse: *N*-Nitrosodi-*n*-butylamine (NDBA) was administered at a concentration of 50 mg/kg of diet to 39 male ICR mice for 12 months; 30 mice received the basal diet only for 15 months. Of the 33 animals that lived for more than 12 months, 27 developed squamous-cell carcinomas and 6, papillomas of the forestomach; 15 animals also developed liver tumours (5 trabecular hepatomas and 10 adenomas). Papillomas of the oesophagus and adenomas of the lung were observed in 4 and 8 mice, respectively. Among the 28 control animals that lived more than 15 months, lung adenomas developed in 2 and a lymphatic leukaemia was observed in 1 other (Takayama & Imaizumi, 1969).

In 2 groups of 50 male and 50 female C57BL/6 mice, continuous administration of 29.1 and 7.6 mg/kg bw/day to males and 30.9 and 8.2 mg/kg bw/day to females in the drinking-water led to the development of squamous-cell carcinomas and papillomas of the oesophagus in almost all animals, together with some tumours of the tongue and the soft palate. With the lower dose, 5 carcinomas of the forestomach occurred also. No liver tumours were seen in this study; however, 44/90 mice given the higher dose level and 19/89 given the lower dose level developed papillomas and multifocal squamous-cell carcinomas of the urinary bladder. Male animals were more sensitive to bladder carcinogenesis than were females (Bertram & Craig, 1970).

The different sensitivity of two strains of mice, BTO and C57BL/60, to NDBA carcinogenicity was reported in an abstract (Akamatsu, 1975). A single gastric intubation of 300 mg/kg bw in saline caused papillomas and carcinomas of the forestomach in 3/39 BTO mice, but tumours of the intestine in 2/11 C57BL/60 mice.

Rat: The carcinogenicity of NDBA in rats was first demonstrated by Druckrey *et al.* (1962, 1967). Four concentrations were administered in the diet to BD rats. In those receiving 75 mg/kg bw/day, liver carcinomas were induced in all 4 surviving rats. In those receiving the lower doses (37.5, 20 or 10 mg/kg bw/day), the incidence of liver cancer was lower, but malignant tumours were observed in the oesophagus and pharynx. Squamous-cell carcinomas of the urinary bladder occurred in 5/16 and 7/10 animals that received 37.4 and 20 mg/kg bw/day.

In Wistar rats, bladder tumours occurred after the administration of 0.01 or 0.05% NDBA in the drinking-water; liver cancers were seen only in those given the higher dose (Okajima *et al.*, 1970). In 30 female Wistar rats given 20 mg/kg bw/day NDBA in the drinking-water, 16 papillomas and 2 carcinomas of the urinary bladder were found (Kunze & Schauer, 1971); Kunze *et al.* (1969, 1971) obtained similar results.

Bladder tumours induced by administration of 0.05% NDBA solution in the drinking-water for 28 weeks in 12/12 male adult Wistar rats were classified histologically as transitional-cell carcinomas (Ito, 1973).

Hamster: Groups of 100 Syrian golden and 66 Chinese male hamsters given weekly doses of 300 mg/kg bw NDBA in olive oil by stomach tube for life showed a low incidence of papillomas and carcinomas of the bladder (11-14%). Syrian hamsters had high incidences of papillomas and carcinomas of the trachea (41/100) and of the lungs (14/100). Chinese hamsters developed papillomas (39/66) and carcinomas (21/66) of the forestomach but no tumours of the trachea or lungs (Althoff *et al.*, 1971). Similar results were obtained by Mohr *et al.* (1970).

Single doses of 400, 800 or 1600 mg/kg bw given by stomach tube to Syrian golden hamsters produced tumours of the respiratory tract in 3/10, 5/10 and 7/10 animals, respectively; the first tumour appeared after 31 weeks (Althoff *et al.*, 1973).

Guinea-pig: A dose of 40 mg/kg bw/day NDBA given 5 times a week in the drinking-water for life induced hepatocellular carcinomas in 15/15 animals that lived longer than 550 days. Cholangiomas were also seen in a few animals; and 3 animals had papillomas and 4, squamous-cell carcinomas of the urinary bladder (Ivankovic & Bücheler, 1968).

(b) Subcutaneous and/or intramuscular administration

Mouse: Twelve-week old IF x C57 mice (30 males and 30 females) were given s.c. injections of 10 µl pure NDBA every two weeks for 40 weeks. Of females that lived 54 weeks, 7/17 had carcinomas of the bladder; and of males that lived 46 weeks, 6/12 had carcinomas and 1, a papilloma of the urinary bladder. Carcinomas were mainly of the transitional-cell type (Wood *et al.*, 1970).

Female (A x IF)F_1 mice were given 13 fortnightly s.c. injections of 5 µl pure NDBA (average survival time, 486 days); bladder carcinomas developed in 12/44, lung carcinomas in 19/44, lung adenomas in 21/44 and mammary carcinomas in 19/44. Mammary carcinomas were also observed in 13/40 untreated controls (Flaks *et al.*, 1973).

Newborn mouse: Benign and malignant liver-cell tumours developed in 36/37 male and 20/24 female IF x C57 mice given 1 µl pure NDBA in 0.05 ml aqueous gelatine subcutaneously on days 1, 8 and 15 of life. A few lung adenomas and carcinomas were observed, but no urinary bladder tumours. No liver or lung tumours were observed in the controls (Wood *et al.*, 1970).

In CDF_1 mice injected subcutaneously with 158 µg NDBA in 0.03 ml of a 1% gelatine solution on days 1, 8, 15 and 22 of life hepatocellular adenomas were found in 20/26 males and 5/22 females, 1 hepatocellular carcinoma was found in 1 male, and lung tumours were found in 38/48 mice (Fujii *et al.*, 1977).

Rat: Weekly s.c. injections of 200 or 400 mg/kg bw NDBA to BD rats for life resulted in the development of carcinomas of the urinary bladder in 18/20 rats, carcinomas of the oesophagus in 3/20 and carcinomas of the liver in 2/20. S.c. administration thus led to a greater incidence of urinary bladder cancer than did oral administration (Druckrey *et al.*, 1967).

The histogenesis of NDBA-induced bladder tumours in rats was reported in an abstract of an electron microscope study (Levin, 1973).

Weekly injections of 200 mg/kg bw NDBA in sunflower oil were given to 60 male and 30 female 'non-bred' rats for 11 months. Of 25 male and 6 female rats still alive at the appearance of the first tumour (a lung adenocarcinoma), the total numbers of animals with tumours were 17 males and 4 females; the average latent period for tumour induction was 472 days. Papillomas of the bladder occurred in 11/25 males and 3/6 females, pulmoadenocarcinomas in 9 males and squamous-cell papillomas of the oesophagus in 3 males and 1 female (Vlasov *et al.*, 1973).

Lung tumours (adenomas, adenocarcinomas, squamous-cell carcinomas) were induced in 23/24 male SIV-50 rats given weekly s.c. injections of 200 or 400 mg/kg bw NDBA in 0.5 ml dimethylsulphoxide for 26 weeks. Tumours of the urinary bladder were also observed in 18 animals. The animals died or were killed within 420 days (Sander *et al.*, 1974).

Hamster: Of 25 Syrian golden hamsters given weekly s.c. doses of 300 mg/kg bw NDBA in olive oil, 21 developed tracheal papillomas and carcinomas, 4 developed urinary bladder papillomas and 6, bladder carcinomas. Of 16 Chinese hamsters treated similarly, 9 developed forestomach papillomas and 1, a forestomach carcinoma. One papilloma and two carcinomas of the urinary bladder were found, but no tumours developed in the respiratory tract (Althoff *et al.*, 1971). Mohr *et al.* (1970) obtained similar results. Single s.c. doses of 150, 300, 600 and 1200 mg/kg bw given to 4 groups of 10 Syrian golden hamsters produced tumours of the respiratory tract in 3, 4, 5 and 7 animals, respectively; the first tumour appeared after 19 weeks (Althoff *et al.*, 1973).

After treatment of 55 European hamsters with 1/50-1/3 of the LD_{50} (LD_{50}: 2500 in males and 1900 mg/kg bw in females) once weekly for life, all animals that survived longer than 20 weeks developed benign and malignant tumours in more than one organ. The majority of neoplasms (papillary polyps, papillomas, squamous-cell carcinomas, adenocarcinomas) were found in the respiratory tract (up to 100% at high dose levels), in the digestive system, mainly forestomach (20-60%), and in the urinary bladder (20-60%).

The average latent period was 36 weeks. A dose-response relationship with regard to survival times and to weight was observed in both sexes. Two transitional-cell carcinomas of the urinary bladder were found to have metastasized to the lungs and one to the liver (Althoff *et al.*, 1974).

An electron microscope study of pulmonary adenocarcinomas induced in European hamsters by NDBA showed cells that resembled alveolar epithelial cells type II. A possible bronchiolar origin of the neoplasms was suggested (Reznik-Schüller & Mohr, 1975). The ultrastructural characteristics of NDBA-induced adenocarcinomas and squamous-cell carcinomas of the nasal cavity in European hamsters suggest that the adenocarcinomas originate from goblet cells and the squamous-cell carcinomas from squamous metaplastic or adenomatous areas (Reznik-Schüller & Mohr, 1976). An ultrastructural study of transitional-cell and squamous-cell carcinomas of the urinary bladder induced in European hamsters by s.c. injection of NDBA suggests that these tumours represent developmentally different stages of the same type of tumour rather than two fundamentally different types of neoplasms (Reznik-Schüller & Mohr, 1977).

When NDBA in commercial vegetable oil was injected subcutaneously into groups of 20 male and 20 female Chinese hamsters at several different dose levels (1/5, 1/10, 1/20 LD_{50}: 284, 142, 71 mg/kg bw), weekly for 18 weeks, a similar organotropy to that seen in Syrian golden and European hamsters was produced: mainly benign lung tumours were found. In contrast to the controls, which received vegetable oil alone, and to the other experimental groups, 7/19 male animals which received the highest dose level developed fibrosarcomas at the injection site (Reznik *et al.*, 1976).

Rabbit: S.c. injections of 400 mg/kg bw NDBA twice weekly, then once weekly, in male rabbits for a period of 21 months resulted in 7/14 bladder tumours (2 papillomas, 2 haemangiomas, 3 transitional-cell carcinomas) and 2/14 pulmonary adenocarcinomas within 8-26 months after the start of treatment (Cohen *et al.*, 1975).

(c) Intraperitoneal administration

Hamster: Single doses of 200, 400 and 800 mg/kg bw NDBA given to 3 groups of 5 male and 5 female Syrian golden hamsters produced tumours of the respiratory tract in 4, 6 and 7 animals, respectively; the first tumour appeared after 17 weeks. Some papillary tumours of the forestomach were also observed (Althoff *et al.*, 1973).

(d) Intravenous administration

Mouse: Twice-weekly injections of 6 µg/animal NDBA in 0.1 ml saline for 25-30 weeks to 43 male and 46 female CBA/H-T_6T_6 mice resulted in acute leukaemia of the reticulum-cell type in 13/39 males and 17/37 females within 92-218 days. No leukaemias were observed in 51 control animals (Emura, 1970).

(e) Other experimental systems

Comparative routes

After treatment with single i.p., s.c. or i.g. doses of 150-1600 mg/kg bw, mainly papillary tumours of the trachea were observed in groups of 5 male and 5 female Syrian golden hamsters. The average survival times were 74 weeks for males and 53 weeks for females. Tumour incidence was dependent only on the administered dose and not on the route of application or sex of the animal (Althoff *et al.*, 1973). A combination of tumours in the urinary and respiratory system was observed after weekly i.g. or s.c. administrations of 22-464 mg/kg bw NDBA to groups of 10 male and 10 female Syrian golden hamsters (Althoff, 1974).

Prenatal exposure

Two groups of 40 and 45 female Syrian golden hamsters were injected subcutaneously 2-8 times or with a single injection of 30 mg/kg bw NDBA between days 8-15 of pregnancy. Postnatal mortality in the offspring was high: effective numbers of animals/number of animals at birth were 212/357 and 202/282 after several and single administrations, respectively. Single-dose treatment induced no respiratory tract neoplasms in the parental generation, but a low incidence of tumours of the respiratory tract (7%, 14 tumours) was seen in the F_1 generation. Multiple administrations led to a higher incidence of respiratory tract tumours in the parental generation (22%, 24 tumours) than in the F_1 generation (6%, 17 tumours) (Althoff *et al.*, 1976).

Carcinogenesis in plants

Seeds of hybrids of *Nicotiana* were soaked in 10 mM solutions of NDBA in water for 1 or 2 days; 20 days later, tumours were found on 10.8% of germinated seedlings, but on none of the controls (Andersen, 1973).

(f) Carcinogenicity of metabolites (see also section 3.2 (a))

N-Nitroso-*n*-butyl-*N*-(4-hydroxybutyl)amine

(i) Oral administration

Treatment of 50 male and 50 female C57BL/6 mice with 35 mg/kg bw/day *N*-nitroso-*n*-butyl-*N*-(4-hydroxybutyl)amine in the drinking-water for life induced anaplastic carcinomas of the urinary bladder in all animals reaching autopsy, with average tumour induction times of 190 days for males and 253 for females (Bertram & Craig, 1972).

Daily oral doses of 40 and 20 mg/kg bw *N*-nitroso-*n*-butyl-*N*-(4-hydroxybutyl)amine given to 5 and 20 BD rats in the drinking-water selectively induced multiple carcinomas of the urinary bladder in all animals (Druckrey *et al.*, 1964). Identical results were obtained by Ito *et al.* (1969) in Wistar rats and by Hashimoto *et al.* (1972) in ACI/N rats.

The influence of length of treatment has been investigated in groups of 9-18 male Wistar rats given 0.05% *N*-nitroso-*n*-butyl-*N*-(4-hydroxybutyl)-amine in the drinking-water for 2, 4, 6, 8 and 12 weeks. At the time the animals were sacrificed (40 weeks), a clear dose-response effect was observed in the incidence of bladder papillomas (33-100%) and carcinomas (0-100%) (Ito *et al.*, 1972).

Histological classification of 613 urinary bladder cancers induced in rats by *N*-nitroso-*n*-butyl-*N*-(4-hydroxybutyl)amine showed that the large majority (more than 95%) were transitional-cell carcinomas. The others were squamous-cell carcinomas, undifferentiated carcinomas and carcino-sarcomas. The morphological characteristics of these bladder carcinomas appeared to be similar to those seen in humans (Fukushima *et al.*, 1976).

The histogenesis and progression of the various preneoplastic and neoplastic lesions of the bladder in rats have been described by Kunze *et al.* (1976). Electron microscope investigations of *N*-nitroso-*n*-butyl-*N*-(4-hydroxybutyl)amine-treated rats revealed characteristic surface changes of the preneoplastic epithelium of the urinary bladder, in addition to hyperplasia. Similar changes were observed in treated mice and hamsters but not in guinea-pigs (Shirai *et al.*, 1977).

Significant differences in the induction of urinary bladder tumours by *N*-nitroso-*n*-butyl-*N*-(4-hydroxybutyl)amine were seen in different strains of male rats. The tumour incidence varied from 0% in Lewis rats to 100% in ACI/NC rats, with intermediate values in Sprague-Dawley, BDIX/N and Wistar rats (Ito *et al.*, 1972).

The effect of sex and age and of the dose and period of administration of *N*-nitroso-*n*-butyl-*N*-(4-hydroxbutyl)amine on the incidence of urinary bladder tumours in rats has also been investigated. No sex difference was found; however, the incidence of cancer and of squamous metaplasia in areas of cancerous tissue was much higher in older rats than in younger ones. The minimum carcinogenic dose was 0.005% administered in the drinking-water for 12 weeks (2/13 carcinomas); when this dose was administered for 4 weeks, 1 papilloma was produced in 15 rats. With a 0.1% solution, the minimum period of administration before bladder cancers were produced was 4 weeks (4/12 carcinomas) (Ito *et al.*, 1973, 1975).

(ii) Subcutaneous and/or intramuscular administration

The induction of respiratory and cholangiocellular tumours, in addition to carcinomas of the urinary bladder, was reported in Syrian golden hamsters after s.c. administration of *N*-nitroso-*n*-butyl-*N*-(4-hydroxybutyl)amine (Althoff & Krüger, 1975).

(iii) Intravesicular instillation

Tumours of the urinary bladder were produced in female ACI/N rats given intravesicular instillations of *N*-nitroso-*n*-butyl-*N*-(4-hydroxybutyl)-amine (Hashimoto *et al.*, 1974, 1976).

(iv) Route unspecified

In an abstract, production of bladder carcinomas was reported in dogs given 10 mg/kg bw/day (total dose, 80 mg) or 15 mg/kg bw/day (total dose, 160 mg) *N*-nitroso-*n*-butyl-*N*-(4-hydroxybutyl)amine and observed for 4 or 2 years, respectively (Okajima *et al.*, 1975a).

N-Nitroso-*n*-butyl-*N*-(3-carboxypropyl)amine

This compound is the principal urinary metabolite of NDBA and *N*-nitroso-*n*-butyl-*N*-(4-hydroxybutyl)amine (Okada & Ishidate, 1977).

(i) Oral administration

A total of 8 male ACI/N rats were treated with 0.06% *N*-nitroso-*n*-butyl-*N*-(3-carboxypropyl)amine in the drinking-water for up to 20 weeks. Three animals killed at 14 weeks showed papillomas of the urinary bladder; the remaining 5 animals, which were killed at 28 weeks, all showed transitional-cell carcinomas of the urinary bladder (Hashimoto *et al.*, 1972). The histological type of tumour induced by *N*-nitroso-*n*-butyl-*N*-(3-carboxypropyl)amine was similar to that obtained with NDBA and *N*-nitroso-*n*-butyl-*N*-(4-hydroxybutyl)amine (Okada *et al.*, 1975, 1976).

Other urinary metabolites of NDBA and *N*-nitroso-*n*-butyl-*N*-(4-hydroxybutyl)amine did not produce bladder tumours after their oral administration in rats (Okada *et al.*, 1975, 1976).

(ii) Intravesicular instillation

Tumours of the urinary bladder were produced by intravesicular instillation of *N*-nitroso-*n*-butyl-*N*-(3-carboxypropyl)amine in female ACI/N rats (Hashimoto *et al.*, 1974, 1976).

(g) Factors that modify carcinogenicity in animals

N-Nitrosodi-*n*-butylamine

A combination of X-irradiation with 1000 rads and 13 fortnightly s.c. injections of 5 µl NDBA in female (A x If)F_1 mice markedly reduced the incidence of mammary carcinomas (3/41, compared with 19/44 in mice that received NDBA alone) (Flaks *et al.*, 1973).

When weekly s.c. injections of 200 mg/kg bw NDBA were given in conjunction with a lipotrope (choline)-deficient diet to Sprague-Dawley rats for 15 weeks, the incidence of hepatocarcinomas was enhanced: 16/25, compared with 6/25 in animals given a normal diet (Rogers & Newberne, 1973; Rogers *et al.*, 1974).

A complete inhibition of NDBA tumorigenesis in the liver, but not in the bladder and oesophagus, was achieved in Wistar rats by simultaneous administration of 1.4% DL-tryptophan in the diet and 0.05% NDBA in the drinking-water (Hiramatsu, 1974; Okajima *et al.*, 1971).

Indole (1.6% in the diet), given either *ad libitum* or controlled by pair-feeding, together with 0.02 or 0.05% NDBA in the drinking-water to 75 male and 69 female or 68 male and 68 female Syrian golden hamsters significantly suppressed bladder tumour incidence (Matsumoto *et al.*, 1977).

N-Nitroso-*n*-butyl-*N*-(4-hydroxybutyl)amine

The sex difference observed in C57BL/6 mice in the average induction time for anaplastic carcinomas of the urinary bladder after treatment with 35 mg/kg bw/day *N*-nitroso-*n*-butyl-*N*-(4-hydroxybutyl)amine in the drinking-water (190 days for males and 253 days for females) can be abolished by castrating males or by treating females with testosterone (Bertram & Craig, 1972).

The incidence of tumours of the ureter, which were seen occasionally in Wistar rats treated with *N*-nitroso-*n*-butyl-*N*-(4-hydroxybutyl)amine, was greatly increased after ligation of one ureter; this suggests that the concentration of the carcinogen is an important factor in the induction of tumours in the urinary system (Ito *et al.*, 1971).

The incidence of urinary bladder tumours, but not of papillomas and hyperplasia, induced by *N*-nitroso-*n*-butyl-*N*-(4-hydroxybutyl)amine in Wistar rats was inhibited by treatment with *N*-nitrosopiperidine, *N*-nitrosomorpholine, *N*-nitrosodiethylamine or *N*-2-fluorenylacetamide. Pretreatment with various hepatotoxic and nephrotoxic substances, such as 4-chloroacetanilide and 1-naphthylisothiocyanate, was found to inhibit both urinary bladder cancer and preneoplastic alterations of the urinary bladder epithelium (hyperplasia and papillomas) (Ito *et al.*, 1972, 1975).

A reduction in the incidence of bladder tumours in both castrated and non-castrated male Wistar rats was observed after s.c. implantation of diethylstilboestrol with or after oral administration of 0.05% *N*-nitroso-*n*-butyl-*N*-(4-hydroxybutyl)amine in the drinking-water for 6 weeks. In contrast, administration of testosterone in females, with or without ovariectomy, with or after *N*-nitroso-*n*-butyl-*N*-(4-hydroxybutyl)amine treatment raised the incidence of bladder tumours (Okajima *et al.*, 1975b).

3.2 Other relevant biological data

(a) Experimental systems

Toxic effects

The acute LD_{50} of NDBA in rats was 1200 mg/kg bw after either oral or s.c. administration (Druckrey *et al.*, 1967). In Syrian golden hamsters it was 1200 mg/kg bw (i.p.), 1750 mg/kg bw (s.c.) and 2150 mg/kg bw (i.g.) (Althoff *et al.*, 1973). In European hamsters, the s.c. LD_{50} was 2500 mg/kg bw in males and 1900 mg/kg bw in females (Althoff *et al.*, 1974). In Chinese hamsters, the s.c. LD_{50} in males and females was 1420 mg/kg bw (Reznik *et al.*, 1976).

Haematuria was observed at 28 weeks in 3/30 male mice given 10 µl pure NDBA subcutaneously every 2 weeks for 40 weeks (Wood *et al.*, 1970).

A dose of 500 mg/kg bw NDBA induced a 56% inhibition of thymidine incorporation into DNA of mouse testis 3.5 hours after administration of the carcinogen (Friedman & Staub, 1976).

Embryotoxicity and teratogenicity

No teratogenic effects were observed in rats when a single maximum tolerated dose of 1000 mg/kg bw NDBA was given intraperitoneally or when 1200 mg/kg bw were given orally during pregnancy. An increase in foetal mortality was noted, with peaks of susceptibility on days 3 and 9 and of high susceptibility on days 10 and 12 of gestation (Napalkov & Alexandrov, 1968).

Metabolism

Available evidence suggests that NDBA requires metabolic activation to form the proximate and/or ultimate carcinogen (Druckrey *et al.*, 1967; Magee & Barnes, 1967; Okada *et al.*, 1975). The main metabolites that have been identified in the urine of rats treated with the carcinogen are *N*-nitroso-*n*-butyl-*N*-(4-hydroxybutyl)amine and *N*-nitroso-*n*-butyl-*N*-(3-carboxypropyl)amine; also found are *N*-nitroso-*n*-butyl-*N*-(2-hydroxy-3-carboxypropyl)amine, *N*-nitroso-*n*-butyl-*N*-(carboxymethyl)amine, *N*-nitroso-*n*-butyl-*N*-(2-hydroxypropyl)amine, *N*-nitroso-*n*-butyl-*N*-(2-oxopropyl)amine, *N*-nitroso-*n*-butyl-*N*-(3-hydroxypropyl)amine, *N*-nitroso-*n*-butyl-*N*-(3-oxo-propyl)amine, *N*-nitroso-*n*-butyl-*N*-(2-carboxyethyl)amine and the glucuronides of the hydroxy compounds (Blattmann & Preussmann, 1974, 1975; Okada & Ishidate, 1977; Okada *et al.*, 1975). The two major metabolites were also excreted by mice, hamsters, guinea-pigs and dogs after oral administration of NDBA; in guinea-pigs, the glucuronide of *N*-nitroso-*n*-butyl-*N*-(3-hydroxy-butyl)amine and traces of *N*-nitroso-*n*-butyl-*N*-(2-hydroxy-3-carboxypropyl)-amine were also excreted (Okada & Ishidate, 1977).

It has been suggested that the induction of bladder tumours by NDBA or by *N*-nitroso-*n*-butyl-*N*-(4-hydroxybutyl)amine may be due to their common major urinary metabolite, *N*-nitroso-*n*-butyl-*N*-(3-carboxypropyl)amine (Okada *et al.*, 1975); about 45% of a dose of the latter compound given orally to rats was recovered unchanged in the urine after 48 hours (Okada & Suzuki, 1972).

NDBA is oxidized to form *n*-butyraldehyde and small amounts of propion-aldehyde and acetaldehyde *in vitro* in rat liver microsomal fractions (Blattmann & Preussmann, 1973, 1977).

Incubation of NDBA with a rat liver microsomal system and 3,4-dichloro-thiophenol as a trapping agent yields methyl- and butyl-thioethers (Preussmann *et al.*, 1976).

Following administration of di[1-^{14}C]-NDBA, rat liver RNA contained labelled 7-*n*-butylguanine and 7-methylguanine (Krüger, 1971, 1972).

Mutagenicity and other short-term tests

NDBA, in the presence of a liver microsomal fraction from Kanechlor 500- or phenobarbital-treated rats, induced reverse mutations in *Salmonella typhimurium* strains TA 100, TA 1530 and TA 1535 and in *Escherichia coli* (Bartsch *et al.*, 1976; Nagao *et al.*, 1977; Nakajima *et al.*, 1974). No mutagenic effect was detected in *S. typhimurium* strain TA 1530 with microsomal fractions from human liver biopsies (Bartsch *et al.*, 1976).

N-Nitroso-*n*-butyl-*N*-(4-hydroxybutyl)amine, *N*-nitroso-*n*-butyl-*N*-(3-carboxypropyl)amine, *N*-nitroso-*n*-butyl-*N*-(2-oxopropyl)amine and *N*-nitroso-*n*-butyl-*N*-(2-carboxyethyl)amine were mutagenic in *S. typhimurium* TA 100 and TA 1535 in the presence of a liver microsomal fraction from rats treated with Kanechlor 500 (Nagao *et al.*, 1977).

N-Nitroso-*n*-butyl-*N*-(α-acetoxy-*n*-butyl)amine, a synthetic model compound which is readily converted into the unstable α-hydroxybutyl derivative, is mutagenic in *S. typhimurium* strain TA 1530 in the absence of microsomal activation (Camus *et al.*, 1978).

In the presence of a liver microsomal system from phenobarbital-treated rats, NDBA induced 8-azaguanine resistant mutants in Chinese hamster V79 cells (Kuroki *et al.*, 1977).

Epithelial cells of the bladder of adult rats were transformed *in vitro* when treated with urea and *N*-nitroso-*n*-butyl-*N*-(4-hydroxybutyl)-amine or *N*-nitroso-*n*-butyl-*N*-(3-carboxypropyl)amine. After their s.c. or i.p. injection, or their injection into the bladder wall of rats, the transformed cells developed into transitional-cell carcinomas (Hashimoto & Kitagawa, 1974).

(b) Humans

No data were available to the Working Group.

3.3 Case reports and epidemiological studies

No data were available to the Working Group.

4. Summary of Data Reported and Evaluation

4.1 Experimental data

N-Nitrosodi-*n*-butylamine is carcinogenic in all animal species tested: mice, rats, Syrian golden, Chinese and European hamsters, rabbits and guinea-pigs, after its oral, subcutaneous, intraperitoneal or intravenous administration. It produces benign and malignant tumours in the urinary bladder, oesophagus, liver, respiratory tract, stomach and intestine, and also leukaemia; it is particularly effective as a bladder carcinogen. It is carcinogenic following its administration prenatally and in single doses.

The two metabolites, *N*-nitroso-*n*-butyl-*N*-(4-hydroxybutyl)amine and *N*-nitroso-*n*-butyl-*N*-(3-carboxypropyl)amine, are also carcinogenic, the first in mice, rats, hamsters and dogs and the second in rats. When given orally to mice, *N*-nitroso-*n*-butyl-*N*-(4-hydroxybutyl)amine produces carcinomas of the urinary bladder; when given orally or intravesicularly to rats, it produces papillomas and carcinomas of the urinary bladder; when given subcutaneously to hamsters, it produces tumours of the urinary bladder and respiratory tract and cholangiocellular tumours; and when given subcutaneously to dogs, it produces urinary bladder tumours. *N*-Nitroso-*n*-butyl-*N*-(3-carboxypropyl)amine produces tumours of the urinary bladder in rats after its oral administration or intravesicular instillation.

4.2 Human data

No case reports or epidemiological studies were available to the Working Group. Available information on occurrence suggests that the general population may be exposed sporadically to low levels of *N*-nitrosodi-*n*-butylamine; however, no exposed group suitable for an epidemiological investigation has yet been identified.

4.3 Evaluation

There is *sufficient evidence* of a carcinogenic effect of *N*-nitrosodi-*n*-butylamine in several experimental animal species. Although no epidemiological data were available, *N*-nitrosodi-*n*-butylamine should be regarded for practical purposes as if it were carcinogenic to humans.

5. References

Akamatsu, Y. (1975) Carcinogenicity of *N*-nitro[so]diethylamine (DEN), *N*-nitrosodi-*N*-butylamine (DBN), and *N*-methyl-*N*-nitro-*N*-nitrosoguanidine (MNG) in strains of mice: single intragastric treatment of 10 times maximum tolerated dose (MTD) (Abstract No. 645). Proc. Amer. Ass. Cancer Res., 16, 162

Alliston, T.G., Cox, G.B. & Kirk, R.S. (1972) The determination of steam-volatile *N*-nitrosamines in foodstuffs by formation of electron-capturing derivatives from electrochemically derived amines. Analyst, 97, 915-920

Althoff, J. (1974) Simultaneous tumors in the respiratory system and urinary bladder of Syrian golden hamsters. Z. Krebsforsch., 82, 153-158

Althoff, J. & Krüger, F.W. (1975) Carcinogenicity of 4-hydroxybutyl-butylnitrosamine in Syrian hamsters. Cancer Lett., 1, 15-19

Althoff, J., Krüger, F.W., Mohr, U. & Schmähl, D. (1971) Dibutylnitrosamine carcinogenesis in Syrian golden and Chinese hamsters. Proc. Soc. exp. Biol. (N.Y.), 136, 168-173

Althoff, J., Pour, P., Cardesa, A. & Mohr, U. (1973) Comparative studies of neoplastic response to a single dose of nitroso compounds. II. The effect of *N*-dibutylnitrosamine in the Syrian golden hamster. Z. Krebsforsch., 79, 85-89

Althoff, J., Mohr, U., Page, N. & Reznik, G. (1974) Carcinogenic effect of dibutylnitrosamine in European hamsters (*Cricetus cricetus*). J. nat. Cancer Inst., 53, 795-800

Althoff, J., Pour, P., Grandjean, C. & Eagen, M. (1976) Transplacental effects of nitrosamines in Syrian hamsters. I. Dibutylnitrosamine and nitrosohexamethyleneimine. Z. Krebsforsch., 86, 69-75

Andersen, R.A. (1973) Carcinogenicity of phenols, alkylating agents, urethan, and a cigarette-smoke fraction in *Nicotiana* seedlings. Cancer Res., 33, 2450-2455

Archer, M.C. & Wishnok, J.S. (1976) Nitrosamine formation in corrosion-inhibiting compositions containing nitrite salts of secondary amines. J. environm. Sci. Hlth, A11, 583-590

Bartsch, H., Camus, A. & Malaveille, C. (1976) Comparative mutagenicity of *N*-nitrosamines in a semi-solid and in a liquid incubation system in the presence of rat or human tissue fractions. Mutation Res., 37, 149-162

Bertram, J.S. & Craig, A.W. (1970) Induction of bladder tumours in mice with dibutylnitrosamine. Brit. J. Cancer, 24, 352-359

Bertram, J.S. & Craig, A.W. (1972) Specific induction of bladder cancer in mice by butyl-(4-hydroxybutyl)nitrosamine and the effects of hormonal modifications on the sex difference in response. Europ. J. Cancer, 8, 587-594

Blattmann, L. & Preussmann, R. (1973) Struktur von Metaboliten carcinogener Dialkylnitrosamine im Rattenurin. Z. Krebsforsch., 79, 3-5

Blattmann, L. & Preussmann, R. (1974) Biotransformation von carcinogenen Dialkylnitrosaminen. Weitere Urinmetaboliten von Di-*n*-butyl- und Di-*n*-pentyl-nitrosamin. Z. Krebsforsch., 81, 75-78

Blattmann, L. & Preussmann, R. (1975) Metaboliten von (2-Hydroxybutyl)-*n*-butylnitrosamin im Rattenurin. Z. Krebsforsch., 83, 125-127

Blattmann, L. & Preussmann, R. (1977) Oxidative biotransformation of di-*n*-butylnitrosamine. Formation *in vitro* of aldehydes in the presence of rat liver microsomes. Z. Krebsforsch., 88, 311-314

Camus, A.-M., Wiessler, M., Malaveille, C. & Bartsch, H. (1978) High mutagenicity of *N*-(α-acyloxy)alkyl-*N*-alkylnitrosamines in *S. typhimurium*: model compounds for metabolically activated *N,N*-dialkylnitrosamines. Mutation Res., 49, 187-194

Cerutti, G., Zappavigna, R. & Santini, P.L. (1975) *N*-Alkylnitrosamines in domestic and imported cheeses. Latte, 3, 224-227 [Chem. Abstr., 83, 130147c]

Cohen, A.E., Weisburger, E.K., Weisburger, J.H., Ward, J.M. & Putnam, C.L. (1975) Cystoscopy of chemically induced bladder neoplasms in rabbits administered the carcinogen dibutylnitrosamine. Invest. Urol., 12, 262-266

Cohen, J.B. & Bachman, J.D. (1978) Measurement of environmental nitrosamines. In: Walker, E.A., Castegnaro, M., Griciute, L. & Lyle, R.E., eds, Environmental Aspects of *N*-Nitroso Compounds, Lyon (IARC Scientific Publications No. 19) (in press)

Derr, P.F. (1960) Reduction of nitrosamines. US Patent 2,961,467, 22 November (to Food Machinery and Chemical Corp.) [Chem. Abstr., 55, 9280-9281]

Druckrey, H., Preussmann, R., Schmähl, D. & Müller, M. (1962) Erzeugung von Blasenkrebs an Ratten mit *N,N*-Dibutylnitrosamin. Naturwissenschaften, 49, 19

Druckrey, H., Preussmann, R., Ivankovic, S., Schmidt, C.H., Mennel, H.D. & Stahl, K.W. (1964) Selektive Erzeugung von Blasenkrebs an Ratten durch Dibutyl- und *N*-Butyl-*N*-butanol(4)-nitrosamin. Z. Krebsforsch., 66, 280-290

Druckrey, H., Preussmann, R., Ivankovic, S. & Schmähl, D. (1967) Organotrope carcinogene Wirkungen bei 65 verschiedenen *N*-Nitroso-Verbindungen an BD-Ratten. Z. Krebsforsch., 69, 103-201

Eisenbrand, G. & Preussmann, R. (1970) Eine neue Methode zur kolorimetrischen Bestimmung von Nitrosaminen nach Spaltung der *N*-Nitrosogruppe mit Bromwasserstoff in Eisessig. Arzneimittel-Forsch., 20, 1513-1517

Eisenbrand, G., Hodenberg, A. von & Preussmann, R. (1970) Trace analysis of *N*-nitroso compounds. II. Steam distillation at neutral, alkaline and acid pH under reduced and atmospheric pressure. Z. analyt. Chem., 251, 22-24

Eisenbrand, G., Spiegelhalder, B., Janzowski, C., Kann, J. & Preussmann, R. (1978) Volatile and non-volatile *N*-nitroso compounds in foods and other environmental media. In: Walker, E.A., Castegnaro, M., Griciute, L. & Lyle, R.E., eds, Environmental Aspects of *N*-Nitroso Compounds, Lyon (IARC Scientific Publications No. 19) (in press)

Emura, M. (1970) Some histologic and cytologic features of leukemias induced by dibutylnitrosamine in CBA/H-T_6T_6 mice. Jap. J. Genet., 45, 71-78

Flaks, A., Hamilton, J.M., Clayson, D.B. & Burch, P.R.J. (1973) The combined effect of radiation and chemical carcinogens in female AxIF mice. Brit. J. Cancer, 28, 227-231

Fridman, A.L., Mukhametshin, F.M. & Novikov, S.S. (1971) Advances in the chemistry of aliphatic *N*-nitrosamines. Russ. chem. Rev., 40, 34-50

Friedman, M.A. & Staub, J. (1976) Inhibition of mouse testicular DNA synthesis by mutagens and carcinogens as a potential simple mammalian assay for mutagenesis. Mutation Res., 37, 67-76

Fujii, K., Odashima, S. & Okada, M. (1977) Induction of tumours by administration of *N*-dibutylnitrosamine and derivatives to infant mice. Brit. J. Cancer, 35, 610-614

Fukushima, S., Hirose, M., Tsuda, H., Shirai, T., Hirao, K., Arai, M. & Ito, N. (1976) Histological classification of urinary bladder cancers in rats induced by *N*-butyl-*N*-(4-hydroxybutyl)nitrosamine. Gann, 67, 81-90

Gough, T.A. (1978) An examination of some foodstuff for trace amounts of volatile nitrosamines using the thermal energy analyser. In: Walker, E.A., Castegnaro, M., Griciute, L. & Lyle, R.E., eds, Environmental Aspects of *N*-Nitroso Compounds, Lyon (IARC Scientific Publications No. 19) (in press)

Hashimoto, Y. & Kitagawa, H.S. (1974) *In vitro* neoplastic transformation of epithelial cells of rat urinary bladder by nitrosamines. Nature (Lond.), 252, 497-499

Hashimoto, Y., Suzuki, E. & Okada, M. (1972) Induction of urinary bladder tumors in ACI/N rats by butyl(3-carboxypropyl)nitrosoamine, a major urinary metabolite of butyl(4-hydroxybutyl)nitrosoamine. Gann, 63, 637-638

Hashimoto, Y., Suzuki, K. & Okada, M. (1974) Induction of urinary bladder tumors by intravesicular instillation of butyl(4-hydroxybutyl)nitrosoamine and its principal urinary metabolite, butyl(3-carboxypropyl)-nitrosoamine in rats. Gann, 65, 69-73

Hashimoto, Y., Kitagawa, H.S. & Ogura, K. (1976) *In vivo* and *in vitro* aspects of carcinogenesis of the urinary bladder by nitrosamines. In: Magee, P.N., Takayama, S., Sugimura, T. & Matsushima, T., eds, Fundamentals in Cancer Prevention, Tokyo, University of Tokyo Press, pp. 267-280

Havery, D.C., Fazio, T. & Howard, J.W. (1978) Survey of cured meat products for volatile *N*-nitrosamines: comparison of two analytical methods. In: Walker, E.A., Castegnaro, M., Griciute, L. & Lyle, R.E., eds, Environmental Aspects of *N*-Nitroso Compounds, Lyon (IARC Scientific Publications No. 19) (in press)

Hedler, L., Kaunitz, H., Marquardt, P., Fales, H. & Johnson, R.E. (1972) Detection of *N*-nitroso compounds by gas chromatography (nitrogen detector) in soyabean oil extract. In: Bogovski, P., Preussmann, R. & Walker, E.A., eds, *N*-Nitroso Compounds, Analysis and Formation, Lyon (IARC Scientific Publications No. 3), pp. 71-73

Hiramatsu, T. (1974) Effect of DL-tryptophan on tumorigenesis in the urinary bladder and liver of rats treated with *N*-nitrosodibutylamine. J. Nara med. Ass., 25, 101-112

IARC (1974) IARC Monographs on the Evaluation of Carcinogenic Risk of Chemicals to Man, 4, Some Aromatic Amines, Hydrazine and Related Substances, *N*-Nitroso Compounds and Miscellaneous Alkylating Agents, Lyon, pp. 197-210

IARC (1977) Annual Report 1977, Lyon, International Agency for Research on Cancer, p. 63

Ito, N. (1973) Experimental studies on tumors of the urinary system of rats induced by chemical carcinogens. Acta path. Jap., 23, 87-109

Ito, N., Hiasa, Y., Tamai, A., Okajima, E. & Kitamura, H. (1969) Histogenesis of urinary bladder tumors induced by *N*-butyl-*N*-(4-hydroxybutyl)nitrosamine in rats. Gann, 60, 401-410

Ito, N., Makiura, S., Yokota, Y., Kamamoto, Y., Hiasa, Y. & Sugihara, S. (1971) Effect of unilateral ureter ligation on development of tumors in the urinary system of rats treated with *N*-butyl-*N*-(4-hydroxybutyl)-nitrosoamine. Gann, 62, 359-365

Ito, N., Hiasa, Y., Toyoshima, K., Okajima, E., Kamamoto, Y., Makiura, S., Yokota, Y., Sugihara, S. & Matayoshi, K. (1972) Rat bladder tumors induced by *N*-butyl-*N*-(4-hydroxybutyl)nitrosamine. In: Nakahara, W., Takayama, S., Sugimura, T. & Odashima, S., eds, Topics in Chemical Carcinogenesis, Tokyo, University of Tokyo Press, pp. 175-197

Ito, N., Matayoshi, K., Arai, M., Yoshioka, Y., Kamamoto, Y., Makiura, S. & Sugihara, S. (1973) Effect of various factors on induction of urinary bladder tumors in animals by *N*-butyl-*N*-(4-hydroxybutyl)nitrosoamine. Gann, 64, 151-159

Ito, N., Arai, M., Sugihara, S., Hirao, K., Makiura, S., Matayoshi, K. & Denda, A. (1975) Experimental urinary bladder tumors induced by *N*-butyl-*N*-(4-hydroxybutyl)nitrosamine. Gann Monogr. Cancer Res., 17, 367-381

Ivankovic, S. & Bücheler, J. (1968) Leber- und Blasen-Carcinome beim Meerschweinchen nach Di-*n*-butylnitrosamin. Z. Krebsforsch., 71, 183-185

Joffe, B.V. (1958) Synthesis of unsymmetric dialkylhydrazines. Zh. obsch. Khim., 28, 1296-1302

Krüger, F.W. (1971) Metabolismus von Nitrosaminen *in vivo*. I. Über die β-Oxidation aliphatischer Di-*n*-alkylnitrosamine: die Bildung von 7-Methylguanin neben 7-Propyl- bzw. 7-Butylguanin nach Applikation von Di-*n*-propyl- oder Di-*n*-butylnitrosamin. Z. Krebsforsch., 76, 145-154

Krüger, F.W. (1972) New aspects in metabolism of carcinogenic nitrosamines. In: Nakahara, W., Takayama, S., Sugimura, T. & Odashima, S., eds, Topics in Chemical Carcinogenesis, Tokyo, University of Tokyo Press, pp. 213-235

Kunze, E. & Schauer, A. (1971) Enzymhistochemische und autoradiographische Untersuchungen an Dibutylnitrosamin-induzierten Harnblasenpapillomen der Ratte. Z. Krebsforsch., 75, 146-160

Kunze, E., Schauer, A. & Calvoer, R. (1969) Zur Histochemie von Harnblasen-Papillomen der Ratte, induziert durch Dibutylnitrosamin. Naturwissenschaften, 56, 639

Kunze, E., Schauer, A. & Spielmann, J. (1971) Autoradiographische Untersuchungen über den RNS-Stoffwechsel während der Entwicklung von Dibutylnitrosamin-induzierten Harnblasentumoren der Ratte. Z. Krebsforsch., 76, 236-248

Kunze, E., Schauer, A. & Schatt, S. (1976) Stages of transformation in the development of *N*-butyl-*N*-(4-hydroxybutyl)-nitrosamine-induced transitional cell carcinomas in the urinary bladder of rats. Z. Krebsforch., 87, 139-160

Kuroki, T., Drevon, C. & Montesano, R. (1977) Microsome-mediated mutagenesis in V79 Chinese hamster cells by various nitrosamines. Cancer Res., 37, 1044-1050

Levin, S. (1973) Ultrastructural pathogenesis of urinary bladder neoplasms induced by dibutylnitrosamine (Abstract No. 3426). Fed. Proc., 32, 826

Magee, P.N. & Barnes, J.M. (1967) Carcinogenic nitroso compounds. Adv. Cancer Res., 10, 163-246

Matsumoto, M., Oyasu, R., Hopp, M.L. & Kitajima, T. (1977) Suppression of dibutylnitrosamine-induced bladder carcinomas in hamsters by dietary indole. J. nat. Cancer Inst., 58, 1825-1829

McCormick, A., Nicholson, M.J., Baylis, M.A. & Underwood, J.G. (1973) Nitrosamines in cigarette smoke condensate. Nature (Lond.), 244, 237-238

Mohr, U., Althoff, J., Schmähl, D. & Krüger, F.W. (1970) The carcinogenic effect of dibutylnitrosamine in Syrian and Chinese hamsters. Z. Krebsforsch., 74, 112-113

Nagao, M., Suzuki, E., Yasuo, K., Yahagi, T., Seino, Y., Sugimura, T. & Okada, M. (1977) Mutagenicity of *N*-butyl-*N*-(4-hydroxybutyl)nitrosamine, a bladder carcinogen, and related compounds. Cancer Res., 37, 399-407

Nakajima, T., Tanaka, A. & Tojyo, K.-I. (1974) The effect of metabolic activation with rat liver preparations on the mutagenicity of several *N*-nitrosamines on a streptomycin-dependent strain of *Escherichia coli*. Mutation Res., 26, 361-366

Napalkov, N.P. & Alexandrov, V.A. (1968) On the effects of blastomogenic substances on the organism during embryogenesis. Z. Krebsforsch., 71, 32-50

Okada, M. & Ishidate, M. (1977) Metabolic fate of *N*-*n*-butyl-*N*-(4-hydroxybutyl)nitrosamine and its analogues. Selective induction of urinary bladder tumours in the rat. Xenobiotica, 7, 11-24

Okada, M. & Suzuki, E. (1972) Metabolism of butyl(4-hydroxybutyl)-nitrosoamine in rats. Gann, 63, 391-392

Okada, M., Suzuki, E., Aoki, J., Iiyoshi, M. & Hashimoto, Y. (1975) Metabolism and carcinogenicity of *N*-butyl-*N*-(4-hydroxybutyl)nitrosamine and related compounds, with special reference to induction of urinary bladder tumors. Gann, 17, 161-176

Okada, M., Suzuki, E. & Hashimoto, Y. (1976) Carcinogenicity of *N*-nitrosamines related to *N*-butyl-*N*-(4-hydroxybutyl)nitrosamine and *N*,*N*-dibutylnitrosamine in ACI/N rats. Gann, 67, 825-834

Okajima, E., Hiramatsu, T., Motomiya, Y., Iriya, K., Ijuin, M. & Ito, N. (1970) Bladder carcinogenesis with di-*n*-butylnitrosamine in the rat (Abstract No. 142). In: Proceedings of the Japanese Cancer Association, 29th Annual Meeting, Tokyo, The Japanese Cancer Association, p. 73

Okajima, E., Hiramatsu, T., Motomiya, Y., Iriya, K., Ijuin, M. & Ito, N. (1971) Effect of DL-tryptophan on tumorigenesis in the urinary bladder and liver of rats treated with *N*-nitrosodibutylamine. Gann, 62, 163-169

Okajima, E., Motomiya, Y., Ijuin, M., Matsushima, S., Hirao, Y., Yamada, K., Ohara, S., Shiomi, T., Oishi, H. & Hosoki, Y. (1975a) Development of urinary bladder tumours in dogs induced by *N*-butyl-*N*-(4-hydroxybutyl)-nitrosamine (BBN) (Abstract No. 41). In: Proceedings of the Japanese Cancer Association, 34th Annual Meeting, Tokyo, The Japanese Cancer Association, p. 22

Okajima, E., Hiramatsu, T., Iriya, K., Ijuin, M., Matsushima, S. & Yamada, K. (1975b) Effects of sex hormones on development of urinary bladder tumours in rats induced by *N*-butyl-*N*-(4-hydroxybutyl)nitrosamine. Urol. Res., 3, 73-79

Pensabene, J.W., Fiddler, W., Dooley, C.J., Doerr, R.C. & Wasserman, A.E. (1972) Spectral and gas chromatographic characteristics of some *N*-nitrosamines. J. agric. Fd Chem., 20, 274-277

Prager, B., Jacobson, P., Schmidt, P. & Stern, D., eds (1922) Beilsteins Handbuch der Organischen Chemie, 4th ed., Vol. 4, Syst. No. 337, Berlin, Springer, p. 158

Preussmann, R., Arjungi, K.N. & Ebers, G. (1976) *In vitro* detection of nitrosamines and other indirect alkylating agents by reaction with 3,4-dichlorothiophenol in the presence of rat liver microsomes. Cancer Res., 36, 2459-2462

Preussmann, R., Walker, E.A., Wasserman, A.E. & Castegnaro, M., eds (1978) Environmental Carcinogens - Selected Methods of Analysis, Vol. 1, Nitrosamines, Lyon (IARC Scientific Publications No. 18) (in press)

Rainey, W.T., Christie, W.H. & Lijinsky, W. (1978) Mass spectrometry of *N*-nitrosamines. Biomed. Mass Spectrom. (in press)

Reznik, G., Mohr, U. & Kmoch, N. (1976) Carcinogenic effects of different nitroso-compounds in Chinese hamsters: *N*-dibutylnitrosamine and *N*-nitrosomethylurea. Cancer Lett., 1, 183-188

Reznik-Schüller, H. & Mohr, U. (1975) The ultrastructure of *N*-dibutylnitrosamine induced pulmonary tumours (adenocarcinomata) in European hamsters. Brit. J. Cancer, 32, 230-238

Reznik-Schüller, H. & Mohr, U. (1976) Ultrastructure of *N*-nitrosodibutylamine-induced tumors of the nasal cavity in the European hamster. J. nat. Cancer Inst., 57, 401-407

Reznik-Schüller, H. & Mohr, U. (1977) Ultrastructure of *N*-dibutylnitrosamine-induced tumors of the urinary bladder in European hamsters. J. nat. Cancer Inst., 58, 1383-1385

Rogers, A.E. & Newberne, P.M. (1973) Effect of diet on carcinogenesis by nitrosamines or dimethylhydrazine (Abstract No. 24). Toxicol. appl. Pharmacol., 25, 448

Rogers, A.E., Sanchez, O., Feinsod, F.M. & Newberne, P.M. (1974) Dietary enhancement of nitrosamine carcinogenesis. Cancer Res., 34, 96-99

Sander, J., Bürkle, G. & Bürkle, V. (1974) Induktion von Lungentumoren und Harnblasentumoren bei Ratten durch Di-*n*-butylnitrosamin in Dimethylsulfoxid (DMSO). Z. Krebsforsch., 82, 83-89

Sen, N.P., Donaldson, B.A., Seaman, S., Iyengar, J.R. & Miles, W.F. (1978) Recent studies in Canada on the analysis and occurrence of volatile and non-volatile *N*-nitroso compounds in foods. In: Walker, E.A., Castegnaro, M., Griciute, L. & Lyle, R.E., eds, Environmental Aspects of *N*-Nitroso Compounds, Lyon (IARC Scientific Publications No. 19) (in press)

Shirai, T., Murasaki, G., Tatematsu, M., Tsuda, H., Fukushima, S. & Ito, N. (1977) Early surface changes of the urinary bladder epithelium of different animal species induced by *N*-butyl-*N*-(4-hydroxybutyl)nitrosamine. Gann, 68, 203-212

Stephany, R.W., Freudenthal, J. & Schuller, P.L. (1976) Quantitative and qualitative determination of some volatile nitrosamines in various meat products. In: Walker, E.A., Bogovski, P. & Griciute, L., eds, Environmental *N*-Nitroso Compounds Analysis and Formation, Lyon (IARC Scientific Publications No. 14), pp. 343-354

Takayama, S. & Imaizumi, T. (1969) Carcinogenic action of *N*-nitrosodibutylamine in mice. Gann, 60, 353

Vlasov, N.N., Dzhioev, F.K. & Pliss, G.B. (1973) On peculiarities of a carcinogenic action of dibutyl nitrosamine. Vop. Onkol., 19, 55-59

Wood, M., Flaks, A. & Clayson, D.B. (1970) The carcinogenic activity of dibutylnitrosamine in IF x C_{57} mice. Europ. J. Cancer, 6, 433-440

1. Chemical and Physical Data

1.1 Synonyms and trade names

Chem. Abstr. Services Reg. No.: 1116-54-7

Chem. Abstr. Name: 2,2'-(Nitrosoimino)bis-ethanol

Diethanolnitrosamine; NDELA; *N*-nitroso-bis(2-hydroxyethyl)amine; nitrosoimino diethanol

1.2 Structural and molecular formulae and weight

$$O{=}N{-}N(CH_2{-}CH_2OH)_2$$

$C_4H_{10}N_2O_3$ Mol. wt: 134.1

1.3 Chemical and physical properties of the pure substance

(a) Description: Yellow, viscous oil

(b) Boiling-point: 114°C (1.5 mm); decomposes at approximately 200°C (14 mm)

(c) Refractive index: n_D^{20} 1.4540

(d) Spectroscopy data: λ_{max} 234 and 345 nm (E_1^1 = 470.7 and 5.3) in water (Druckrey *et al.*, 1967); mass spectrometry data are given by Fan *et al.* (1977a).

(e) Solubility: Miscible with water in all proportions; soluble in polar organic solvents; insoluble in non-polar organic solvents

(f) Volatility: Not steam-volatile

(g) Stability: Stable at room temperature for more than 14 days in neutral or alkaline aqueous solutions in the dark; slightly less stable in acidic solutions; light-sensitive, especially to ultra-violet light

(h) Reactivity: Can be reduced to the corresponding hydrazine and/or amine; cyclized by sulphuric acid at 155°C to form *N*-nitrosomorpholine (Fan *et al.*, 1977b)

1.4 Technical products and impurities

No data were available to the Working Group.

2. Production, Use, Occurrence and Analysis

2.1 Production and use

(a) Production

N-Nitrosodiethanolamine (NDELA) has been prepared by the reaction of sodium nitrite with diethanolamine dissolved with dilute hydrochloric acid (Jones & Wilson, 1949). No evidence was found that NDELA has been produced commercially; it is difficult to prepare and purify.

(b) Use

No data were available to the Working Group.

2.2 Occurrence

(a) Tobacco

Schmeltz *et al.* (1977) found 0.1-173 μg/kg NDELA in tobacco. The source was believed to be a maleic hydrazide herbicide formulated as the diethanolamine salt, which had been used on the tobacco.

(b) Cutting fluids

Cutting fluids are widely used to reduce the temperature of the metal-tool interface during metal cutting or grinding. The may be synthetic (water, sodium nitrite and triethanolamine), semi-synthetic (water, oil, emulsifier) or pure oil (Bureau of National Affairs, 1976). In Europe and the US, most cutting fluid concentrates are synthetic, containing up to 45% triethanolamine and 18% sodium nitrite in water, and are diluted for final use (Fan *et al.*, 1977b).

Zingmark & Rappe (1976) reported initially that NDELA was not found in a freshly prepared nitrite-triethanolamine-based cutting fluid; however, on standing for 5-7 months, the fluid was found to contain 400-800 mg/l NDELA (colorimetric and gas chromatographic quantification) (Rappe & Zingmark, 1978; Zingmark & Rappe, 1977). Fan *et al.* (1977b) found that even when the pH of the fluids was in the range of 9-11, all cutting fluids examined contained NDELA at concentrations varying from 0.02-3%.

(c) Pesticides

An atrazine formulation emulsified with triethanolamine was reported to contain 0.5 mg/kg NDELA[1] (Cohen *et al.*, 1978).

(d) Cosmetics

NDELA was found in all of 7 facial cosmetic formulations at levels of 42-49,000 μg/kg and in 12/13 hand and body lotions (<10-140 μg/kg) and in 8/9 hair shampoos (<10-260 μg/kg) (Fan *et al.*, 1977a).

2.3 Analysis

For the analysis of NDELA in cutting fluids, pesticides and cosmetics, samples are extracted with ethyl acetate in the presence of ammonium sulphamate, washed off a silica column with acetone and analysed by thermal energy analyser-high-pressure liquid chromatography using a μ Porasil column with 2 ml/min of 40% acetone and 60% hexane (Cohen *et al.*, 1978; Fan *et al.*, 1977a,b).

Gas chromatography can also be used for analysis of NDELA in pesticides (Cohen *et al.*, 1978); for cutting fluids, conversion to the *O*-methyl ether followed by gas chromatography (Fan *et al.*, 1977b) or a colorimetric method (Rappe & Zingmark, 1978) can be used. Analysis of NDELA in tobacco is described by Schmeltz *et al.* (1977).

---

[1]This result was not confirmed by mass spectroscopy (see also 'General Remarks on the Substances Considered', p. 40).

3. Biological Data Relevant to the Evaluation of Carcinogenic Risk to Man

3.1 Carcinogenicity and related studies in animals

(a) Oral administration

Rat: A group of 20 BD rats was given *N*-nitrosodiethanolamine (NDELA) in the drinking-water at concentrations equivalent to 600-1000 mg/kg bw/day, up to a total dose of 150-300 g/kg bw. All 20 animals developed hepatocellular carcinomas between 242-325 days after the start of treatment; 4 rats also had renal adenomas (Druckrey *et al.*, 1967) [The Working Group noted that the dose required to produce the effects was very much higher than that of other carcinogenic nitrosamines].

(b) Subcutaneous administration

Hamster: Two groups of 15 male and 15 female Syrian golden hamsters received either 7 twice weekly s.c. injections each of 2260 mg/kg bw NDELA (1/5 of the LD_{50}) or 27 injections of 565 mg/kg bw (1/20 of the LD_{50}) over 45 weeks; in the latter case, several injection-free intervals of 1-2 weeks were required due to local necrosis. Total doses were approximately 15 g/kg bw; all surviving animals were killed at 78 weeks. In the first group, 28/30 animals were still alive at the appearance of the first tumour (33 weeks), and 20 developed tumours, including 10 adenocarcinomas of the nasal cavity, 8 papillary tumours of the trachea and 3 hepatocellular adenomas. In the second group, 27/30 animals survived 33 weeks, and 19 developed tumours, including 12 adenocarcinomas of the nasal cavity, 7 papillary tumours of the trachea and 3 fibrosarcomas at the injection site. Of 27 effective controls, 3 developed 1 thyroid carcinoma, 1 haemangioendothelioma of the spleen and 2 adenomas of the adrenal gland (Hilfrich *et al.*, 1978) [The Secretariat became aware of this paper subsequent to the meeting of the Working Group].

3.2 Other relevant biological data

(a) Experimental systems

The s.c. LD_{50} of NDELA in Syrian golden hamsters was 11.3 g/kg bw (Hilfrich *et al.*, 1978). NDELA was not lethal when given as a single oral dose of 7.5 g/kg bw to rats (Druckrey *et al.*, 1967).

No data on the metabolism, mutagenicity, embryotoxicity or teratogenicity of this compound were available to the Working Group.

(b) Humans

No data were available to the Working Group.

3.3 Case reports and epidemiological studies

No data were available to the Working Group.

4. Summary of Data Reported and Evaluation

4.1 Experimental data

N-Nitrosodiethanolamine is carcinogenic in rats after its oral administration and in hamsters after its subcutaneous injection. It produces hepatocellular carcinomas and renal adenomas in rats, and adenocarcinomas of the nasal cavity, papillary tumours of the trachea, hepatocellular adenomas and local fibrosarcomas in hamsters.

4.2 Human data

No case reports or epidemiological studies were available to the Working Group. *N*-Nitrosodiethanolamine has been found in variable concentrations in tobacco, one pesticide formulation, some cosmetic preparations and, in much higher concentrations (0.02-3%), in cutting fluids. These reports should permit the identification of exposed groups.

4.3 Evaluation

There is *sufficient evidence* of a carcinogenic effect of *N*-nitrosodiethanolamine in two experimental animal species. In view of the widespread exposure to appreciable concentrations of *N*-nitrosodiethanolamine, efforts should be made to obtain epidemiological information. Although no epidemiological data were available, *N*-nitrosodiethanolamine should be regarded for practical purposes as if it were carcinogenic to humans.

5. References

Bureau of National Affairs (1976) Procedures for reducing exposure to cutting oils are issued by NIOSH. Occupational Safety and Health Reporter, Washington DC, US Government Printing Office, pp. 565-566

Cohen, S.Z., Bontoyan, W.R. & Zweig, G. (1978) Analytical determination of *N*-nitroso compounds in pesticides by the United States Environmental Protection Agency. In: Walker, E.A., Castegnaro, M., Griciute, L. & Lyle, R.E., eds, Environmental Aspects of *N*-Nitroso Compounds, Lyon (IARC Scientific Publications No. 19) (in press)

Druckrey, H., Preussmann, R., Ivankovic, S. & Schmähl, D. (1967) Organotrope carcinogene Wirkungen bei 65 verschiedenen *N*-Nitroso-Verbindungen an BD-Ratten. Z. Krebsforsch., 69, 103-201

Fan, T.-Y., Goff, U., Song, L., Fine, D.H., Arsenault, G.P. & Biemann, K. (1977a) *N*-Nitrosodiethanolamine in cosmetics, lotions and shampoos. Fd Cosmet. Toxicol., 15, 423-430

Fan, T.-Y., Morrison, J., Rounbehler, D.P., Ross, R., Fine, D.H., Miles, W. & Sen, N.P. (1977b) *N*-Nitrosodiethanolamine in synthetic cutting fluids: a part-per-hundred impurity. Science, 196, 70-71

Hilfrich, J., Schmeltz, I. & Hoffmann, D. (1978) Effects of *N*-nitrosodiethanolamine and 1,1-diethanolhydrazine in Syrian golden hamsters. Cancer Lett. (in press)

Jones, E.R.H. & Wilson, W. (1949) The preparation of some chloroalkylamino-compounds. J. chem. Soc., 547-552

Rappe, C. & Zingmark, P.-A. (1978) Formation of *N*-nitrosamines in cutting fluids. In: Walker, E.A., Castegnaro, M., Griciute, L. & Lyle, R.E., eds, Environmental Aspects of *N*-Nitroso Compounds, Lyon (IARC Scientific Publications No. 19) (in press)

Schmeltz, I., Abidi, S. & Hoffmann, D. (1977) Tumorigenic agents in unburned processed tobacco: *N*-nitrosodiethanolamine and 1,1-dimethylhydrazine. Cancer Lett., 2, 125-132

Zingmark, P.-A. & Rappe, C. (1976) On the formation of *N*-nitrosodiethanolamine from a grinding fluid under simulated gastric conditions. Ambio, 5, 80-81

Zingmark, P.-A. & Rappe, C. (1977) On the formation of *N*-nitrosodiethanolamine in a grinding fluid concentrate after storage. Ambio, 6, 237-238

N-NITROSODIETHYLAMINE

This substance was considered previously by an IARC Working Group, in December 1971 (IARC, 1972). Since that time new data have become available, and these have been incorporated into the monograph and taken into account in the present evaluation.

1. Chemical and Physical Data

1.1 Synonyms and trade names

Chem. Abstr. Services Reg. No.: 55-18-5

Chem. Abstr. Name: *N*-Ethyl-*N*-nitroso-ethanamine

DEN; DENA; *N,N*-diethylnitrosamine; diethylnitrosamine; nitrosodiethylamine; NDEA

1.2 Structural and molecular formulae and weight

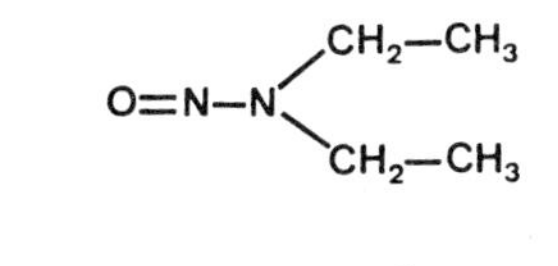

$C_4H_{10}N_2O$ Mol. wt: 102.1

1.3 Chemical and physical properties of the pure substance

(a) Description: Yellow, volatile liquid

(b) Boiling-point: 177°C (760 mm); 64-65°C (17 mm) (Druckrey *et al.*, 1967)

(c) Density: d_4^{20} 0.9422

(d) Refractive index: n_D^{20} 1.4386

(e) Spectroscopy data: λ_{max} 230 and 340 nm (E_1^1 = 726.7 and 8.3) in water (Druckrey *et al.*, 1967); mass spectroscopy data are given by Pensabene *et al.* (1972) and Rainey *et al.* (1978).

(f) Solubility: Soluble in water (approximately 10%) (Druckrey *et al.*, 1967) and in organic solvents and lipids

(g) Volatility: Can be steam-distilled quantitatively (Eisenbrand *et al.*, 1970)

(h) Stability: Stable at room temperature for more than 14 days in neutral or alkaline aqueous solutions in the dark (Druckrey *et al.*, 1967); slightly less stable in acidic solutions; light-sensitive, especially to ultra-violet light

(i) Reactivity: Strong oxidants (peracids) oxidize it to the corresponding nitramine; can be reduced to the corresponding hydrazine and/or amine; relatively resistant to hydrolysis but can easily be split by hydrogen bromide in acetic acid (Eisenbrand & Preussmann, 1970). Photochemically reactive (Fridman *et al.*, 1971). A description of the preparation of various derivatives is available (Preussmann *et al.*, 1978).

1.4 Technical products and impurities

No data were available to the Working Group.

2. Production, Use, Occurrence and Analysis

2.1 Production and use

For background information on this section, see preamble, p. 22.

(a) Production

N-Nitrosodiethylamine (NDEA) was first prepared in 1863 by Geuther & Kreutzhage (Prager *et al.*, 1922). It can be made by the reaction of diethylamine and nitrous acid (Druckrey *et al.*, 1967).

Although NDEA is available in small quantities for research purposes, no evidence was found that it has been manufactured commercially.

(b) Use

No data were available to the Working Group.

2.2 Occurrence

(a) Air

When the air of a number of major US cities was examined for *N*-nitrosamines, NDEA (200 mg/m^3)[1] was found only in one area of Baltimore (Fine *et al.*, 1976a,b). Levels of <10 ng/m^3[1] have been found in the smoking compartment of a train (Brunnemann & Hoffman, 1978).

(b) Tobacco smoke

McCormick *et al.* (1973) reported NDEA in tobacco smoke condensate at a level of 1-28 ng/cigarette. The mainstream smoke of a blended cigarette without filter tip (85 mm; 0.9% nitrate; 2.05% nicotine) was reported to contain <5 ng NDEA/cigarette (Hoffmann *et al.*, 1974). Klimsch *et al.* (1976) reported trace levels in 9 types of tobacco smoke, and 1 ng/cigarette in one sample. Up to 8.3 ng/cigarette were found in the mainstream smoke of 19 commercial and experimental cigarettes; far greater concentrations (8-73 ng/cigarette) were found in sidestream smoke (Brunnemann & Hoffmann, 1978; Brunnemann *et al.*, 1977).

(c) Water

NDEA was found at the 0.010 μg/l[1] level in high-nitrate well-water used for drinking (Fine, 1978). Fiddler *et al.* (1977) reported 0.33 and 0.83 μg/l NDEA in deionized water. Levels of 0.07 and 0.24 μg/l[1] were found in the waste-water from 2/19 chemical plants (Cohen & Bachman, 1978).

(d) Food and feed

Cheese: NDEA was detected in a sample of Cheddar cheese in trace amounts (>0.5 μg/kg but <1.0 μg/kg) and in Cheshire cheese at a level of 1.5 μg/kg[1] (Alliston *et al.*, 1972). It was found in 1/16 cheese samples at a level of 20-30 μg/kg[1] (Cerutti *et al.*, 1975). Sen *et al.* (1978) reported 2-20 μg/kg NDEA in 10/63 cheeses. Eisenbrand *et al.* (1978) found 3 μg/kg in 1/173 cheeses.

---

[1]These results were not confirmed by mass spectroscopy (see also 'General Remarks on the Substances Considered', p. 40).

Vegetables and vegetable oils: NDEA has been detected in beans at a level of 0.2 μg/kg[1] (Roach, 1972), and in five samples of freshly expressed soya bean oil at a level of 4 μg/kg[1] (Hedler & Marquardt, 1974).

Cereal products: In earlier work using inadequate methodology, conflicting reports were made about the presence of NDEA in cereal products. Hedler & Marquardt (1968), Heyns & Röper (1974), Kroeller (1967), Marquardt & Hedler (1966), Roach (1972), Sen *et al.* (1969), Thewlis (1967) and studies in Iran (Joint Iran-IARC Study Group, 1977) found no evidence of NDEA in such products.

Fish: NDEA has been found at levels of less than 1 μg/kg in spotted catfish, cod, coalfish, greater silver smelt, grenadier, herring, pollock, redfish and torsk; haddock was found to contain up to 4 μg/kg (Telling *et al.*, 1974). In another study, cod was found to contain up to 50 μg/kg[1] in salted samples, 39 μg/kg[1] in samples in tomato sauce, 1 μg/kg[1] in frozen samples and none in smoked samples. The same study reported that dwarf herring contained 147 μg/kg[1] in baked samples, 2 μg/kg[1] in fresh samples and 1 μg/kg[1] in smoked samples. Herring was found to contain 108 μg/kg[1] in pickled samples, 27 μg/kg[1] in samples in tomato sauce and 4 μg/kg[1] in smoked samples (Kann *et al.*, 1976). Earlier studies reported a level of 1.5 μg/kg[1] in both uncooked and fried stale cod (Alliston *et al.*, 1972) and traces[1] of NDEA in samples of pickled but not frozen herring (Sen *et al.*, 1969). Levels of 1.2-21.0 mg/kg[1] have been reported in Cantonese salt-dried fish (Fong & Walsh, 1971).

NDEA has also been detected[1] in salted salmon roe which contained sodium nitrite (Sakai & Tanimura, 1971). Iyengar *et al.* (1976) found 4-14 μg/kg NDEA in halibut, salmon, cod, sole, ocean perch and scallops only after frying or baking.

Meat products: A maximum of 40 μg/kg[1] NDEA was reported in cured meats (Freimuth & Glaeser, 1970). Less than 1 μg/kg was detected in 1/24 samples of fried bacon, and 1-4 μg/kg were found in a sample of chopped

---

[1]These results were not confirmed by mass spectroscopy (see also 'General Remarks on the Substances Considered', p. 40).

pork (Crosby *et al.*, 1972). In the UK, 1.5 μg/kg[1] NDEA was found in fried back bacon and in uncooked pig's liver (Alliston *et al.*, 1972). Levels of 2-25 μg/kg were found in 11/298 samples (Sen *et al.*, 1974) and in 9/80 samples of various meat products (Panalaks *et al.*, 1974). Trace amounts[1] of NDEA were reported in samples of tea sausage, smoked 'Krekovi' sausage and smoked 'Servelaad' sausage (Kann *et al.*, 1976). Samples of uncooked bacon were found to contain 0.3 μg/kg, and cooked bacon samples contained 2.0 μg/kg[1] (Fine & Rounbehler, 1976).

Sen *et al.* (1976) found 10 μg/kg in pepperoni, 3-10 μg/kg in bologna, 7 μg/kg in wieners, 10 μg/kg in mock chicken, 16 μg/kg in meatloaf and 5 μg/kg in ham sausage. Groenen *et al.* (1976) found 7 and 91 μg/kg in two samples of smoked meat and 4-43 μg/kg in fried and unfried bacon. Stephany *et al.* (1976) found a mean of 0.1-0.6 μg/kg in meat products, with up to 2.8 μg/kg in cooked and smoked ham; and Groenen *et al.* (1977) found 0.1-0.8 μg/kg in 11/47 samples of processed meats.

Havery *et al.* (1978) and Eisenbrand *et al.* (1978) found no evidence of NDEA in a large number of meat products. Gough (1978) found 0.05 μg/kg[1] in 1/13 prepared meals, <0.03 μg/kg[1] in 3/36 pastry foods and up to 0.2 μg/kg[1] in cured meats.

Feed: A level of 1 μg/kg NDEA was found in 4/6 samples of fishmeal (Mirna *et al.*, 1976), and 28 and 36 μg/kg were found in 2/16 samples (Juszkiewicz & Kowalski, 1976). Kann *et al.* (1978) reported <1.0 μg/kg in 3/46 samples of animal feed. Levels of 0-17 μg/kg have been found in experimental animal feed (IARC, 1977a).

(e) Alcoholic beverages

NDEA has been detected in a number of alcoholic beverages, including apple brandy, ciders, cognac, armagnac, rum and whiskey. The average level was 0.1 μg/kg (IARC, 1977b).

---

[1]These results were not confirmed by mass spectroscopy (see also 'General Remarks on the Substances Considered', p. 40).

(f) *In vivo*

NDEA was present in human blood both before and after the ingestion of a meal: the level in the blood increased from 0.09 μl/l[1] before to 0.46 μg/l[1] following the meal (Fine *et al.*, 1977). Lakritz *et al.* (1978) reported the presence of 5-30 μg/kg NDEA in the stomachs of 4/35 fasting patients [No adequate precautions were taken to prevent nitrosamine formation during storage of the samples].

2.3 Analysis

An IARC Manual gives selected methods for the analysis of volatile *N*-nitrosamines, including NDEA (Preussmann *et al.*, 1978).

On 29 September 1977, the US Environmental Protection Agency issued a notice requiring all registrants of pesticide products that are potentially contaminated with *N*-nitroso compounds to analyse commercial samples which have been stored for at least 18 days to determine the extent of contamination. This notice prescribes in general terms the types of analytical methods to be used for volatile *N*-nitroso compounds (e.g., gas chromatography plus mass spectrometry or thermal energy analysis, and others) as well as for nonvolatile *N*-nitroso compounds (e.g., high-pressure liquid chromatography plus ultra-violet spectroscopy). Confirmation of positive results by gas chromatography and mass spectrometry or by valid independent methods is required when possible (US Environmental Protection Agency, 1977).

3. Biological Data Relevant to the Evaluation of Carcinogenic Risk to Man

3.1 Carcinogenicity and related studies in animals

(a) Oral administration

Mouse: Several studies on different strains have demonstrated the carcinogenicity of *N*-nitrosodiethylamine (NDEA) in this species. In the

[1]These results were not confirmed by mass spectroscopy (see also 'General Remarks on the Substances Considered', p. 40).

liver, mainly haemangioendotheliomas (Schmähl & Thomas, 1965a; Schmähl *et al.*, 1963a) and adenomas (Takayama & Oota, 1965), but also hepatomas (Clapp & Craig, 1967; Clapp *et al.*, 1970; Schmähl *et al.*, 1963a), were produced. Squamous-cell carcinomas of the oesophagus and forestomach were also found (Clapp & Craig, 1967; Clapp *et al.*, 1970, 1971; Shvemberger, 1965; Takayama & Oota, 1965). An increased incidence of lung adenomas has also been observed (Clapp & Craig, 1967; Clapp *et al.*, 1970; Mirvish & Kaufman, 1970). The site and histological type of the tumours depended to a certain extent on the mouse strain used (Clapp *et al.*, 1971). Tumour frequency was usually very high, approaching in many cases 100%, in mice given a dosage of 2-13 mg/kg bw/day. Some indication of a dose-response relationship has been reported by Clapp *et al.* (1970) and Schmähl & Thomas (1965a).

It was reported in an abstract that single i.g. doses of 60 mg/kg bw NDEA produced 7/24 hepatomas and 7/24 lung adenomas in BTO mice; no significant increase was seen in C57BL/60 mice (Akamatsu, 1975).

Rat: Following the first report of liver carcinogenesis by NDEA in rats (Schmähl *et al.*, 1960), many laboratories confirmed and enlarged this finding using different strains and conditions (Grundmann & Sieburg, 1962; Lacassagne *et al.*, 1967; Reid *et al.*, 1963; Takayama *et al.*, 1975; Thomas, 1961). In most cases, hepatocellular tumours have been observed, often with lung metastases; in some cases, cholangiomas have also been described (Argus & Hoch-Ligeti, 1961; Hoch-Ligeti *et al.*, 1964). In lifetime feeding studies with daily doses of between 1 and 10 mg/kg bw, tumour yields approaching 100% have been found. While most investigations have shown no sex difference, Reuber & Lee (1968) reported an increased sensitivity in young females. The same authors also reported that four-week-old animals were more sensitive than older animals. Feeding for only 82 days increased the latent period and reduced the tumour yield as compared with lifetime feeding (Rajewsky *et al.*, 1966). With lower daily dosages (0.15-0.6 mg/kg bw), squamous-cell carcinomas of the oesophagus were obtained in addition to liver tumours (Druckrey *et al.*, 1963a). A single dose of 280 mg/kg bw induced liver and kidney tumours, and 4 weekly doses of 25 or 35 mg/kg bw induced tumours of the liver, the oesophagus and the kidney (Druckrey *et al.*, 1963b, 1964).

In a dose-response study (Table 1), the mean total dose administered in drinking-water until appearance of the first tumour ranged from 56-965 mg/kg bw, and the induction time for tumours between 68 and 750 days. All dosages higher than 0.15 mg/kg bw/day gave a tumour yield of 100%; 0.15 mg/kg bw/day gave a tumour yield of 27/30. At a dose of 0.075 mg/kg bw/day, 20 rats lived for more than 600 days (40/60 died from pneumonia); at 750 days, 16 were dead and 1 animal had a hepatoma, 3 had multiple papillomas of the oesophagus, and 3 had a squamous-cell carcinoma of the nasal cavity. The four animals given this dose level that lived at least until 940 days of age (850 days of the experiment) all had tumours: 3 had hepatomas (one of these also had a jaw carcinoma) and one had a hepatocellular carcinoma; 2 sarcomas were seen also (Druckrey *et al.*, 1963a).

Liver tumours, including 13 hepatocellular carcinomas, 9 haemangiosarcomas and 1 unclassified blastoma, were induced in 23/25 16-week-old male Wistar rats by daily administration of 1 mg NDEA in the drinking-water, up to a total dose of 134 mg/animal (Hadjiolov, 1972).

Carcinomas of the oesophagus were induced in 9/14 male and 5/14 female 12-week-old Buffalo rats after feeding 0.0114% NDEA in the diet for 26 weeks. Animals survived an average of 28 weeks (Reuber, 1975).

It was reported in an abstract that nasal and other tumours (unspecified) occurred after the tenth month of life in the offspring of a female rat given NDEA during nursing (route unspecified); the mother developed a kidney tumour and died after 9 months (Schoental & Appleby, 1973).

Hamster: The i.g. administration of 0.4 ml of a dilute aqueous solution of NDEA (1:250) twice weekly induced tumours of the trachea and/or lung in 37/68 Syrian golden hamsters (Dontenwill & Mohr, 1961; Dontenwill *et al.*, 1962). In another study, malignant liver-cell tumours and tumours of the nasal cavity and bronchi were also induced (Herrold & Dunham, 1963).

Tumours of the forestomach and oesophagus developed in all of 20 male and 20 female inbred Chinese hamsters that received 40 mg/l NDEA in

Table 1[a]

N-Nitrosodiethylamine dose-response

Daily dose mg/kg bw	Number of animals alive at appearance of first malignant liver tumour	Number of animals with malignant tumours of the liver and/ or oesophagus	Number of malignant liver tumours	Number of lung metastases	Number of oesophageal tumours	
					Papillomas	Carcinomas
14.2	5	5	5			
9.6	25	25	25	4		
4.8	25	25	25	4		
2.4	34	34	34	7		
1.2	36	36	36	10		
0.6	49	49	49	8	4	5
0.3	67	62	4	4	7	23
0.15	30	27	18	2	13	9
0.075	4	1	1		3	

[a]From Druckrey *et al.*, 1963*a*

drinking-water for 17-26 weeks. Squamous-cell carcinomas accounted for 23% of the stomach tumours and for 15% of those of the oesophagus. Hepatocellular carcinomas also occurred in 5 animals (Baker *et al.*, 1974).

Guinea-pig: NDEA administered in the drinking-water as 5 mg/kg bw/day induced hepatocellular carcinomas and liver adenocarcinomas, some metastasizing into the lungs, in all of 11 treated animals. The median total dose was 1200 mg/kg bw (Druckrey & Steinhoff, 1962). With a dose of 3 mg/kg bw/day, 7/8 animals had liver tumours (Thomas & Schmähl, 1963). In another study, hepatocellular carcinomas were again the main tumour type induced in 14/15 animals that lived more than 16 weeks (Argus & Hoch-Ligeti, 1963). In a dose-response study, NDEA was given in the drinking-water for periods of 4, 8, 12 and 24 weeks; with an average daily intake of 1.2 mg/animal (total dose, <75 mg/animal), no tumours were observed after one year. With a higher daily intake, treatment for 12 weeks gave a 21% tumour yield and treatment for 24 weeks a 100% yield (Arcos *et al.*, 1969).

Rabbit: Daily doses of 3.4 mg/kg bw NDEA given continuously in the drinking-water induced liver-cell carcinomas in 2/2 treated rabbits (Schmähl & Thomas, 1965b). In another experiment, all 13 animals that received NDEA continuously in the drinking-water (0.042 g/l) on 6 days a week died with metastasizing hepatic carcinomas; one animal had an adenocarcinoma of the lung (Rapp *et al.*, 1965).

Dog: Primary hepatic neoplasms of various types were induced in 14/14 adult male mongrel dogs given 50, 100 or 500 mg/l NDEA in the drinking-water for 2-50 weeks; these consisted of 3 fibromas, 4 leiomyomas, 1 haemangioma, 10 haemangioendotheliomas, 4 fibrosarcomas, 2 leiomyosarcomas, 1 hepatocellular carcinoma, 1 cholangiocarcinoma and 1 undifferentiated-cell carcinoma. Six dogs developed squamous-cell carcinomas of the nasal cavity (Hirao *et al.*, 1974).

Pig: Various tumours of the liver, 1 adenoma of the kidney and 1 squamous-cell carcinoma of the ethmoid were induced by daily doses of 4.4 mg/kg bw NDEA to 4 pigs (Schmähl *et al.*, 1967). In another study, 2 pigs treated with 1.5 mg/kg bw for 11 months and then 3 mg/kg bw until death developed a hepatoma and a kidney adenoma, respectively (total doses, 750 mg/kg bw for the pig that died after 470 days and 1090 mg/kg bw for the one that died after 594 days) (Schmähl *et al.*, 1969).

A group of 6 Göttingen mini-pigs received doses of 0.4 mg/kg bw NDEA in aqueous solution 5 times/week for 42 weeks/year. After 5 years, 3 long-term survivors died (total dose, 420 mg/kg bw), and 2 others were killed. All 5 mini-pigs had a hepatocellular adenoma. Four animals had hepatocellular carcinomas; one of these animals also had a Kupffer-cell sarcoma, and in another metastases of the hepatocellular carcinoma were found in the lung. In addition, 1 renal carcinoma and 1 brain tumour were observed (Graw & Berg, 1977).

Monkey: It was reported in an abstract that after oral administration of NDEA, beginning 12 hours after birth, at a dosage varying from 2-30 mg/kg bw/day, hepatocellular carcinomas were induced in 3/15 rhesus and cynomolgus monkeys (O'Gara & Kelly, 1965). Hepatocellular carcinomas were induced in 6/15 rhesus and cebus monkeys treated with various doses of NDEA for more than a year; treatment of newborn or young animals was with 2 mg/kg bw, and the dose was gradually increased up to 30 mg/kg bw. The cumulative oral dosage ranged from 6-26 g/monkey, and the induction time varied between 14 and 24 months (Kelly *et al.*, 1966).

(b) Skin application

Mouse: Twice-weekly skin application of two drops of a 0.2% solution of NDEA in acetone for 10 months induced squamous-cell carcinomas of the nasal cavity in 17/24 animals; no local skin tumours were observed (Hoffmann & Graffi, 1964a). Daily treatment with three drops of 0.2% solution, or twice-weekly treatment with two drops, induced squamous-cell carcinomas of the nasal cavity in almost all treated animals after application of more than 8 mg/animal (Hoffmann & Graffi, 1964b).

Hamster: In 6/8 Syrian hamsters, skin painting with NDEA in water produced epithelial papillomas of the nasal cavity, but no skin tumours (Herrold, 1964a,b).

(c) Inhalation and/or intratracheal administration

Rat: Spray inhalation of a dilute aqueous solution of NDEA (1:250) for 4 months produced liver carcinomas in 8/17 animals, but no lung tumours (Dontenwill & Mohr, 1962).

Hamster: Spray inhalation of 1-2 mg NDEA twice weekly for 5 months produced tumours of the trachea and/or lungs in 18/33 Syrian golden hamsters (Dontenwill *et al.*, 1962). The weekly intratracheal instillation of 0.05 ml of an aqueous solution (1:14) for a period of up to 6 months induced tumours in the trachea in 14/14 and in the bronchi in 10/14 animals, but no liver tumours (Herrold & Dunham, 1963).

(d) Subcutaneous and/or intramuscular administration

Mouse: S.c. doses of 50 mg/kg bw once or twice weekly, up to a total dose of 200 or 400 mg/kg bw, significantly increased the frequency of lung adenomas from 15% in untreated controls to 25-90% in treated animals (Hilfrich *et al.*, 1971).

Groups of 20 male and 20 female 8-week-old Swiss mice were treated with single s.c. injections of 0, 2, 4, 8, 16 or 32 mg/kg bw NDEA. In treated animals, the incidences of lung tumours (including adenomas and carcinomas) were 16/39, 18/38, 24/39, 25/39 and 21/40, compared with 33/218 in controls; 3 treated mice developed s.c. sarcomas (average survival, 88 weeks) (Cardesa *et al.*, 1974).

Newborn mouse: Treatment of newborn mice with a single s.c. dose of 50 mg/kg bw caused a significant increase in the number of lung adenomas. Most of the animals also developed hepatomas within 6 months (Gargus *et al.*, 1969).

Hamster: Several experiments with Syrian golden hamsters have shown that NDEA produces carcinomas and papillomas of the upper and lower respiratory tract (nasal cavity, bronchi, trachea, lungs) and, much less frequently, tumours of the liver (Dontenwill *et al.*, 1962; Herrold, 1964b,c). A positive dose-response relationship for tumour induction in the upper respiratory tract, but not for that in the lower respiratory tract (where tumour frequency was low), was observed after 12 weekly s.c. doses of

0.5, 1, 2 or 4 mg/animal; tumour yields in the nasal cavity and the larynx ranged from 17-72% and in the trachea from 88-100%; one liver tumour was observed (Montesano & Saffiotti, 1968). Six different single doses, ranging from 0.75-4 mg/animal, produced papillomas in the trachea, while lower doses, down to 0.03 mg/animal, were without effect when the animals were killed at 25 weeks (Mohr *et al.*, 1966a). A smaller dose (4.6-9.3 mg/kg bw) was found to give a 10% yield of tracheal papillomas in hamsters observed for their lifespan (Dontenwill, 1968).

Twice-weekly s.c. injections of 20 mg/kg bw NDEA to 40 Syrian golden hamsters resulted in 18 neoplasms of the nasal cavity (squamous-cell carcinomas, adenocarcinomas, 'neurogenic tumours'), 31 papillomas of the trachea and 19 tumours of the liver (hepatomas, hepatocellular carcinomas, cholangiocarcinomas); the medium induction time was 190±21.4 days (Mennel *et al.*, 1974).

Daily s.c. injections of 5-20 mg/kg bw NDEA to 3 groups of 5 nursing Syrian golden hamsters for 30 days, commencing on the first day after delivery, caused papillomas in the respiratory tracts (trachea, larynx, bronchi, nasal cavity, lung) of mothers and their offspring. The tumour frequency in the F_1 generation was dependent upon the dose the mother received; the findings indicated that the carcinogen or its metabolites were transmitted to the offspring during lactation (Mohr *et al.*, 1972a).

Tracheal tissue from Syrian golden hamsters pretreated twice weekly with 18 mg/kg bw NDEA for 20 weeks was implanted into their mothers' spleens, and the mothers were subsequently given 18 mg/kg bw NDEA subcutaneously twice weekly for 20 weeks. Tracheal tumours developed within the spleen in the mothers (16/22); three of the tumours were squamous-cell carcinomas (Mohr *et al.*, 1976).

The consistent affinity of NDEA for the respiratory tract was not observed in experiments with Chinese hamsters. A s.c. dose of 77 mg/kg bw, given once weekly for up to 22 weeks to 132 animals, resulted in 82% multiple papillomas of the forestomach and 30% papillomas of the oesophagus; squamous metaplasia but no tumours was observed in the respiratory tract (Mohr *et al.*, 1967).

In three groups of 40 Chinese hamsters, s.c. treatment with 1/5, 1/10 or 1/20 LD_{50} NDEA (LD_{50}: 230 mg/kg bw) once a week for life produced squamous-cell papillomas of the cheek pouch, tongue, pharynx, oesophagus and forestomach in up to 100% of animals. Carcinomas were also seen occasionally at these sites (Reznik *et al.*, 1976).

Once-weekly s.c. injection of 20 mg/kg bw NDEA for life to 10 wild male European hamsters yielded tumours of the respiratory system in all animals; the main target organ was the nasal cavities. Squamous-cell papillomas were seen in the larynx, trachea and stem bronchi (Mohr *et al.*, 1972b).

Newborn hamster: A single s.c. dose of 0.015, 0.03, 0.09 or 0.15 mg/animal given to newborn hamsters produced tumours of the upper respiratory tract in 30-65% of the animals, but very few tumours were observed in the lungs and bronchi. One liver-cell carcinoma and 1 hepatoma were seen in 144 animals (Montesano & Saffiotti, 1970).

Gerbil: When groups of 40 or 120 gerbils (*Meriones unguiculatus*) were given once-weekly s.c. injections of 6, 12 or 24 mg/kg bw NDEA for life, high incidences (66-80%) of multifocal tumours of the nasal cavity were observed. In addition, papillomas of the tracheobronchial system, adenomas and carcinomas of the lung, as well as cholangiocellular and hepatocellular carcinomas were seen (Cardesa *et al.*, 1976; Haas *et al.*, 1975).

Guinea-pig: S.c. administration of total doses of between 341 and 1310 mg/kg bw produced malignant liver-cell tumours and some benign or malignant tumours in the trachea and ethmoidal region of guinea-pigs (Lombard, 1965).

Hedgehog: S.c. administration of NDEA to Algerian hedgehogs (*Erinaceus*) (total dose, 375-1050 mg/kg bw) resulted in necrosis of the liver parenchyma and benign and malignant tumours of the liver and lung (Graw *et al.*, 1974).

Bird: Grass parakeets were injected intramuscularly once weekly with 100 mg/kg bw for 19 weeks and then once every second week, to a total dose of 2500±600 mg/kg bw; 6/9 birds that survived the treatment died with malignant hepatic tumours (Schmähl *et al.*, 1966).

(e) Intraperitoneal administration

Mouse: Two i.p. injections of 100 mg/kg bw produced lung adenomas in 28/29 SWR mice (Mirvish & Kaufman, 1970).

A strain-specific susceptibility to NDEA carcinogenesis was identified by Diwan & Meier (1976a). A single i.p. injection of 90 mg/kg bw led predominantly to lung adenomas (24% *versus* 0% in controls) and leukaemia (68% in both experimental and control animals) in 25 AKR/J mice, to lung adenomas (70% *versus* 22% in controls) and leukaemia (28% *versus* 18% in controls) in 25 SWR/J mice and to 6 hepatomas and 1 bile-duct adenoma in 21 C57BL/6J mice. No liver tumours were seen in 20 C57BL/6J control mice.

Studies on the metastatic tendency of NDEA-induced liver tumours in $(C57BL/6JxC3HeB/FeJ)F_1$ mice revealed metastatic foci in the lungs in 22% (Kyriazis *et al.*, 1974) and 38% of the animals (route unspecified) (Koka & Vesselinovitch, 1974).

Rat: A daily i.p. dose of 0.55 mg/animal for 12 or 23 weeks produced hepatomas in more than 80% of F-344 rats treated (Svoboda & Higginson, 1968).

Hamster: An i.p. dose of 2 mg/animal once a week for 4-7 months produced squamous-cell papillomas of the trachea, epithelial papillomas, carcinomas and neuroepithelial tumours of the nasal cavity, squamous-cell papillomas of the bronchi and hepatic carcinomas (Herrold, 1964b).

Monkey: Two *Ceropethicus aethiops* (green) monkeys treated with 20-40 mg/kg bw every two weeks for 26 months developed hepatic-cell carcinomas (Kelly *et al.*, 1966). It was reported in an abstract that hepatomas and hepatocellular carcinomas were produced by i.p. administration of 40 mg/kg bw once every two weeks for 15 months or longer in all 25 monkeys treated; 17 of these had metastases (O'Gara *et al.*, 1970).

It was reported in an abstract that i.p. administration of NDEA resulted in liver tumours within 8-27 months in rhesus and cynomolgus monkeys. This was preceded by a significant increase in the *alpha*-foeto-protein levels in serum between the third and sixth months (Adamson *et al.*, 1973).

Mucoepidermoid carcinomas in the nasal cavities occurred in 10/14 prosimian primates (*Galago crassicaudatus*) treated by i.p. injection every 2 weeks with 10-30 mg/kg bw NDEA; 2/10 animals also had primary carcinomas of the liver (Dalgard *et al.*, 1975, 1976).

Newborn monkey: It was reported in an abstract that i.p. injections of NDEA every other week to newborn rhesus monkeys resulted in 100% liver tumour incidence within 10-15 months (Adamson *et al.*, 1974).

(f) Intravenous administration

Rat: A single i.v. injection of 280 mg/kg bw NDEA to 4 rats produced kidney tumours in all animals and one carcinoma of the ovary (Druckrey *et al.*, 1963b, 1964).

The effect upon the kidneys of a single i.v. injection of 1.25-160 mg/kg bw NDEA was studied in groups of 10 male and 10 female Sprague-Dawley rats (Table 2). One female given 1.25 mg/kg bw developed an adenoma of the kidney. Dose levels of 40 mg/kg bw and above increased the tumour incidence and decreased survival time (Mohr & Hilfrich, 1972, 1974).

Gerbil: Single i.v. injections of 50 or 100 mg/kg bw NDEA to groups of 10 male gerbils resulted in the development of carcinomas of the nasal cavities; the tumours originated mainly from the respiratory-olfactory mucosal junction (Cardesa *et al.*, 1976).

(g) Other experimental systems

Prenatal exposure

Pregnant NMRI mice were given NDEA in s.c. doses of 80-240 mg/kg bw from the 15th to the 20th day of gestation; their offspring were killed after 8 or 12 months. A significant increase (up to 63%) in the occurrence of multiple pulmonary adenomas was observed (Mohr & Althoff, 1965a). In addition to lung adenomas, benign and malignant tumours of the liver, oesophagus and forestomach were observed in the offspring of pregnant random-bred or C3H mice treated with NDEA during the last days of pregnancy (Likhachev, 1971, 1974). After treatment with 50 mg/kg bw NDEA on day 18 of gestation, 87% of the offspring of (AKR/JxSWR/J)F_1 mice developed pulmonary adenomas (Diwan & Meier, 1976b).

Table 2[a]

Dose mg/kg bw	Females			Males		
	Survival (weeks)	Number of rats with tumours	Number and type of tumours	Survival (weeks)	Number of rats with tumours	Number and type of tumours
1.25	117	1	1 Adenoma	99	-	- -
2.5	108	1	1 Adenoma	98	1	1 Adenoma
5	110	2	2 Adenomas	105	1	1 Adenoma
10	93	-	- -	98	3	3 Adenomas
20	112	1	1 Adenoma	81	-	- -
40	82	3(1)[b]	3 Adenomas 1 Carcinoma	77	3	2 Adenomas 1 Carcinoma
80	72	6(5)	10 Adenomas 9 Carcinomas 1 Malignant mesen-chymal tumour	87	3(3)	8 Adenomas 1 Carcinoma
160	67	8(7)	13 Adenomas 15 Carcinomas	61	3(2)	4 Adenomas 1 Carcinoma

[a] From Mohr & Hilfrich, 1972

[b] Figures in parentheses are numbers of rats with tumours in both kidneys.

Daily s.c. doses of 4 or 8 mg/animal were given to female Sprague-Dawley rats from the 10th to the 21st day of pregnancy; 14/26 of the mothers showed kidney tumours after 1 year, 5 of which were carcinomas. Some kidney tumours were observed in the offspring at one year of age (Wrba *et al.*, 1967). Under similar conditions, oral or s.c. administration to pregnant Wistar rats of varying doses of NDEA produced benign and malignant tumours, mainly thymomas and adenomas of the mammary gland, in the offspring. Treated female rats died with carcinomas and adenomas of the kidneys and liver (Thomas & Bollmann, 1968). Daily oral doses of 1 mg/animal given to female rats before and during pregnancy, up to a total dose of 60-90 mg/animal, did not result in an increased tumour rate in the offspring during lifetime observation; however, 5 carcinomas of the kidney were observed in 3/4 of the mothers that received a total dose of 60 mg (Sydow, 1970).

Daily s.c. doses of 2 mg/animal were given to Syrian golden hamsters for 1-7 days during the second half of the gestation period. Multiple tracheal papillomas were found in 42% of the young 25 weeks after birth, and the first tumours appeared when they were between 8 and 12 weeks of age (Mohr *et al.*, 1965). When 4 mg were given for 2-5 days to mothers, 75% tracheal papillomas were found in the young at 25 weeks (Mohr & Althoff, 1965b). Of the treated mothers, 73% developed tracheal papillomas (Mohr *et al.*, 1966b). When Syrian golden hamsters were treated with a single dose of 45 mg/kg bw NDEA on one of the last four days of pregnancy (12-15 days), the offspring showed an incidence of up to 95% respiratory tract tumours, whereas treatment of the mothers during the first 11 days of pregnancy resulted in no respiratory tract tumours in the offspring (Mohr *et al.*, 1975).

Oral and subcutaneous administration

The oral administration to a dog of 3 mg/kg bw NDEA, followed by weekly s.c. injections of the same dose, to a total dose of 565 mg/kg bw, induced a large leiomyosarcoma of the liver (Schmähl *et al.*, 1964).

Intrarecetal administration

Twice-weekly treatment of 14 albino rats with 11.2 mg/kg bw for life-time produced hepatocellular carcinomas in all treated animals (Schmähl *et al.*, 1963b).

Intradermal administration

Weekly injections of 3.5 mg NDEA in water for 5-6 months produced epithelial papillomas of the nasal cavity in 10/19 Syrian hamsters; no local tumours were observed (Herrold, 1964a,b).

Immersion

Exposure of the aquarium fish, *Brachydanio rerio*, to 10-100 mg/l NDEA in the tank-water for 8 weeks resulted in hepatomas or cholangiomas in 17/63 animals (Stanton, 1965). Treatment of guppies (*Lebistes reticulatus*) with 13.3-100 mg/l NDEA in the aquarium-water resulted in neoplastic changes in the liver. After 7-8 weeks, 23% of the fish exhibited liver-cell adenomas, cholangiomas, cholangiocarcinomas or hepatocellular carcinomas (Khudoley, 1971, 1973).

In another study, 60/224 guppies had tumours after application of 26-100 mg/l NDEA in the water for 4-8 weeks. The average latent period was 18 weeks. In the high-dose group (those treated with 100 mg/l for 56 days), mortality was 40-46%; in the low-dosage groups (26-32 mg/l), mortality was 20-28%. Females were more resistant to the toxic effects of NDEA than males (Pliss & Khudoley, 1975).

Levels of 15-135 mg/l NDEA in tank-water for 8 weeks resulted in hepatomas in 21/32 medakas (*Oryzias latipes*) within the subsequent 5 weeks (Ishikawa *et al.*, 1975).

NDEA in tank-water (50 mg/l) induced hepatocellular carcinomas and adenomas and tumours of the haematopoietic system in 41/94 exposed frogs (Khudoley, 1977).

Carcinogenesis in plants

Seeds of hybrids of *Nicotiana* were soaked in 10 mM solutions of NDEA in water for 1 or 2 days, and tumours were found on 7.8% of germinated seedlings 20 days later, compared with 2.1% on controls (Andersen, 1973).

(h) Carcinogenicity of metabolites (see also section 3.2 (a))

N-Nitroso-*N*-ethyl-*N*-(2-hydroxyethyl)amine, which has been detected in the urine of rats treated with NDEA (Blattmann & Preussmann, 1973), produced tumours of the liver and a few oesophageal tumours when given orally to rats (Druckrey *et al.*, 1967).

(i) Factors that modify carcinogenicity in animals

Phenobarbital was reported to decrease the carcinogenic effect of NDEA and to increase the survival time when the two compounds were administered concomitantly to NMRI mice. No such effect was observed when halothane or methoxyflurane were administered together with NDEA, although changes in the ratio of types of tumours (haemangioendotheliomas and liver-cell carcinomas) induced by NDEA were observed (Kunz *et al.*, 1969).

A decreased incidence of hepatomas was observed in CF-1 mice given NDEA neonatally if the neonatal treatment was preceded by prenatal exposure to methylcholanthrene (Turusov *et al.*, 1973).

In Porton rats, a single i.p. dose of 50-114 mg/kg NDEA 0-2 hours after partial hepatectomy induced 4/9 liver tumours; 2/9 liver tumours were induced by 100-130 mg/kg NDEA in intact animals (Craddock 1975). A high incidence of kidney tumours and a short survival time were observed in Wistar rats treated with 80 mg/kg bw NDEA 4, 16 or 24 hours after partial hepatectomy (Meister & Rabes, 1973).

In male Fischer rats, combined treatment with phenobarbital and NDEA reduced the incidence of hepatocellular carcinomas induced by NDEA, whereas an opposite effect was observed if phenobarbital was administered one week after cessation of the hepatocarcinogen. This increased effect was not modified by concomitant treatment with an antilymphocytic serum (Weisburger *et al.*, 1975). Treatment of Fischer rats with dibenamine [*N*-(2-chloroethyl)dibenzylamine] during chronic oral treatment with NDEA resulted in a decreased number of hepatocellular carcinomas but not of oral, pharnygeal or oesophageal tumours seen at 25 weeks, when the animals were killed (Weisburger *et al.*, 1974).

Simultaneous administration to Sprague-Dawley rats of disulfiram (500 mg/kg bw/week) and NDEA (20 mg/kg bw/week) resulted in a significant decrease in the number of liver tumours and in an increased number of tumours of the oesophagus and nasal cavities, as compared with rats treated with NDEA alone (Schmähl *et al.*, 1976). Combined treatment of rats with NDEA and ethanol resulted in an increased number of tumours of the oesophagus and forestomach but no change in the induction of hepatomas (Gibel, 1967).

Cyclopropenoid fatty acids have no effect on the carcinogenic response of rats treated with NDEA (Nixon *et al.*, 1974). A large reduction in the incidence of liver tumours induced by NDEA was observed in rats when Kanechlor 500 was administered together with the nitrosamine (Makiura *et al.*, 1974); no such reduction was observed with 3-methylcholanthrene or 1-naphthyl isothiocyanate (Makiura *et al.*, 1973).

The incidence of hepatocellular carcinomas induced in rats by NDEA was reduced by supplementing a marginally deficient diet with lipotropes or amino acids (both containing methionine) (Rogers, 1977), but was enhanced by a diet high in fat and marginally deficient in lipotropes (Rogers *et al.*, 1974).

In Syrian golden hamsters given benzo[*a*]pyrene and ferric oxide intratracheally, followed by s.c. administration of NDEA, a higher incidence of squamous-cell carcinomas of the tracheobronchial tract was found as compared with hamsters treated with the carcinogens singly (Montesano *et al.*, 1974).

3.2 Other relevant biological data

(a) Experimental systems

Toxic effects

The acute oral or i.v. LD_{50} of NDEA in rats was 280 mg/kg bw (Druckrey *et al.*, 1967). The s.c. LD_{50} was 250 mg/kg bw in European hamsters (Mohr *et al.*, 1972b) and 230 mg/kg bw in Chinese hamsters (Reznik *et al.*, 1976).

Toxic doses of NDEA produce acute haemorrhagic centrilobular necrosis of the liver. The toxicity and the inhibitory effects on protein and nucleic acid synthesis in the liver and other organs have been reviewed (Magee & Barnes, 1967; Magee & Swann, 1969; Magee *et al.*, 1976; Witschi, 1973).

Feeding of NDEA to rats resulted in the development of histologically distinct foci in the liver, referred to as 'enzyme-deficient islands' (Friedrich-Freksa *et al.*, 1969a,b; Schauer & Kunze, 1968). These islands are considered to be precursors of liver-cell carcinomas. NDEA induces a a hepatocellular population which is resistant to the necrogenic effect of a second carcinogen, 2-acetylaminofluorene (Solt & Farber, 1976).

Embryotoxicity and teratogenicity

Teratogenic effects were not observed in rats given single doses of 180 mg/kg bw intraperitoneally or 200 mg/kg bw orally during pregnancy. An increase in foetal mortality was noted when the substance was administered on days 3, 9, 10 or 12 of gestation. Similar foetal mortality was observed after an intraplacental injection of 0.1-0.3 mg NDEA to every embryonic chamber on day 13 of gestation (Alexandrov, 1974; Napalkov & Alexandrov, 1968).

Absorption, distribution and excretion

In goats, one hour after oral administration of 30 mg/kg bw NDEA, there were 11.4 mg/kg NDEA in the milk and 11.9 mg/kg in the blood. Only traces were found in the milk and none in the blood after 24 hours (Juszkiewicz & Kowalski, 1974).

Metabolism

Available evidence suggests that NDEA requires metabolic activation in order to exert its carcinogenic and toxic effects. Such activation has been demonstrated both *in vitro* and *in vivo*. Tissue distribution and blood concentration have been followed in rats (Magee & Barnes, 1967; Rajewsky & Dauber, 1970); and metabolism has been monitored by measurement of the rate of loss from the blood and by $^{14}CO_2$ exhalation after administration of ^{14}C-NDEA (Heath, 1962; Mundt & Hadjiolov, 1974). A dose of 200 mg/kg bw was metabolized in rats during 24 hours (Heath, 1962).

N-Nitrosoethyl-*N*-(2-hydroxyethyl)amine and *N*-nitrosoethyl-*N*-(carboxymethyl)amine have been detected in the urine of rats given NDEA (Blattmann & Preussmann, 1973).

Oxidative *N*-deethylation of NDEA accounts for the production of CO_2 and alkylating species *in vivo* (Heath, 1962; Swann & Magee, 1971). The rate of metabolism of NDEA by slices of organs from rats and hamsters *in vitro* has been measured, and a correlation made between the degree of metabolism and the distribution of induced tumours (Montesano & Magee, 1974).

After administration of NDEA to rats or hamsters, several ethylated derivatives were produced in liver and kidney nucleic acids. These included 7-ethylguanine, O^6-ethylguanine and 3-ethyladenine (Magee & Lee, 1964; Montesano & Bartsch, 1976; Pegg, 1977; Swann & Magee, 1971).

Treatment with aminoacetonitrile reduced the ethylation of liver RNA and the exhalation of $^{14}CO_2$ after a single i.p. injection of ^{14}C-NDEA (Mundt & Hadjiolov, 1974).

NDEA incubated in the presence of a rat liver microsomal system and 3,4-dichlorothiophenol as a trapping agent yields the corresponding methyl and ethyl thioethers (Preussmann *et al.*, 1976).

Mutagenicity and other short-term tests

The genetic effects of NDEA have been reviewed (Montesano & Bartsch, 1976).

NDEA, in the presence of microsomal fractions from mouse liver or with Udenfriend's oxidation system, caused forward mutations in *Saccharomyces cerevisiae* and *Neurospora crassa* (Malling, 1966; Mayer, 1971). It produced reverse mutations in *Salmonella typhimurium* strains TA 100 and TA 1530 (Bartsch *et al.*, 1975; Sugimura *et al.*, 1976) and in *Escherichia coli* in the presence of a rat liver microsomal fraction from phenobarbital- or polychlorinated biphenyl-treated rats (Nakajima *et al.*, 1974).

N-Nitrosoethyl-*N*-(α-acetoxyethyl)amine, which is readily converted into the unstable α-hydroxyethyl derivative, is mutagenic in *Drosophila melanogaster* (Fahmy & Fahmy, 1976) and in *S. typhimurium* TA 1530 in the absence of a liver activation system (Camus *et al.*, 1978).

In host-mediated assays in mice given doses of 50 mg/kg, tests on *S. typhimurium* demonstrated mutagenic effects (Malling, 1974).

In the presence of a liver microsomal fraction from phenobarbital-treated rats, NDEA caused 8-azaguanine-resistant mutants in Chinese hamster V79 cells (Kuroki *et al.*, 1977).

NDEA was mutagenic in the recessive lethal test in *Drosophila melanogaster* (Pasternak, 1963). The induction of point mutations was a function of concentrations over more than two orders of magnitude. The ability of NDEA to produce more than one point mutation per germ cell contrasts with the lack of dominant lethals, translocations and chromosome loss seen with concentrations below toxic levels (LD_{60}-LD_{90}) (Fahmy *et al.*, 1966; Vogel & Leigh, 1975).

Dominant lethal mutations were not observed in mice treated with 13.5 mg/kg bw NDEA (Propping *et al.*, 1972).

In the presence of a rat liver microsomal system *in vitro*, 4-200 mM NDEA induced chromosomal aberrations as well as sister chromatid exchanges in Chinese hamster cells (Natarajan *et al.*, 1976).

NDEA did not induce transformation of hamster embryo cells; however, treatment of the embryo by transplacental administration of NDEA led to the appearance of transformed cells in the primary culture. These transformed cells were produced at a much higher frequency than in control cultures from untreated embryos, and they produced tumours (fibrosarcomas) when injected back into animals (DiPaolo *et al.*, 1972; Evans & DiPaolo, 1975).

(b) Humans

No data were available to the Working Group.

3.3 Case reports and epidemiological studies

No data were available to the Working Group.

4. Summary of Data Reported and Evaluation

4.1 Experimental data

N-Nitrosodiethylamine is carcinogenic in all animal species tested: mice, rats, Syrian golden, Chinese and European hamsters, guinea-pigs, rabbits, dogs, gerbils, pigs, monkeys, hedgehogs, various fish, frogs and birds. It induces benign and malignant tumours after its administration by various routes, including ingestion, parenteral injection, inhalation and rectal instillation. The major target organs are the liver, respiratory and upper digestive tracts and kidney. It is carcinogenic following its administration prenatally and in single doses. In several studies, dose-response relationships were established.

N-Nitroso-*N*-ethyl-*N*-(2-hydroxyethyl)amine, a metabolite of *N*-nitrosodiethylamine, produced mainly liver tumours after its oral administration to rats.

4.2 Human data

No case reports or epidemiological studies were available to the Working Group. Available information on occurrence suggests that the general population may be exposed to low levels of *N*-nitrosodiethylamine; however, no exposed group suitable for an epidemiological investigation has yet been identified.

4.3 Evaluation

There is *sufficient evidence* of a carcinogenic effect of *N*-nitrosodiethylamine in many experimental animal species. Although no epidemiological data were available, *N*-nitrosodiethylamine should be regarded for practical purposes as if it were carcinogenic to humans.

5. References

Adamson, R.H., Correa, P., Smith, C.F., Yancey, S.T. & Dalgard, D.W. (1973) Induction of tumors in monkeys by chemical carcinogens - correlation of serum *alpha*-fetoprotein and appearance of liver tumors (Abstract No. 168). Proc. Amer. Ass. Cancer Res., 14, 42

Adamson, R.H., Correa, P. & Dalgard, D.W. (1974) Induction of tumors in non-human primates with various chemical carcinogens (Abstract No. 45). Toxicol. appl. Pharmacol., 29, 93

Akamatsu, Y. (1975) Carcinogenicity of *N*-nitrosodiethylamine (DEN), *N*-nitrosodi-*N*-butylamine (DBN), and *N*-methyl-*N*-nitro-*N*-nitrosoguanidine (MNG) in strains of mice: single intragastric treatment of 10 times maximum tolerated dose (MTD) (Abstract No. 645). Proc. Amer. Ass. Cancer Res., 16, 162

Alexandrov, V.A. (1974) Embryotoxic and transplacental oncogenic action of symmetrical dialkylnitrosamines on the progeny of rats. Bull. exp. Biol. Med., 78, 1308-1310

Alliston, T.G., Cox, G.B. & Kirk, R.S. (1972) The determination of steam-volatile *N*-nitrosamines in foodstuffs by formation of electron-capturing derivatives from electrochemically derived amines. Analyst, 97, 915-920

Andersen, R.A. (1973) Carcinogenicity of phenols, alkylating agents, urethan, and a cigarette-smoke fraction in *Nicotiana* seedlings. Cancer Res., 33, 2450-2455

Arcos, J.C., Argus, M.F. & Mathison, J.B. (1969) Hepatic carcinogenesis threshold and biphasic mitochondrial swelling response in the guinea-pig during diethylnitrosamine administration. Experientia, 25, 296-298

Argus, M.F. & Hoch-Ligeti, C. (1961) Comparative study of the carcinogenic activity of nitrosamines. J. nat. Cancer Inst., 27, 695-709

Argus, M.F. & Hoch-Ligeti, C. (1963) Induction of malignant tumors in the guinea-pig by oral administration of diethylnitrosamine. J. nat. Cancer Inst., 30, 533-543

Baker, J.R., Mason, M.M., Yerganian, G., Weisburger, E.K. & Weisburger, J.H. (1974) Induction of tumors of the stomach and esophagus in inbred Chinese hamsters by oral diethylnitrosamine. Proc. Soc. exp. Biol. (N.Y.), 146, 291-292

Bartsch, H., Malaveille, C. & Montesano, R. (1975) Differential effect of phenobarbitone, pregnenolone-16α-carbonitrile and aminoacetonitrile on dialkylnitrosamine metabolism and mutagenicity *in vitro*. Chem.-biol. Interact., 10, 377-382

Blattmann, L. & Preussmann, R. (1973) Struktur von Metaboliten carcinogener Dialkylnitrosamine im Rattenurin. Z. Krebsforsch., 79, 3-5

Brunnemann, K.D. & Hoffmann, D. (1978) Chemical studies on tobacco smoke. LIX. Analysis of volatile nitrosamines in tobacco smoke and polluted indoor environments. In: Walker, E.A., Castegnaro, M., Griciute, L. & Lyle, R.E., eds, Environmental Aspects of *N*-Nitroso Compounds, Lyon (IARC Scientific Publications No. 19) (in press)

Brunnemann, K.D., Yu, L. & Hoffmann, D. (1977) Assessment of carcinogenic volatile *N*-nitrosamines in tobacco and in mainstream and sidestream smoke from cigarettes. Cancer Res., 37, 3218-3222

Camus, A.-M., Wiessler, M., Malaveille, C. & Bartsch, H. (1978) High mutagenicity of *N*-(α-acyloxy)alkyl-*N*-alkylnitrosamines in *S. typhimurium*: model compounds for metabolically activated *N,N*-dialkylnitrosamines. Mutation Res., 49, 187-194

Cardesa, A., Pour, P., Althoff, J. & Mohr, U. (1974) Comparative studies of neoplastic response to a single dose of nitroso compounds. IV. The effect of dimethyl- and diethyl-nitrosamine in Swiss mice. Z. Krebsforsch., 81, 229-233

Cardesa, A., Pour, P., Haas, H., Althoff, J. & Mohr, U. (1976) Histogenesis of tumors from the nasal cavities induced by diethylnitrosamine. Cancer, 37, 346-355

Cerutti, G., Zappavigna, R. & Santini, P.L. (1975) *N*-Alkylnitrosamines in domestic and imported cheeses. Latte, 3, 224-227 [Chem. Abstr., 83, 130147c]

Clapp, N.K. & Craig, A.W. (1967) Carcinogenic effects of diethylnitrosamine in RF mice. J. nat. Cancer Inst., 39, 903-916

Clapp, N.K., Craig, A.W. & Toya, R.E., Sr (1970) Diethylnitrosamine oncogenesis in RF mice as influenced by variations in cumulative dose. Int. J. Cancer, 5, 119-123

Clapp, N.K., Tyndall, R.L. & Otten, J.A. (1971) Differences in tumor types and organ susceptibility in BALB/c and RF mice following dimethylnitrosamine and diethylnitrosamine. Cancer Res., 31, 196-198

Cohen, J.B. & Bachman, J.D. (1978) Measurement of environmental nitrosamines. In: Walker, E.A., Castegnaro, M., Griciute, L. & Lyle, R.E., eds, Environmental Aspects of *N*-Nitroso Compounds, Lyon (IARC Scientific Publications No. 19) (in press)

Craddock, V.M. (1975) Effect of a single treatment with the alkylating carcinogens dimethylnitrosamine, diethylnitrosamine and methyl methanesulphonate on liver regenerating after partial hepatectomy. I. Test for induction of liver carcinomas. Chem.-biol. Interact., 10, 313-321

Crosby, N.T., Foreman, J.K., Palframan, J.F. & Sawyer, R. (1972) Estimation of steam-volatile *N*-nitrosamines in foods at the 1 μg/kg level. Nature (Lond.), 238, 342-343

Dalgard, D.W., Correa, P., Waalkes, T.P. & Adamson, R.H. (1975) Induction of mucoepidermoid carcinoma in prosimians with *N*-nitrosodiethylamine (Abstract No. 346). Proc. Amer. Ass. Cancer Res., 16, 87

Dalgard, D.W., Correa, P., Sieber, J.M. & Adamson, R.H. (1976) Induction of tumors in non-human primates with *N*-nitrosodiethylamine (Abstract No. 690). Fed. Proc., 35, 329

DiPaolo, J.A., Nelson, R.L. & Donovan, P.J. (1972) *In vitro* transformation of Syrian hamster embryo cells by diverse chemical carcinogens. Nature (Lond.), 235, 278-280

Diwan, B.A. & Meier, H. (1976a) Carcinogenic effects of a single dose of diethylnitrosamine in three unrelated strains of mice: genetic dependence of the induced tumor types and incidence. Cancer Lett., 1, 249-253

Diwan, B.A. & Meier, H. (1976b) Transplacental carcinogenic effects of diethylnitrosamine in mice. Naturwissenschaften, 63, 487-488

Dontenwill, W. (1968) Experimental studies on the organotropic effect of nitrosamines in the respiratory tract. Fd Cosmet. Toxicol., 6, 571

Dontenwill, W. & Mohr, U. (1961) Carcinome des Respirationstractus nach Behandlung von Goldhamstern mit Diäthylnitrosamin. Z. Krebsforsch., 64, 305-312

Dontenwill, W. & Mohr, U. (1962) Die organotrope Wirkung der Nitrosamine. Z. Krebsforsch., 65, 166-167

Dontenwill, W., Mohr, U. & Zagel, M. (1962) Über die unterschiedliche Lungen-carcinogene Wirkung des Diäthylnitrosamin bei Hamster und Ratte. Z. Krebsforsch., 64, 499-502

Druckrey, H. & Steinhoff, D. (1962) Erzeugung von Leberkrebs an Meerschweinchen. Naturwissenschaften, 49, 497-498

Druckrey, H., Schildbach, A., Schmähl, D., Preussmann, R. & Ivankovic, S. (1963a) Quantitative Analyse der carcinogenen Wirkung von Diäthylnitrosamin. Arzneimittel-Forsch., 13, 841-851

Druckrey, H., Steinhoff, D., Preussmann, R. & Ivankovic, S. (1963b) Krebserzeugung durch einmalige Dosis von Methylnitrosoharnstoff und verschiedenen Dialkyl-nitrosaminen. Naturwissenschaften, 50, 735

Druckrey, H., Steinhoff, D., Preussmann, R. & Ivankovic, S. (1964) Erzeugung von Krebs durch eine einmalige Dosis von Methylnitroso-Harnstoff und verschiedenen Dialkylnitrosaminen an Ratten. Z. Krebsforsch., 66, 1-10

Druckrey, H., Preussmann, R., Ivankovic, S. & Schmähl, D. (1967) Organotrope carcinogene Wirkungen bei 65 verschiedenen *N*-Nitroso-Verbindungen an BD-Ratten. Z. Krebsforsch., 69, 103-201

Eisenbrand, G. & Preussmann, R. (1970) Eine neue Methode zur kolorimetrischen Bestimmung von Nitrosaminen nach Spaltung der *N*-Nitrosogruppe mit Bromwasserstoff in Eisessig. Arzneimittel-Forsch., 20, 1513-1517

Eisenbrand, G., Hodenberg, A. von & Preussmann, R. (1970) Trace analysis of *N*-nitroso compounds. II. Steam distillation at neutral, alkaline and acid pH under reduced and atmospheric pressure. Z. analyt. Chem., 251, 22-24

Eisenbrand, G., Spiegelhalder, B., Janzowski, C., Kann, J. & Preussmann, R. (1978) Volatile and non-volatile *N*-nitroso compounds in foods and other environmental media. In: Walker, E.A., Castegnaro, M., Griciute, L. & Lyle, R.E., eds, Environmental Aspects of *N*-Nitroso Compounds, Lyon (IARC Scientific Publications No. 19) (in press)

Evans, C.H. & DiPaolo, J.A. (1975) Neoplastic transformation of guinea pig fetal cells in culture induced by chemical carcinogens. Cancer Res., 35, 1035-1044

Fahmy, O.G. & Fahmy, M.J. (1976) Mutagenicity of *N*-α-acetoxyethyl-*N*-ethylnitrosamine and *N*,*N*-diethylnitrosamine in relation to the mechanisms of metabolic activation of dialkylnitrosamines. Cancer Res., 36, 4504-4512

Fahmy, O.G., Fahmy, M.J., Massasso, J. & Ondrěj, M. (1966) Differential mutagenicity of the amine and amide derivatives of nitroso compounds in *Drosophila melanogaster*. Mutation Res., 3, 201-217

Fiddler, W., Pensabene, J.W., Doerr, R.C. & Dooley, C.J. (1977) The presence of dimethyl- and diethylnitrosamines in deionized water. Fd Cosmet. Toxicol. , 15, 441-443

Fine, D.H. (1978) An assessment of human exposure to *N*-nitroso compounds. In: Walker, E.A., Castegnaro, M., Griciute, L. & Lyle, R.E., eds, Environmental Aspects of *N*-Nitroso Compounds, Lyon (IARC Scientific Publications No. 19) (in press)

Fine, D.H. & Rounbehler, D.P. (1976) Analysis of volatile *N*-nitroso compounds by combined gas chromatography and thermal energy analysis. In: Walker, E.A., Bogovski, P. & Griciute, L., eds, Environmental *N*-Nitroso Compounds Analysis and Formation, Lyon (IARC Scientific Publications No. 14), pp. 117-127

Fine, D.H., Rounbehler, D.P., Sawicki, E., Krost, K. & DeMarrais, G.A. (1976a) *N*-Nitroso compounds in the ambient community air of Baltimore, Maryland. Analyt. Lett., 9, 595-604

Fine, D.H., Rounbehler, D.P., Belcher, N.M. & Epstein, S.S. (1976b) *N*-Nitroso compounds: detection in ambient air. Science, 192, 1328-1330

Fine, D.H., Ross, R., Rounbehler, D.P., Silvergleid, A. & Song, L. (1977) Formation *in vivo* of volatile *N*-nitrosamines in man after ingestion of cooked bacon and spinach. Nature (Lond.), 265, 753-755

Fong, Y.Y. & Walsh, E.O'F. (1971) Carcinogenic nitrosamines in Cantonese salt-dried fish. Lancet, ii, 1032

Freimuth, U. & Glaeser, E. (1970) Occurrence of nitrosamines in foods. Nahrung, 14, 357-361 [Chem. Abstr., 74, 11971w]

Fridman, A.L., Mukhametshin, F.M. & Novikov, S.S. (1971) Advances in the chemistry of aliphatic *N*-nitrosamines. Russ. chem. Rev., 40, 34-50

Friedrich-Freksa, H., Gössner, W. & Börner, P. (1969a) Histochemische Untersuchungen der Cancerogenese in der Rattenleber nach Dauergaben von Diäthylnitrosamin. Z. Krebsforsch., 72, 226-239

Friedrich-Freksa, H., Papadopulu, G. & Gössner, W. (1969b) Histochemische Untersuchungen der Cancerogenese in der Rattenleber nach zeitlich begrenzter Verabfolgung von Diäthylnitrosamin. Z. Krebsforsch., 72, 240-253

Gargus, J.L., Paynter, O.E. & Reese, W.H., Jr (1969) Utilization of newborn mice in the bioassay of chemical carcinogens. Toxicol. appl. Pharmacol., 15, 552-559

Gibel, W. (1967) Experimentelle Untersuchungen zur Synkarzinogenese beim Ösophaguskarzinom. Arch. Geschwulstforsch., 30, 181-189

Gough, T.A. (1978) An examination of some foodstuff for trace amounts of volatile nitrosamines using the thermal energy analyser. In: Walker, E.A., Castegnaro, M., Griciute, L. & Lyle, R.E., eds, Environmental Aspects of *N*-Nitroso Compounds, Lyon (IARC Scientific Publications No. 19) (in press)

Graw, J.J. & Berg, H. (1977) Hepatocarcinogenic effect of DENA in pigs. Z. Krebsforsch., 89, 137-143

Graw, J.J., Berg, H. & Schmähl, D. (1974) Carcinogenic and hepatotoxic effects of diethylnitrosamine in hedgehogs. J. nat. Cancer Inst., 53, 589

Groenen, P.J., Jonk, R.J.G., van Ingen, C. & ten Noever de Brauw, M.C. (1976) Determination of eight volatile nitrosamines in thirty cured meat products with capillary gas chromatography-high-resolution mass spectrometry: the presence of nitrosodiethylamine and the absence of nitrosopyrrolidine. In: Walker, E.A., Bogovski, P. & Griciute, L., eds, Environmental *N*-Nitroso Compounds Analysis and Formation, Lyon (IARC Scientific Publications No. 14), pp. 321-331

Groenen, P.J., de Cock-Bethbeder, M.W., Jonk, R.J.G. & van Ingen, C. (1977) Further studies on the occurrence of volatile *N*-nitrosamines in meat products by combined gas chromatography and mass spectrometry. In: Tinbergen, B.J. & Krol, B., eds, Proceedings of the 2nd International Symposium on Nitrite in Meat Products, Zeist, 1976, Wageningen, Centre for Agricultural Publishing and Documentation, pp. 227-237

Grundmann, E. & Sieburg, H. (1962) Die Histogenese und Cytogenese des Lebercarcinoms der Ratte durch Diäthylnitrosamin im lichtmikroskopischen Bild. Beitr. path. Anat., 126, 57-90

Haas, H., Kmoch, N., Mohr, U. & Cardesa, A. (1975) Susceptibility of gerbils (*Meriones unguiculatus*) to weekly subcutaneous and single intravenous injections of *N*-diethylnitrosamine. Z. Krebsforsch., 83, 233-238

Hadjiolov, D. (1972) Hemangiothelial sarcomas of the liver in rats induced by diethylnitrosamine. Neoplasma, 19, 111-114

Havery, D.C., Fazio, T. & Howard, J.W. (1978) Survey of cured meat products for volatile *N*-nitrosamines: comparison of two analytical methods. In: Walker, E.A., Castegnaro, M., Griciute, L. & Lyle, R.E., eds, Environmental Aspects of *N*-Nitroso Compounds, Lyon (IARC Scientific Publications No. 19) (in press)

Heath, D.F. (1962) The decomposition and toxicity of dialkylnitrosamines in rats. Biochem. J., 85, 72-90

Hedler, L. & Marquardt, P. (1968) Occurrence of diethylnitrosamine in some samples of food. Fd Cosmet. Toxicol., 6, 341-348

Hedler, L. & Marquardt, P. (1974) Determination of volatile *N*-nitroso compounds, and particularly of nitrosodimethylamine, nitrosodiethylamine and nitrosodipropylamine, in soyabean oil: effect of oil storage period on recovery rates. In: Bogovski, P. & Walker, E.A., eds, *N*-Nitroso Compounds in the Environment, Lyon (IARC Scientific Publications No. 9), pp. 183-191

Herrold, K.M. (1964a) Epithelial papillomas of the nasal cavity: experimental induction in Syrian hamsters. Arch. Path., 78, 189-195

Herrold, K.M. (1964b) Effect of route of administration on the carcinogenic action of diethylnitrosamine (*N*-nitrosodiethylamine). Brit. J. Cancer, 18, 763-767

Herrold, K.M. (1964c) Induction of olfactory neuroepithelial tumors in Syrian hamsters by diethylnitrosamine. Cancer, 17, 114-121

Herrold, K.M. & Dunham, L.J. (1963) Induction of tumors in the Syrian hamster with diethylnitrosamine (*N*-nitrosodiethylamine). Cancer Res., 23, 773-777

Heyns, K. & Röper, H. (1974) Gas chromatographic trace analysis of volatile nitrosamines in various types of wheat flour after application of different nitrogen fertilizers to the wheat. In: Bogovski, P. & Walker, E.A., eds, *N*-Nitroso Compounds in the Environment, Lyon (IARC Scientific Publications No. 9), pp. 166-172

Hilfrich, J., Althoff, J. & Mohr, U. (1971) Untersuchungen zur Stimulation der Lungentumorrate durch Diäthylnitrosamin bei O-20-Mäusen. Z. Krebsforsch., 75, 240-242

Hirao, K., Matsumura, K., Imagawa, A., Enomoto, Y., Hosogi, Y., Kani, T., Fujikawa, K. & Ito, N. (1974) Primary neoplasms in dog liver induced by diethylnitrosamine. Cancer Res., 34, 1870-1882

Hoch-Ligeti, C., Lobl, L.T. & Arvin, J.M. (1964) Effect of nitrosamine derivatives on enzyme concentrations in rat organs during carcinogenesis. Brit. J. Cancer, 18, 271-284

Hoffmann, D., Rathkamp, G. & Liu, Y.Y. (1974) Chemical studies on tobacco smoke. XXVI. On the isolation and identification of volatile and non-volatile *N*-nitrosamines and hydrazines in cigarette smoke. In: Bogovski, P. & Walker, E.A., eds, *N*-Nitroso Compounds in the Environment, Lyon (IARC Scientific Publications No. 9), pp. 159-165

Hoffmann, F. & Graffi, A. (1964a) Carcinome der Nasenhöhle bei Mäusen nach Tropfung der Rückenhaut mit Diäthylnitrosamin. Acta biol. med. germ., 12, 623-625

Hoffmann, F. & Graffi, A. (1964b) Nasenhöhlentumoren bei Mäusen nach percutaner Diäthylnitrosaminapplikation. Arch. Geschwulstforsch., 23, 274-288

IARC (1972) IARC Monographs on the Evaluation of Carcinogenic Risk of Chemicals to Man, 1, Lyon, pp. 107-124

IARC (1977a) Annual Report 1977, Lyon, International Agency for Research on Cancer, p. 63

IARC (1977b) Annual Report 1977, Lyon, International Agency for Research on Cancer, pp. 56-58

Ishikawa, T., Shimamine, T. & Takayama, S. (1975) Histologic and electron microscopy observations on diethylnitrosamine-induced hepatomas in small aquarium fish (*Oryzias latipes*). J. nat. Cancer Inst., 55, 909-916

Iyengar, J.R., Panalaks, T., Miles, W.F. & Sen, N.P. (1976) A survey of fish products for volatile *N*-nitrosamines. J. Sci. Fd Agric., 27, 527-530

Joint Iran-International Agency for Research on Cancer Study Group (1977) Esophageal cancer studies in the Caspian littoral of Iran: results of population studies - a prodrome. J. nat. Cancer Inst., 59, 1127-1138

Juszkiewicz, T. & Kowalski, B. (1974) Passage of nitrosamines from rumen into milk in goats. In: Bogovski, P. & Walker, E.A., eds, *N*-Nitroso Compounds in the Environment, Lyon (IARC Scientific Publications No. 9), pp. 173-176

Juszkiewicz, T. & Kowalski, B. (1976) An investigation of the possible presence or formation of nitrosamines in animal feeds. In: Walker, E.A., Bogovski, P. & Griciute, L., eds, Environmental *N*-Nitroso Compounds Analysis and Formation, Lyon (IARC Scientific Publications No. 14), pp. 375-383

Kann, J., Tauts, O., Raja, K. & Kalve, R. (1976) Nitrosamines and their precursors in some Estonian foodstuffs. In: Walker, E.A., Bogovski, P. & Griciute, L., eds, Environmental *N*-Nitroso Compounds Analysis and Formation, Lyon (IARC Scientific Publications No. 14), pp. 385-394

Kann, J., Spiegelhalder, B., Eisenbrand, G. & Preussmann, R. (1978) Occurrence of volatile *N*-nitrosamines in animal diets. Z. Krebsforsch. (in press)

Kelly, M.G., O'Gara, R.W., Adamson, R.H., Gadekar, K., Botkin, C.C., Reese, W.H., Jr & Kerber, W.T. (1966) Induction of hepatic cell carcinomas in monkeys with *N*-nitrosodiethylamine. J. nat. Cancer Inst., 36, 323-351

Khudoley, V.V. (1971) The induction of hepatic tumors by nitrosamines in aquarium fish (*Lebistes reticulatus*). Vop. Onkol., 12, 67-72

Khudoley, V.V. (1973) Morphological changes in the liver of fish (*Lebistes reticulatus*) under the action of diethyl- and dimethylnitrosamines. Vop. Onkol., 19, 88-94

Khudoley, V.V. (1977) The induction of tumors in *Rana temporaria* with nitrosamines. Neoplasma, 24, 249-251

Klimsch, H.-J., Stadler, L. & Brahm, S. (1976) Quantitative Bestimmung flüchtiger Nitrosamine in Zigarettenrauchkondensat. Z. Lebensmittel-Untersuch., 162, 131-138

Koka, M. & Vesselinovitch, S.D. (1974) High metastic rate of diethylnitrosamine-induced liver tumors in mice (Abstract No. 479). Proc. Amer. Ass. Cancer Res., 15, 120

Kroeller, E. (1967) Detection of nitrosamines in tobacco smoke and food. Dtsch. Lebensmittel.-Rundsch., 63, 303-305 [Chem. Abstr., 67, 115822v]

Kunz, W., Schaude, G. & Thomas, C. (1969) Die Beeinflussung der Nitrosamin-carcinogenese durch Phenobarbital und Halogenkohlenwasserstoffe. Z. Krebsforsch., 72, 291-304

Kuroki, T., Drevon, C. & Montesano, R. (1977) Microsome-mediated mutagenesis in V79 Chinese hamster cells by various nitrosamines. Cancer Res., 37, 1044-1050

Kyriazis, A.P., Koka, M. & Vesselinovitch, S.D. (1974) Metastatic rate of liver tumors induced by diethylnitrosamine in mice. Cancer Res., 34, 2881-2886

Lacassagne, A., Buu-Hoï, N.P., Giao, N.B., Hurst, L. & Ferrando, R. (1967) Comparaison des actions hépatocancérogènes de la diéthylnitrosamine et du *p*-diméthylaminoazobenzène. Int. J. Cancer, 2, 425-433

Lakritz, L., Wasserman, A.E., Gates, R. & Spinelli, A.M. (1978) Preliminary observations on amines and nitrosamines in non-normal human gastric contents. In: Walker, E.A., Castegnaro, M., Griciute, L. & Lyle, R.E., eds, Environmental Aspects of *N*-Nitroso Compounds, Lyon (IARC Scientific Publications No. 19) (in press)

Likhachev, A.J. (1971) Transplacental blastomogenic action of *N*-nitroso-diethyl-amine in mice. Vop. Onkol., 17, 45-50

Likhachev, A.J. (1974) The dependence of the blastomogenic effect on a *N*-nitrosodiethyl amine dose. Vop. Onkol., 20, 60-64

Lombard, C. (1965) Hépatocancérisation du cobaye par la diéthylnitrosamine en injection sous-cutanée. Bull. Cancer, 52, 389-410

Magee, P.N. & Barnes, J.M. (1967) Carcinogenic nitroso compounds. Adv. Cancer Res., 10, 163-246

Magee, P.N. & Lee, K.Y. (1964) Cellular injury and carcinogenesis. Alkylation of ribonucleic acid of rat liver by diethylnitrosamine and *n*-butylmethylnitrosamine *in vivo*. Biochem. J., 91, 35-42

Magee, P.N. & Swann, P.F. (1969) Nitroso compounds. Brit. med. Bull., 25, 240-244

Magee, P.N., Montesano, R. & Preussmann, R. (1976) *N*-Nitroso compounds and related carcinogens. In: Searle, C.E., ed., Chemical Carcinogens (ACS Monograph 173), Washington DC, American Chemical Society, pp. 491-625

Makiura, S., Kamamoto, Y., Sugihara, S., Hirao, K., Hiasa, Y., Arai, M. & Ito, N. (1973) Effect of 1-naphthyl isothiocyanate and 3-methylcholanthrene on hepatocarcinogenesis in rats treated with diethylnitrosamine. Gann, 64, 101-104

Makiura, S., Aoe, H., Sugihara, S., Hirao, K., Arai, M. & Ito, N. (1974) Inhibitory effect of polychlorinated biphenyls on liver tumorigenesis in rats treated with 3'-methyl-4-dimethylaminoazobenzene, *N*-2-fluorenylacetamide and diethylnitrosamine. J. nat. Cancer Inst., 53, 1253-1257

Malling, H.V. (1966) Mutagenicity of two potent carcinogens, dimethylnitrosamine and diethylnitrosamine, in *Neurospora crassa*. Mutation Res., 3, 537-540

Malling, H.V. (1974) Mutagenic activation of dimethylnitrosamine and diethylnitrosamine in the host-mediated assay and the microsomal system. Mutation Res., 26, 465-472

Marquardt, P. & Hedler, L. (1966) Über das Vorkommen von Nitrosaminen in Weizenmehl. Arzneimittel-Forsch., 16, 778-779

Mayer, V.W. (1971) Mutagenicity of dimethylnitrosamine and diethylnitrosamine for *Saccharomyces* in an *in vitro* hydroxylation system. Mol. gen. Genet., 112, 289-294

McCormick, A., Nicholson, M.J., Baylis, M.A. & Underwood, J.G. (1973) Nitrosamines in cigarette smoke condensate. Nature (Lond.), 244, 237-238

Meister, P. & Rabes, H. (1973) Nierentumoren durch Diäthylnitrosamin nach partieller Leberresektion: morphologie und Wachstumsverhalten. Z. Krebsforsch., 80, 169-178

Mennel, H.D., Wechsler, W. & Zülch, K.J. (1974) Morphologie und Morphogenese der durch Diäthylnitrosamin erzeugten Nasenhöhlentumoren beim Goldhamster. Beitr. Path., 151, 134-156

Mirna, A., Harada, K., Rapp, U. & Kaufmann, H. (1976) *N*-Nitrosamine in Futtermitteln. Fleischwirtschaft, 56, 1014

Mirvish, S.S. & Kaufman, L. (1970) A study of nitrosamines and *S*-carboxyl derivatives of cysteine as lung carcinogens in adult SWR mice. Int. J. Cancer, 6, 69-73

Mohr, U. & Althoff, J. (1965a) Die diaplacentare Wirkung des Cancerogens Diäthylnitrosamin bei der Maus. Z. Krebsforsch., 67, 152-155

Mohr, U. & Althoff, J. (1965b) Zum Nachweis der diaplazentaren Wirkung von Diäthylnitrosamin beim Goldhamster. Z. Naturforsch., 20b, 5

Mohr, U. & Hilfrich, J. (1972) Effect of a single dose of *N*-diethylnitrosamine on the rat kidney. J. nat. Cancer Inst., 49, 1729-1731

Mohr, U. & Hilfrich, J. (1974) Tumor induction in the rat kidney with different doses of DEN (diethylnitrosamine): frequency, latency and morphology of the tumors. Recent Results Cancer Res., 44, 130-137

Mohr, U., Althoff, J. & Wrba, H. (1965) Diaplacentare Wirkung des Carcinogens Diäthylnitrosamin beim Goldhamster. Z. Krebsforsch., 66, 536-540

Mohr, U., Wieser, O. & Pielsticker, K. (1966a) Die Minimaldosis für die Wirkung von Diäthylnitrosamin auf die Trachea beim Goldhamster. Naturwissenschaften, 53, 229

Mohr, U., Althoff, J. & Authaler, A. (1966b) Diaplacental effect of the carcinogen diethylnitrosamine in the golden hamster. Cancer Res., 26, 2349-2352

Mohr, U., Pielsticker, K., Wieser, O. & Kinzel, V. (1967) Tumoren im Vormagen des chinesischen Hamsters nach Diäthylnitrosamin-Behandlung. Ein Beitrag zur Frage der Organotropie eines Karcinogens. Europ. J. Cancer, 3, 139-142

Mohr, U., Althoff, J., Emminger, A., Bresch, H. & Spielhoff, R. (1972a) Effect of nitrosamines on nursing Syrian golden hamsters and their offspring. Z. Krebsforsch., 78, 73-77

Mohr, U., Althoff, J. & Page, N. (1972b) Tumors of the respiratory system induced in the common European hamster by *N*-diethylnitrosamine. J. nat. Cancer Inst., 49, 595-597

Mohr, U., Reznik-Schüller, H., Reznik, G. & Hilfrich, J. (1975) Transplacental effects of diethylnitrosamine in Syrian hamsters as related to different days of administration during pregnancy. J. nat. Cancer Inst., 55, 681-683

Mohr, U., Reznik, G. & Emminger, E. (1976) Intrasplenic tumour formation in the Syrian hamster (*Mesocricetus auratus*) after tracheal implants and treatment with diethylnitrosamine. J. nat. Cancer Inst., 56, 811-818

Montesano, R. & Bartsch, H. (1976) Mutagenic and carcinogenic *N*-nitroso compounds: possible environmental hazards. Mutation Res., 32, 179-228

Montesano, R. & Magee, P.N. (1974) Comparative metabolism *in vitro* of nitrosamines in various animal species including man. In: Montesano, R. & Tomatis, L., eds, Chemical Carcinogenesis Essays, Lyon (IARC Scientific Publications No. 10), pp. 39-56

Montesano, R. & Saffiotti, U. (1968) Carcinogenic response of the respiratory tract of Syrian golden hamsters to different doses of diethylnitrosamine. Cancer Res., 28, 2197-2210

Montesano, R. & Saffiotti, U. (1970) Carcinogenic response of the hamster respiratory tract to single subcutaneous administrations of diethylnitrosamine at birth. J. nat. Cancer Inst., 44, 413-417

Montesano, R., Saffiotti, U., Ferrero, A. & Kaufman, D.G. (1974) Synergistic effects of benzo[*a*]pyrene and diethylnitrosamine on respiratory carcinogenesis in hamsters. J. nat. Cancer Inst., 53, 1395-1397

Mundt, D. & Hadjiolov, D. (1974) Effect of aminoacetonitrile on the metabolism of diethylnitrosamine during liver carcinogenesis. J. nat. Cancer Inst., 52, 1515-1520

Nakajima, T., Tanaka, A. & Tojyo, K.-I. (1974) The effect of metabolic activation with rat liver preparations on the mutagenicity of several *N*-nitrosamines on a streptomycin-dependent strain of *Escherichia coli*. Mutation Res., 26, 361-366

Napalkov, N.P. & Alexandrov, V.A. (1968) On the effects of blastomogenic substances on the organism during embryogenesis. Z. Krebsforsch., 71, 32-50

Natarajan, A.T., Tates, A.D., Van Buul, P.P.W., Meijers, M. & De Vogel, N. (1976) Cytogenetic effects of mutagens/carcinogens after activation in a microsomal system *in vitro*. I. Induction of chromosome aberrations and sister chromatid exchanges by diethylnitrosamine (DEN) and dimethylnitrosamine (DMN) in CHO cells in the presence of rat-liver microsomes. Mutation Res., 37, 83-90

Nixon, J.E., Sinnhuber, R.O., Lee, D.J., Landers, M.K. & Harr, J.R. (1974) Effect of cyclopropenoid compounds on the carcinogenic activity of diethylnitrosamine and aflatoxin B_1 in rats. J. nat. Cancer Inst., 53, 453-458

O'Gara, R.W. & Kelly, M.G. (1965) Induction of hepatomas in monkeys given *N*-nitrosodiethylamine (DENA) (Abstract No. 195). Proc. Amer. Ass. Cancer Res., 6, 50

O'Gara, R.W., Adamson, R.H. & Dalgard, D.W. (1970) Induction of tumors in subhuman primates by two nitrosamine compounds (Abstract No. 236). Proc. Amer. Ass. Cancer Res., 11, 60

Panalaks, T., Iyengar, J.R., Donaldson, B.A., Miles, W.F. & Sen, N.P. (1974) Further survey of cured meat products for volatile *N*-nitrosamines. J. Ass. off. analyt. Chem., 57, 806-812

Pasternak, L. (1963) Untersuchungen über die mutagene Wirkung von Nitrosamines und Nitrosomethylharnstoff. Acta biol. med. germ., 10, 436-438

Pegg, A.E. (1977) Formation and metabolism of alkylated nucleosides: possible role in carcinogenesis by nitroso compounds and alkylating agents. Adv. Cancer Res., 25, 195-269

Pensabene, J.W., Fiddler, W., Dooley, C.J., Doerr, R.C. & Wasserman, A.E. (1972) Spectral and gas chromatographic characteristics of some *N*-nitrosamines. J. agric. Fd Chem., 20, 274-277

Pliss, G.B. & Khudoley, V.V. (1975) Tumor induction by carcinogenic agents in aquarium fish. J. nat. Cancer Inst., 55, 129-136

Prager, B., Jacobson, P., Schmidt, P. & Stern, D., eds (1922) Beilsteins Handbuch der Organischen Chemie, 4th ed., Vol. 4, Syst. No. 336, Berlin, Springer, p. 129

Preussmann, R., Arjungi, K.N. & Ebers, G. (1976) *In vitro* detection of nitrosamines and other indirect alkylating agents by reaction with 3,4-dichlorothiophenol in the presence of rat liver microsomes. Cancer Res., 36, 2459-2462

Preussmann, R., Walker, E.A., Wasserman, A.E. & Castegnaro, M., eds (1978) Environmental Carcinogens - Selected Methods of Analysis, Vol. 1, Nitrosamines, Lyon (IARC Scientific Publications No. 18) (in press)

Propping, P., Röhrborn, G. & Buselmaier, W. (1972) Comparative investigations on the chemical induction of point mutations and dominant lethal mutations in mice. Mol. gen. Genet., 117, 197-209

Rainey, W.T., Christie, W.H. & Lijinsky, W. (1978) Mass spectrometry of *N*-nitrosamines. Biomed. Mass Spectrom. (in press)

Rajewsky, M.F. & Dauber, W. (1970) Distribution of bound tritium from ^{3}H-diethylnitrosamine in rat tissues. Int. J. Cancer, 5, 389-393

Rajewsky, M.F., Dauber, W. & Frankenberg, H. (1966) Liver carcinogenesis by diethylnitrosamine in the rat. Science, 152, 83-85

Rapp, H.J., Carleton, J.H., Crisler, C. & Nadel, E.M. (1965) Induction of malignant tumors in the rabbit by oral administration of diethylnitrosamine. J. nat. Cancer Inst., 34, 453-458

Reid, J.D., Riley, J.F. & Shepherd, D.M. (1963) Histological and enzymatic changes in the livers of rats fed the hepatic carcinogen diethylnitrosamine. Biochem. Pharmacol., 12, 1151-1156

Reuber, M.D. (1975) Carcinomas of the esophagus in rats ingesting diethylnitrosamine. Europ. J. Cancer, 11, 97-99

Reuber, M.D. & Lee, C.W. (1968) Effect of age and sex on hepatic lesions in Buffalo strain rats ingesting diethylnitrosamine. J. nat. Cancer Inst., 41, 1133-1140

Reznik, G., Mohr, U. & Kmoch, N. (1976) Carcinogenic effects of different nitroso-compounds in Chinese hamsters. I. Dimethylnitrosamine and *N*-diethylnitrosamine. Brit. J. Cancer, 33, 411-418

Roach, W.A. (1972) The possible presence of nitrosamines in Transkeian Bantu foodstuffs. In: Bogovski, P., Preussmann, R. & Walker, E.A., eds, *N*-Nitroso Compounds Analysis and Formation, Lyon (IARC Scientific Publications No. 3), pp. 74-78

Rogers, A.E. (1977) Reduction of *N*-nitrosodiethylamine carcinogenesis in rats by lipotrope or amino acid supplementation of a marginally deficient diet. Cancer Res., 37, 194-199

Rogers, A.E., Sanchez, O., Feinsod, F.M. & Newberne, P.M. (1974) Dietary enhancement of nitrosamine carcinogenesis. Cancer Res., 34, 96-99

Sakai, A. & Tanimura, A. (1971) Nitrosamines in foods. VII. Nitrosamines detected in foods. Shokuhin Eiseigaku Zasshi, 12, 485-488 [Chem. Abstr., 77, 3925f]

Schauer, A. & Kunze, E. (1968) Enzymhistochemische und autoradiographische Untersuchungen während der Cancerisierung der Rattenleber mit Diäthylnitrosamin. Z. Krebsforsch., 70, 252-266

Schmähl, D. & Thomas, C. (1965a) Dosis-Wirkungs-Beziehungen bei der Erzeugung von Hämangioendotheliomen der Leber bei Mäusen durch Diäthylnitrosamin. Z. Krebsforsch., 66, 533-535

Schmähl, D. & Thomas, C. (1965b) Erzeugung von Leberkrebs beim Kaninchen durch Diäthylnitrosamin. Naturwissenschaften, 52, 165

Schmähl, D., Preussmann, R. & Hamperl, H. (1960) Leberkrebs-erzeugende Wirkung von Diäthylnitrosamin nach oraler Gabe bei Ratten. Naturwissenschaften, 47, 89

Schmähl, D., Thomas, C. & König, K. (1963a) Versuche zur Krebserzeugung mit Diäthylnitrosamin bei Mäusen. Naturwissenschaften, 50, 407

Schmähl, D., Thomas, C. & König, K. (1963b) Leberkrebs erzeugende Wirkung von Diäthylnitrosamin nach rectaler Applikation bei Ratten. Z. Krebsforsch., 65, 529-530

Schmähl, D., Thomas, C. & Scheld, G. (1964) Cancerogene Wirkung von Diäthylnitrosamin beim Hund. Naturwissenschaften, 51, 466-467

Schmähl, D., Osswald, H. & Karsten, C. (1966) Leberkrebserzeugung durch Diäthylnitrosamin bei Wellensittichen. Naturwissenschaften, 53, 437

Schmähl, D., Osswald, H. & Mohr, U. (1967) Hepatotoxische und cancerogene Wirkung von Diäthylnitrosamin bei Schweinen. Naturwissenschaften, 54, 341

Schmähl, D., Osswald, H. & Goerttler, K. (1969) Cancerogene Wirkung von Diäthylnitrosamin bei Schweinen. Z. Krebsforsch., 72, 102-104

Schmähl, D., Krüger, F.W., Habs, M. & Diehl, B. (1976) Influence of disulfiram on the organotrophy of the carcinogenic effect of dimethylnitrosamine and diethylnitrosamine in rats. Z. Krebsforsch., 85, 271-276

Schoental, R. & Appleby, E.C. (1973) The development of tumours in a female rat and her offspring, following administration of diethylnitrosamine to the mother during nursing (Abstract). Brit. J. Cancer, 28, 84

Sen, N.P., Smith, D.C., Schwinghamer, L. & Marleau, J.J. (1969) Diethylnitrosamine and other *N*-nitrosamines in foods. J. Ass. off. analyt. Chem., 52, 47-52

Sen, N.P., Iyengar, J.R., Donaldson, B.D., Panalaks, T. & Miles, W.F. (1974) The analysis and occurrence of volatile nitrosamines in cured meat products. In: Bogovski, P. & Walker, E.A., eds, *N*-Nitroso Compounds in the Environment, Lyon (IARC Scientific Publications No. 9), pp. 49-52

Sen, N.P., Iyengar, J.R., Miles, W.F. & Panalaks, T. (1976) Nitrosamines in cured meat products. In: Walker, E.A., Bogovski, P. & Griciute, L., eds, Environmental *N*-Nitroso Compounds Analysis and Formation, Lyon (IARC Scientific Publications No. 14), pp. 333-342

Sen, N.P., Donaldson, B.A., Seaman, S., Iyengar, J.R. & Miles, W.F. (1978) Recent studies in Canada on the analysis and occurrence of volatile and non-volatile *N*-nitroso compounds in foods. In: Walker, E.A., Castegnaro, M., Griciute, L. & Lyle, R.E., eds, Environmental Aspects of *N*-Nitroso Compounds, Lyon (IARC Scientific Publications No. 19) (in press)

Shvemberger, I.N. (1965) Induction of malignant tumours of oesophagus and stomach in C_3HA mice with *N*-nitrosodiethylamine. Vop. Onkol., 11, 74-77

Solt, D. & Farber, E. (1976) New principle for the analysis of chemical carcinogenesis. Nature (Lond.), 263, 701-703

Stanton, M.F. (1965) Diethylnitrosamine-induced hepatic degeneration and neoplasia in the aquarium fish, *Brachydanio rerio*. J. nat. Cancer Inst., 34, 117-130

Stephany, R.W., Freudenthal, J. & Schuller, P.L. (1976) Quantitative and qualitative determination of some volatile nitrosamines in various meat products. In: Walker, E.A., Bogovski, P. & Griciute, L., eds, Environmental *N*-Nitroso Compounds Analysis and Formation, Lyon (IARC Scientific Publications No. 14), pp. 343-354

Sugimura, T., Yahagi, T., Nagao, M., Takeuchi, M., Kawachi, T., Hara, K., Yamasaki, E., Matsushima, T., Hashimoto, Y. & Okada, M. (1976) Validity of mutagenicity tests using microbes as a rapid screening method for environmental carcinogens. In: Montesano, R., Bartsch, H. & Tomatis, L., eds, Screening Tests in Chemical Carcinogenesis, Lyon (IARC Scientific Publications No. 12), pp. 81-101

Svoboda, D. & Higginson, J. (1968) A comparison of ultrastructural changes in rat liver due to chemical carcinogens. Cancer Res., 28, 1703-1733

Swann, P.F. & Magee, P.N. (1971) Nitrosamine-induced carcinogenesis. The alkylation of *N*-7 of guanine of nucleic acids of the rat by diethylnitrosamine *N*-ethyl-*N*-nitrosourea and ethyl methanesulphonate. Biochem. J., 125, 841-847

Sydow, G. (1970) Untersuchungen über die diaplazentare teratogene, karzinogene und mutagene Wirkung von Diäthylnitrosamin (DÄNA) nach oraler Applikation bei der Ratte. Arch. Geschwulstforsch., 36, 331-334

Takayama, S. & Oota, K. (1965) Induction of malignant tumors in various strains of mice by oral administration of *N*-nitrosodimethylamine and *N*-nitrosodiethylamine. Gann, 56, 189-199

Takayama, S., Hitachi, M. & Yamada, K. (1975) Histological and cytological studies on hepatocarcinogenesis in rats by administration of diethylnitrosamine. Gann Monogr. Cancer Res., 17, 343-354

Telling, G.M., Bryce, T.A., Hoar, D., Osborne, D. & Welti, D. (1974) Progress in the analysis of volatile *N*-nitroso compounds. In: Bogovski, P. & Walker, E.A., eds, *N*-Nitroso Compounds in the Environment, Lyon (IARC Scientific Publications No. 9), pp. 12-17

Thewlis, B.H. (1967) Testing of wheat flour for the presence of nitrite and nitrosamines. Fd Cosmet. Toxicol., 5, 333-337

Thomas, C. (1961) Zur Morphologie der durch Diäthylnitrosamin erzeugten Leberveränderungen und Tumoren bei der Ratte. Z. Krebsforsch., 64, 224-233

Thomas, C. & Bollmann, R. (1968) Untersuchungen zur diaplacentaren krebserzeugenden Wirkung des Diäthylnitrosamins an Ratten. Z. Krebsforsch., 71, 129-134

Thomas, C. & Schmähl, D. (1963) Zur Morphologie der durch Diäthylnitrosamin erzeugten Lebertumoren bei der Maus und dem Meerschweinchen. Z. Krebsforsch., 65, 531-536

Turusov, V., Tomatis, L., Guibbert, D., Duperray, B. & Pacheco, H. (1973) The effect of prenatal exposure of mice to methylcholanthrene combined with the neonatal administration of diethylnitrosamine. In: Tomatis, L. & Mohr, U., eds, Transplacental Carcinogenesis, Lyon (IARC Scientific Publications No. 4), pp. 84-91

US Environmental Protection Agency (1977) Requirement for certain pesticide registrants and applicants for registration to submit analyses of pesticides for *N*-nitroso contaminants. Fed. Regist., 42, 51640-51641

Vogel, E. & Leigh, B. (1975) Concentration-effect studies with MMS, TEB, 2,4,5-TriCl-PDMT, and DEN on the induction of dominant and recessive lethals, chromosome loss and translocations in *Drosophila* sperm. Mutation Res., 29, 383-396

Weisburger, E.K., Ward, J.M. & Brown, C.A. (1974) Dibenamine: selective protection against diethylnitrosamine-induced hepatic carcinogenesis but not oral, pharyngeal and esophageal carcinogenesis. Toxicol. appl. Pharmacol., 28, 477-484

Weisburger, J.H., Madison, R.M., Ward, J.M., Viguera, C. & Weisburger, E.K. (1975) Modification of diethylnitrosamine liver carcinogenesis with phenobarbital but not with immunosuppression. J. nat. Cancer Inst., 54, 1185-1188

Witschi, H. (1973) The effects of diethylnitrosamine on ribonucleic acid and protein synthesis in the liver and lung of the Syrian golden hamster. Biochem. J., 136, 789-794

Wrba, H., Pielsticker, K. & Mohr, U. (1967) Die diaplazentar-carcinogene Wirkung von Diäthylnitrosamin bei Ratten. Naturwissenschaften, 54, 47

N-NITROSODIMETHYLAMINE

This substance was considered previously by an IARC Working Group, in December 1971 (IARC, 1972). Since that time new data have become available, and these have been incorporated into the monograph and taken into account in the present evaluation.

1. Chemical and Physical Data

1.1 Synonyms and trade names

Chem. Abstr. Services Reg. No.: 62-75-9

Chem. Abstr. Name: *N*-Methyl-*N*-nitrosomethanamine

N,N-Dimethylnitrosamine; dimethylnitrosamine; DMN; DMNA; NDMA

1.2 Structural and molecular formulae and weight

O=N—N(CH$_3$)$_2$

$C_2H_6N_2O$ Mol. wt: 74.1

1.3 Chemical and physical properties of the pure substance

(a) Description: Yellow, oily liquid (Magee & Barnes, 1967)

(b) Boiling-point: 50-52°C (14 mm); 151°C (760 mm) (Druckrey *et al.*, 1967)

(c) Density: d_4^{20} 1.0061

(d) Refractive index: n_D^{20} 1.4368

(e) Spectroscopy data: λ_{max} 230 and 332 nm (E^1_1 = 978.9 and 12.8) in water (Druckrey *et al.*, 1967); mass spectroscopy data are given by Pensabene *et al.* (1972) and Rainey *et al.* (1978).

(f) Solubility: Soluble in water, organic solvents and lipids

(g) Volatility: Volatile; can be steam-distilled quantitatively (Eisenbrand *et al.*, 1970)

(h) Stability: Stable at room temperature for more than 14 days in neutral or alkaline aqueous solutions in the dark (Druckrey *et al.*, 1967); slightly less stable in acidic solutions; sensitive to ultra-violet light

(i) Reactivity: Strong oxidants (peracids) oxidize it to the corresponding nitramine; can be reduced to the corresponding hydrazine and/or amine; relatively resistant to hydrolysis but can be easily split by hydrogen bromide in acetic acid (Eisenbrand & Preussmann, 1970). Photochemically reactive (Fridman *et al.*, 1971). The preparation of various derivatives has been discussed (Preussmann *et al.*, 1978).

1.4 Technical products and impurities

No data were available to the Working Group.

2. Production, Use, Occurrence and Analysis

2.1 Production and use

For background information on this section, see preamble, p. 22.

(a) Production

N-Nitrosodimethylamine (NDMA) was first prepared in 1895 by Renouf by the reaction of sodium nitrite with an acidified solution of dimethylamine hydrochloride (Prager *et al.*, 1922). Essentially the same procedure is believed to have been used for its commercial production (Getz, 1960).

Production of NDMA has not been reported to the US International Trade Commission; however, prior to 1 April 1976, one US company produced it as an intermediate in the manufacture of 1,1-dimethylhydrazine[1] (unsymmetrical dimethylhydrazine) (Anon., 1975). Prior to closing of this plant, annual production of NDMA is believed to have been less than 500 thousand kg per year. Production of 1,1-dimethylhydrazine was first reported to the US International Trade Commission in 1956 (IARC, 1974). 1,1-Dimethyl-

---

[1]See IARC (1974).

hydrazine is also believed to have been produced in Germany in the early 1940's, but no information is available about the route of synthesis. No evidence was found that NDMA has been produced commercially in Japan, and it is not known if it is produced in other countries.

(b) Use

Prior to 1 April 1976, NDMA was used in the US as an intermediate in the production of 1,1-dimethylhydrazine, a storable liquid rocket fuel which is believed to have contained up to 0.1% NDMA as an impurity. No evidence was found that NDMA is used at present, except for research purposes.

Regulations in the US concerning NDMA designate strict procedures to avoid worker contact. Mixtures containing 1.0% or more NDMA must be maintained in isolated or closed systems, employees must observe special personal hygiene rules, and certain procedures must be followed for movement of the material and in case of accidental spills and emergencies (US Occupational Safety and Health Administration, 1976).

2.2 Occurrence

(a) Air

Bretschneider & Matz (1974, 1976) reported levels of 1-430 ng/m^3 [1] NDMA inside a factory using dimethylamine. Fine *et al.* (1976a) reported its presence as an air pollutant in Baltimore, Maryland and in Belle, West Virginia (USA). In Baltimore, the prime source was found to be a chemical plant which was manufacturing 1,1-dimethylhydrazine using NDMA as a precursor. Typical NDMA levels were between 6000 and 36,000 ng/m^3 on the site of the factory, about 1000 ng/m^3 in residential neighbourhoods adjacent to the factory, and about 100 ng/m^3 two miles away in downtown Baltimore (Fine, 1978; Fine *et al.*, 1976b,c, 1977a; Pellizzari *et al.*, 1976). Following this study, in April 1976, the factory was closed down. In Belle, the source of the NDMA was found to be a chemical factory manufacturing and

[1] This result was not confirmed by mass spectroscopy (see also 'General Remarks on the Substances Considered', p. 40).

using dimethylamine; the NDMA was being produced as an unwanted byproduct. Typical levels in downtown Belle and Charleston ranged from 1-40 ng/m^3 (Fine, 1978). Similar levels[1] were found by Cohen & Bachman (1978) on the site of several chemical factories making or using dimethylamine. In extensive studies in New York City, Boston and New Jersey, NDMA was found at 3/40 sites at levels above the detection limit of 10 ng/m^3 (Fine, 1977, 1978). Gough *et al.* (1976) and Sen *et al.* (1976a) have found that during the frying of bacon, 70% of NDMA volatilized in the fumes.

(b) Tobacco smoke

Johnson & Rhoades (1972) and Rhoades & Johnson (1972) claimed to have found 0-140 ng/cigarette NDMA [One of these results was confirmed by high-resolution mass spectrometry]. Similar results were reported by McCormick *et al.* (1973), using high-resolution mass spectrometry. Klimsch *et al.* (1976) reported 9.5-91 ng/cigarette.

NDMA was present in the mainstream smoke of non-filtered cigarettes at a level of 13-65 ng/cigarette, and 5.7-43 ng/cigarette were found in filtered cigarettes. In the sidestream smoke, the levels were 680-823 ng/cigarette in non-filtered cigarettes and 1040-1770 ng/cigarette in filtered cigarettes. In smoke-filled rooms, such as bars and discotheques, 90-240 ng/m^3 NDMA[1] were found in the air. In residences, the levels[1] were <5 ng/m^3 (Brunnemann & Hoffmann, 1978; Brunnemann *et al.*, 1977). Walker & Castegnaro (IARC, 1977c) found NDMA in all of 10 samples of scrapings from pipes used for smoking tobacco in the Transkei; these are believed to be consumed by the local inhabitants. The levels ranged from 45-340 μg/kg.

(c) Water

NMDA was present in sea-water adjacent to a 1,1-dimethylhydrazine chemical factory in Baltimore which was emitting NDMA into the air; the levels varied from 0.08-0.25 μg/l (Fine & Rounbehler, 1976). NDMA was also reported at a level of 3.0 μg/l in an adjacent sewage-treatment facility.

---

[1]These results were not confirmed by mass spectroscopy (see also 'General Remarks on the Substances Considered', p. 40).

On the site of the Baltimore factory, water in a drainage ditch contained 6 μg/l and that in a mud puddle 200 and 6000 μg/l (Fine *et al.*, 1977a). Industrial waste-water from chemical factories was found to contain 0.2-5 μg/l (Fine, 1978); that from 8/19 chemical factories contained 0.08-3.3 μg/l NDMA (Cohen & Bachman, 1978).

Cohen & Bachman (1978)[1], Gough (1978)[1] and Fiddler *et al.* (1977) found 0.012-0.34 μg/l in deionized water; the source of the NDMA was shown to be the ion-exchange resin. Fine (1978) reported <0.01 μg/l[1] NDMA in high-nitrate well-water. Cohen & Bachman (1978) also reported that chlorination of drinking-water can result in NDMA levels of 0.02-0.82 μg/l[1].

(d) Soil

Soil samples taken from several locations near industrial plants in New Jersey contained NDMA at levels ranging from 0-15.1 ng/g; in West Virginia, near Belle and Charleston, soil samples contained 0.2-5.4 ng/g; and in the New York City area, soil samples contained 0-0.32 ng/g (Fine, 1977).

(e) Food and feed

Cheese: Various cheeses have been analysed for NDMA. Havery *et al.* (1976) found none, and Alliston *et al.* (1972) found only a trace. However, Sen *et al.* (1978) found 2-68 μg/kg NDMA in 20/63 samples of 26 different cheeses. Eisenbrand *et al.* (1978) found that 78/173 cheeses were positive for NDMA, and levels of 1-6 μg/kg were confirmed in 20 of these samples. Gough (1978) found up to 0.2 μg/kg in 13/20 samples, and 3/16 samples of other dairy products contained NDMA at levels of <0.1 μg/kg.

Vegetables and vegetable oils: Telling *et al.* (1974) found no NDMA in raw or cooked vegetables, and Gough (1978) found no NDMA in 16 different vegetable samples. None was found in baby food or lard (Havery *et al.*, 1976), but freshly refined soya bean oil was found to contain levels of 0-20 μg/kg[1] (Hedler *et al.*, 1976).

---

[1]These results were not confirmed by mass spectroscopy (see also 'General Remarks on the Substances Considered', p. 40).

NDMA was found in 5/12 samples of tinned fruit at a level of <0.1 μg/kg (Gough, 1978) and in the fruit of a solanaceous bush, *Solanum incanum*, used in the Transkei for the preparation of foodstuffs (Du Plessis *et al.*, 1969)[1].

In a dietary survey to compare levels of nitrosamines in regions of high and low incidence of oesophageal cancer, no significant difference in NDMA levels was found among 179 samples. Levels were mostly <5 μg/kg[1] (IARC, 1975; Joint Iran-IARC Study Group, 1977).

Meat and fish: The presence of NDMA in meat and fish products has been demonstrated in a number of studies (Table 1).

Spices: Sen *et al.* (1974) found 0-850 μg/kg NDMA in spices used for meat curing, and Havery *et al.* (1976) reported 29-343 μg/kg in spice cures. No nitrosamines were found in the mixtures when the spices and nitrite and/or nitrate salts were packaged separately.

Feed: Among the first reports of nitrosamines in the environment were those of Sakshaug *et al.* (1965) and Ender *et al.* (1964), who found high levels of NDMA in fishmeal, using thin-layer chromatography. Mirna *et al.* (1976) reported 2, 3, 8, 18, 205 and 315 μg/kg NDMA. Fishmeal not treated with nitrate or nitrite was found to contain between 150 and 1000 μg/kg NDMA (Hurst, 1976). Skaare & Dahle (1975) reported 100-2000 μg/kg NDMA, and Juszkiewicz & Kowalski (1976) 5-417 μg/kg[1].

Levels of 0-42 μg/kg NDMA have been found in a number of experimental animal feeds which contain fishmeal (IARC, 1977a). Kann *et al.* (1978) reported NDMA in 37/46 animal feeds: 23 samples contained 1-10 μg/kg and 14, more than 10 μg/kg (one of these had 79 μg/kg).

(f) Alcoholic beverages

Examination of over 100 apple brandies has shown that NDMA was present in a majority of samples. The average level found was 0.5 μg/kg with a maximum of 10 μg/kg. NDMA was also found in a number of ciders, cognacs,

---

[1]These results were not confirmed by mass spectroscopy (see also 'General Remarks on the Substances Considered', p. 40).

Table 1

Levels of *N*-nitrosodimethylamine in various foods from several countries[1]

Product	Country	No. of samples	Number positive	Level (μg/kg)	Reference
Various meat products	Canada	59	5	10-80	Sen (1972)
" " "	"	197	57	2-12	Panalaks *et al.* (1973)
" " "	"	80	29	2-35	" " (1974)
" " "	"	100	26	5-48	Sen *et al.* (1976b)
Bacon (fried)	"	8	7	2-5	" " (1973)
Fish (fresh)	"	18	11	3-18	Iyengar *et al.* (1976)
" (processed)	"	11	3	3-6	" " "
Cured meats (raw)	FRG	34	26	<1-2.4	Eisenbrand *et al.* (1978)
" " (cooked)	"	34	20	<1-1.7	" " "
Bacon (raw)	"	5	5	1-3	" " (1977)
" (cooked)	"	5	5	1-4	" " "
Liver, meatloaf (raw)	"	4	4	1-8	" " "
" " (cooked)	"	4	2	1	" " "
Pepper, salami (raw)	"	5	3	1-10	" " "
" " (cooked)	"	5	5	1-12	" " "
Ham (raw)	"	6	5	1-54	" " "
" (cooked)	"	4	4	1-6	" " "
Salted fish	Hong Kong	21	8	1-35	Huang *et al.* (1978a,b)
Fish products	" "	61	27	1-15	Fong & Chan (1977)
Croakers (fish)	" "	2	1	20-30[2]	" " (1973)

[1]No data were available to the Working Group from other countries.
[2]These results were not confirmed by mass spectroscopy (see also 'General Remarks on the Substances Considered', p. 40).

Product	Country	No. of samples	Number positive	Level (μg/kg)	Reference
Cured meats	The Netherlands	5	5	0.0-27.3	Stephany *et al.* (1976)
" "	"	30	7	2-6	Groenen *et al.* (1976)
Bacon (fried)	"	5	2	2-4	" " "
" "	"	5	5	0.3-1.1	Stephany *et al.* (1976)
Meat (fried)	"	5	5	0.0-0.4	" " "
Bacon (raw)	"	8	7	0.9-9.5	Groenen *et al.* (1977)
" (fried)	"	7	7	1.2-7.5	" " "
Minced meat (raw)	"	5	0	-	" " "
" " (fried)	"	5	5	0.4-1.9	" " "
Cured meats	"	22	22	0.1-15.5	" " "
Stale cod	UK	2	2	1[2]	Alliston *et al.* (1972)
Bacon (grilled/fried)	"	29	NR[3]	>1-3	Telling *et al.* (1974)
" (cooked)	"	16	NR	<0.1-6	Gough & Walters (1976)
" (cooked-out fat)	"	42	NR	<0.2-10	Telling *et al.* (1974)
" " " "	"	16	NR	<0.1-28	Gough & Walters (1976)
Spiced tinned meat	"	NR	5	3-5	Gough (1978)
Various meat products	"	35	NR	<0.2-<1	Telling *et al.* (1974)
" " "	"	6	NR	<0.5[2]	Alliston *et al.* (1972)
Sausages (smoked)	"	4	NR	<0.2-<1	Telling *et al.* (1974)
Ham (tinned)	"	2	NR	<0.2	" " "
Bacon (raw)	"	2	NR	<0.5[2]	Alliston *et al.* (1972)
" "	"	10	NR	<0.2	Telling *et al.* (1974)
" (grilled/fried)	"	24	5	1-4	Crosby *et al.* (1972)
" (fried)	"	8	8	1-10	Gough (1978)
" (grilled/fried)	"	46	13	1-5	Gough *et al.* (1977)

[2]These results were not confirmed by mass spectroscopy (see also 'General Remarks on the Substances Considered', p. 40).
[3]NR = not reported

Product	Country	No. of samples	Number positive	Level (μg/kg)	Reference
Cured meat (tinned)	UK	34	9	1-10	Gough *et al.* (1977)
Salami, sausage	"	22	2	1-5	" " "
Poultry (cooked)	"	9	1	1-5	" " "
Fish (uncooked)	"	61	23	1-10	" " "
" (cooked)	"	9	0	<1[4]	" " "
Cheese	"	58	10	1-15	" " "
Yoghurt and dessert dishes	"	16	0	<1[4]	" " "
Fish (fresh)	"	85	NR[3]	<0.2-9	Telling *et al.* (1974)
" (tinned)	"	16	NR	<0.2-2.5	" " "
" and fish products	"	35	15	1-9	Crosby *et al.* (1972)
" " " " "	"	20	10	up to 0.2[2]	Gough (1978)
Japanese salmon (raw)	USA	24	0	<5[4]	Gadbois *et al.* (1976)
Fin fish	"	26	0	<10[4]	Havery & Fazio (1977)
Shellfish	"	52	0	<10[4]	" " "
Fish and fish products	"	26	22	4-26	Fazio *et al.* (1971a)
Various meat products	"	51	1	5	" " (1971b)
Frankfurters	"	40	3	0-84	Wasserman *et al.* (1972)
Souse, jellied cured meats	"	10	8	3-63	Fiddler *et al.* (1975)
Various cured meats	"	39	0	<10[4]	Havery *et al.* (1976)
Bacon (raw and fried)	"	22	0	<10[4]	" " "
Various cured meats	"	106	some	<1	" " (1978)
Sausages	USSR	12	9	1-13[2]	Kann *et al.* (1976)
Fish (fresh and processed)	"	19	18	6-177[2]	" " "

[2]These results were not confirmed by mass spectroscopy (see also 'General Remarks on the Substances Considered', p. 40).
[3]NR = not reported
[4]Detection limited

armagnacs, rums and whiskeys; average levels ranged from 0.1-0.4 μg/kg with a maximum of 1.6 μg/kg.

In 27 beers examined, the average level was 2 μg/kg, with a maximum of 7 μg/kg (IARC, 1977b). NDMA was detected in 3/18 samples of maize beer at levels of 1.0, 1.5 and 7.5 μg/kg (IARC, 1976).

(g) Pesticides

Fine *et al.* (1978) reported 190-640 mg/l (ppm) NDMA in dimethylamine formulations of 2,3,6-trichlorobenzoic acid; 300 μg/l NDMA were also found in 1/3 herbicide mixtures formulated as dimethylamine salts. Cohen *et al.* (1978) reported levels ranging from 0.1-335 mg/kg (ppm) NDMA in 7/8 dimethylamine salts of various herbicides.

(h) Drugs

Eisenbrand *et al.* (1978) found NDMA in all samples of 68 drugs formulated with aminopyrine, including tablets, suppositories, injections, drops and syrups. The concentration varied within wide limits (<10-371 μg/kg): 35 samples contained 1-10 μg/kg, 27 samples contained 10-50 μg/kg, 5 samples contained 50-100 μg/kg and 1 sample (a tablet) contained 371 μg/kg.

(i) *In vivo* formation

NDMA was formed in laboratory mice *in vivo* following gavage with 250 ng sodium nitrite then 50 ng dimethylamine hydrochloride (Rounbehler *et al.*, 1977).

NDMA has been reported to be present in man *in vivo*. Harington *et al.* (1973) claimed that NDMA was present in vaginal fluids [Confirmation was by low-resolution mass spectrometry, and the results have not been reported elsewhere. No adequate precautions were taken to prevent nitrosamine formation during analysis].

Eisenbrand *et al.* (1976) reported the presence of 10 and 100 μg/l NDMA in 2/8 urine samples from patients with urinary tract infections; Hicks *et al.* (1978) reported traces in the urine of some patients with chronic bladder infections (detection limit, 1 μg/kg); Stephany & Schuller (1978) reported levels of <1 μg/kg in the urine of hospital patients treated with potassium nitrate; and similar results[1] have been reported by Brooks *et al.* (1972) and Radomski & Hearn (1976) [In none of this work were adequate precautions taken to prevent nitrosamine formation during storage and analysis].

Lakritz *et al.* (1978) reported the presence of 2 μg/kg NDMA in the gastric juice from 2/35 fasting patients [No adequate precautions were taken to prevent nitrosamine formation during storage and analysis].

Fine *et al.* (1977c) found more NDMA in human blood immediately after ingestion of a meal containing spinach, bacon, tomato, bread and beer than was present before. Ingestion of ascorbate reduced the background amount to a non-detectable level.

2.3 Analysis

An IARC Manual gives selected methods for the analysis of volatile *N*-nitrosamines, including NDMA (Preussmann *et al.*, 1978). Four techniques have been used for trapping NDMA during air monitoring: charcoal traps (Bretschneider & Matz, 1974), Tenax GC cartridges (Issenberg & Sornson, 1976; Pellizzari *et al.*, 1976), cryogenic traps (Fine *et al.*, 1976c) and ambient temperature alkali traps (Fine *et al.*, 1977a).

On 29 September 1977, the US Environmental Protection Agency issued a notice requiring all registrants of pesticide products that are potentially contaminated with *N*-nitroso compounds to analyse commercial samples which have been stored for at least 18 days to determine the extent of contamination. This notice prescribes in general terms the types of analytical methods to be used for volatile *N*-nitroso compounds (e.g., gas chromatography plus mass spectrometry or thermal energy analysis and others) as well as for nonvolatile *N*-nitroso compounds (e.g., high-pressure liquid chromatography plus ultra-violet spectroscopy). Confirmation of positive results by gas chromatography and mass spectrometry or by valid independent methods is required when possible (US Environmental Protection Agency, 1977).

---

[1]These results were not confirmed by mass spectroscopy (see also 'General Remarks on the Substances Considered', p. 40).

3. Biological Data Relevant to the Evaluation of Carcinogenic Risk to Man

3.1 Carcinogenicity and related studies in animals

(a) Oral administration

Mouse: Several studies on different strains of mice have demonstrated that *N*-nitrosodimethylamine (NDMA) produces haemangiomas, haemangioendotheliomas, haemangioendothelial sarcomas, adenomas and hepatocellular carcinomas of the liver, as well as adenomas and adenocarcinomas of the lung. Kidney adenomas have also been observed in some strains (Clapp & Toya, 1970; Clapp *et al.*, 1968, 1971; Den Engelse *et al.*, 1969/1970; Kuwahara *et al.*, 1972; Otsuka & Kuwahara, 1971; Shabad & Savluchinskaya, 1971; Takayama & Oota, 1963, 1965; Terracini *et al.*, 1966; Toth *et al.*, 1964; Zwicker *et al.*, 1972). A concentration of 50 mg/l NDMA in the drinking-water for one week was sufficient to induce tumours in the kidney and lung (Terracini *et al.*, 1966). The lowest dose tested in long-term studies, a concentration in the drinking-water that corresponded to a dose of 0.4 mg/kg bw/day (total dose, 89 mg/kg bw), produced 13/17 lung adenomas and 2/10 haemangiocellular tumours in male RF mice (Clapp & Toya, 1970).

Rat: The carcinogenicity of NDMA has been demonstrated in several different strains of rat. Although differences have been seen in target organs, a consistent observation has been that long-term treatment with doses compatible with good survival rates, i.e., not more than 50-100 mg/kg in the diet or drinking-water, or 4 mg/kg bw/day, leads to the development of high incidences of hepatocellular carcinomas and cholangiocellular tumours (Argus & Hoch-Ligeti, 1961; Geil *et al.*, 1968; Magee & Barnes, 1956, 1962; Schmähl & Preussmann, 1959; Terracini *et al.*, 1967). Haemangioendothelial sarcomas of the liver have also been observed (Hadjiolov & Markow, 1973; Taylor *et al.*, 1974). Short-term or single-dose treatment with high doses (100-500 mg/kg of diet, or up to 30 mg/kg bw) produces kidney tumours (Magee & Barnes, 1959, 1962; Riopelle & Jasmin, 1969; Shinohara *et al.*, 1976; Terracini *et al.*, 1969; Zak *et al.*, 1960); the histology of these tumours has been described in detail (Ireton *et al.*,

1972; Ito, 1973; Ito *et al.*, 1971; Jasmin & Cha, 1969; Jasmin & Riopelle, 1968, 1969; McGiven & Ireton, 1972). Lung adenocarcinomas and squamous-cell carcinomas have been seen occasionally after NDMA treatment (Argus & Hoch-Ligeti, 1961; Zak *et al.*, 1960).

A dose-response study has been carried out in Porton rats in which NDMA in oil solution was added to the diet. After an observation time of up to 120 weeks, the following frequencies of liver tumours (mainly liver-cell carcinomas) were observed (Table 2) (Terracini *et al.*, 1967):

Table 2[a]

Dose-response study with *N*-nitrosodimethylamine in rats

NDMA mg/kg of diet	Number of rats initially	Number of rats with liver tumours
0 (control)	41	0
2	37	1
5	68	5
10	5	2
20	23	15
50	12	10

[a]From Terracini *et al.*, 1967

Treatment of Sprague-Dawley rats with 0.4 mg/rat 5 times weekly for 24 weeks (total dose, 48 mg/rat) induced liver tumours (3 liver-cell carcinomas, 2 sarcomas) in 5/19 animals (Hoch-Ligeti *et al.*, 1968).

Hexadeutero-NDMA, at a level of 5 mg/l in the drinking-water, induced a 3% incidence of liver carcinomas, while NDMA under identical conditions induced 26% (Keefer *et al.*, 1973).

Hamster: Administration by stomach tube of 1.6, 1.0 and 1.0 mg/animal NDMA over 5 weeks, or of 1 dose of 1.6 mg/animal, to Syrian golden hamsters induced cholangioadenomas, cholangiocarcinomas and haemangiosarcomas as well as haemangioendotheliomas of the liver (Tomatis & Cefis, 1967). Liver-cell carcinomas, cholangiocarcinomas and haemangioendotheliomas were obtained by giving 25 mg/l NDMA in the drinking-water for 11 weeks (Kowalewski & Todd, 1971; Tomatis *et al.*, 1964). Administration of 1 mg/l NDMA in the drinking-water to inbred Syrian hamsters (strain B10® 87.29) for 60 weeks induced 1 adenocarcinoma of the glandular stomach in 40 animals (Homburger *et al.*, 1976).

Guinea-pig: Male guinea-pigs given 25 or 50 mg NDMA/kg of diet for 6-49 weeks developed papillary cholangiomas and liver-cell carcinomas (Le Page & Christie, 1969a).

Rabbit: Doses of 25 and 50 mg NDMA/kg of diet given to rabbits for 17-60 weeks resulted in hepatocellular carcinomas with lung metastases and benign papillary cholangiomas (Le Page & Christie, 1969b).

Duck: It was reported in an abstract that treatment with diet containing 50 mg NDMA/kg of diet to male Peking ducks for 8-10 months resulted in an incidence of 71% anaplastic haemangiosarcomas of the liver after 9 months (McCracken *et al.*, 1973).

Fish: Doses of 300, 1200, 4800 and 19,200 mg NDMA/kg of diet given to rainbow trout for more than 6 months induced adenomas and adenocarcinomas of the liver (Ashley & Halver, 1968). Guppies (*Lebistes reticulatus*) received 4.8 g NDMA/kg of diet for several months; after 13 months, 2/20 developed hepatic nodules, described as liver tumours, and a leiomyosarcoma in the mesentery (Sato *et al.*, 1973).

(b) Inhalation and/or intratracheal administration

Mouse: BALB/c mice were exposed daily to 0.005 or 0.2 mg/m^3 NDMA for 17 months. Tumours were observed earlier and in larger amounts in the lung, liver and kidney only in those given the higher concentration (Moiseev & Benemansky, 1975).

Rat: Twice-weekly inhalation of NDMA at a concentration corresponding to 4 mg/kg bw for 30 minutes induced tumours (aesthesioneuroepitheliomas and squamous-cell carcinomas) of the ethmoturbinals in 4/6 BD rats. With half the concentration, 8/12 rats developed tumours of the nasal cavity

(Druckrey *et al.*, 1967). In Wistar rats exposed daily by inhalation to 0.005 or 0.2 mg/m^3 NDMA for 25 months, those given the higher level had tumours in the lung, kidney and liver earlier and in larger amounts than in controls (Moiseev & Benemansky, 1975).

(c) Subcutaneous and/or intramuscular administration

Mouse: Weekly injections to DD, BALB/c and SJL/J strain mice of 0.15 mg NDMA in 0.2 ml saline for 1-25 weeks (total dose, 0.15-3.75 mg/animal) induced haemangioendothelial sarcomas of the liver and of the retroperitoneal and abdominal soft tissues, and adenomas or adenocarcinomas of the lung (Kuwahara *et al.*, 1972; Otsuka & Kuwahara, 1971). After single s.c. administrations of NDMA, a dose-response relationship was seen for lung tumours (adenomas and carcinomas): 1 mg/kg bw = 29%, 2 mg/kg bw = 35%, 4 mg/kg bw = 39% and 8 mg/kg bw = 67% (Cardesa *et al.*, 1974a).

Newborn and suckling mouse: Following single s.c. injections of 15-75 μg/animal, mice developed parenchymal-cell and vascular tumours of the liver as well as lung adenomas (Terracini *et al.*, 1966; Toth & Shubik, 1967; Toth *et al.*, 1964).

Rat: Injections of 10, 20 or 30 mg/rat at day 21 or 70 after birth produced 38% kidney tumours after median latent periods of 286-369 days; 41% of kidney tumours were of the renal cell type and 59% were stromal nephromas. No control rats developed kidney tumours (Campbell *et al.*, 1974).

Newborn and suckling rat: Single doses of 0.125 mg NDMA/animal induced tumours of the kidney and hepatocellular carcinomas (Terracini & Magee, 1964; Terracini *et al.*, 1969).

Forty weekly s.c. injections to Wistar rats of 0.1 mg/rat, beginning at birth, induced 6/11 kidney tumours, mainly nephroblastomas, adenomas and clear-cell carcinomas (Ito, 1973). Single injections to Wistar rats of 0.125 mg/rat at 1 day of age and 0.125 or 10 mg/rat at day 7 induced 63% kidney tumours after median induction times of 218-237 days; 92% of the induced neoplasms were stromal nephromas (Campbell *et al.*, 1974).

Hamster: Weekly s.c. injections of 0.5-1.0 mg NDMA for 6-20 weeks (total dose, 6-14 mg/animal) caused haemangioendothelial sarcomas and cholangiocarcinomas in the liver and aesthesioneuroepitheliomas of the nasal cavity in Syrian golden hamsters (Herrold, 1967). Lifetime weekly injections of approximately 6, 3 and 1.5 mg/kg to groups of 32, 32 and 30 Syrian golden hamsters (males and females) led mainly to liver tumours: 3, 10 and 8 in males, and 4, 4 and 2 in females, respectively. The liver tumours were: hepatocellular carcinomas (6), hepatomas (8) and cholangiocarcinomas (17). Only a few tumours were seen in the respiratory tract (3), the kidney (1) and the forestomach (1) (Haas *et al.*, 1973). Similar results were obtained in another study (Stenback *et al.*, 1973).

In Chinese hamsters, weekly injections of 0.89, 1.77 or 3.54 mg/kg bw NDMA for lifetime (total doses, about 32, 54 or 104 mg/kg bw, respectively) caused mainly liver haemangioendotheliomas (70-100%). Only 3/108 hamsters had adenocarcinomas in the endoturbinals of the nasal cavity (Reznik, 1975; Reznik *et al.*, 1976).

In 60 European hamsters, weekly s.c. injections of 1.4-8.6 mg/kg bw NDMA induced mainly malignant haemangioendotheliomas of the liver and kidney, hepatocellular carcinomas and 1 cholangiocellular carcinoma. No such tumours were seen in 20 controls (Mohr *et al.*, 1974).

Mastomys: Twice-weekly s.c. injections of 0.1 mg NDMA/animal for 10-44 weeks induced liver tumours in 6/36 males: 2 cholangiomas, 2 cholangiocarcinomas, 1 haemangioendothelioma and 1 hepatic-cell carcinoma; none were seen in the females. In controls, 4/82 liver tumours were seen in females and none in males (Fujii & Sato, 1970).

(d) Intraperitoneal administration

Mouse: A single dose of 7 or 14 mg/kg bw NDMA given to GR or CFW/D mice resulted in lung adenomas (Den Engelse *et al.*, 1969/1970; Frei, 1970). Single doses of 5, 10 or 15 mg/kg bw NDMA to RF mice induced 9/18, 16/19 and 4/5 lung tumours (adenomas, papillary carcinomas), as compared with 25/52 in controls. The incidence of leukaemia was not significantly different from that in controls (Clapp, 1973). Weekly injections of 6 mg/kg bw for 10 weeks in female Swiss mice resulted in a significantly increased incidence ($P<0.001$) of vascular tumours (40%), mainly of the retroperitoneum, while the incidence in males was only 15%. There was a low incidence of hepatic vascular tumours in both sexes (Cardesa *et al.*, 1973). Single doses of 7.5 or 15 mg/kg bw NDMA given to NZO/Bl mice at 60 days of age induced a large increase in the incidence of lung tumours in males and females (76-100%, compared with 19-25% in controls) and of kidney adenomas and carcinomas in males (33% (7/21) in the lower dose group and 56% (10/33) in the higher dose group, compared with only 1/268 in controls) (Noronha, 1975). In adult C3Hf mice, a single dose of 7 mg/animal induced hepatomas in 38% of males but none in females (Den Engelse *et al.*, 1974). A positive dose-response relationship was seen in Swiss mice with regard to lung adenoma incidence: 0 mg/kg (control), 15%; 0.5, 17%; 1.0, 29%; 2.0, 35%; 4.0, 39%; and 8.0, 67%. No clear relationships between applied dose and tumour rate was apparent for other tumour sites and in other strains (ASW/SN and A) (Ii *et al.*, 1976).

Newborn and suckling mouse: Single i.p. injections of 8 mg/kg bw NDMA to newborn mice resulted in hepatomas (hepatocellular type) and lung adenomas (Frei, 1970). Six i.p. injections of 1-4 mg/kg bw to 7-day-old mice resulted in hepatomas, hepatocarcinomas, lung adenomas and haemangiomas (Vesselinovitch, 1969).

Rat: A single i.p. injection of 18 mg/kg bw NDMA to Wistar rats induced kidney tumours (Murphy *et al.*, 1966). In 80-day-old NZR rats, starved for 48 hours, a single i.p. dose of 20 mg/kg induced squamous-cell carcinomas of the nasal cavity (Noronha & Goodall, 1972).

The morphogenesis of kidney tumours induced by i.p. injections of NDMA in rats has been described by Hard & Butler (1971a) and Hard *et al.* (1977).

Newt: While single doses of up to 16 g/kg bw NDMA did not induce tumours, 6-7 injections of 16 g/kg bw within 3-4 weeks induced liver tumours (described as anaplastic and hepatic-cell tumours) in 3 newts surviving more than 3 months (Ingram, 1972).

(e) Other experimental systems

Various injections: Rats given a single injection of 18 mg/kg bw NDMA, either intramuscularly, retroperitoneally, or directly into the kidney, developed kidney tumours (Murphy *et al.*, 1966).

Prenatal exposure: In mice, single or repeated injections of 12.5-75 mg/kg bw NDMA during the last days of pregnancy resulted in lung adenomas and hepatomas in the offspring (Smetanin, 1971). NDMA induced a low frequency of kidney tumours in the offspring of pregnant rats treated during the last week or during the whole of pregnancy (total dose, 11 mg) (Alexandrov, 1968).

Immersion: In 50 guppies exposed for 7 weeks to 100 mg/l NDMA dissolved in aquarium water, an incidence of 6/44 liver tumours was observed (Khudoley, 1973; Pliss & Khudoley, 1975). In frogs (*Rana temporaria*), 5 mg/l NDMA in tank-water induced 19/43 tumours: hepatocellular carcinomas and adenomas and tumours of the haematopoietic system (Khudoley, 1977).

Carcinogenesis in plants: Seeds of hybrids of *Nicotiana* were soaked in 10 or 1 mM solutions of NDMA in water for 1 or 2 days, and tumours were found on 6.5-12.8% of germinated seedlings 20 days later, as compared with 1-2% on controls (Andersen, 1973).

(f) Carcinogenicity of precursors

Administration of 0.1 or 0.025% aminopyrine together with 0.1 or 0.025% sodium nitrite in the drinking-water of Sprague-Dawley rats for 30 weeks produced haemangioendothelial sarcomas in the liver in 29/30 and 26/30 rats, while 0.1% aminopyrine alone was inactive; 0.1% oxytetracycline and 0.1% sodium nitrite administered in a similar protocol induced 4/30 liver tumours (3 hepatocellular carcinomas and 1 cholangioma) (Taylor & Lijinsky, 1975). NDMA is the known reaction product of both interactions in the animal body (Lijinsky & Greenblatt, 1972).

(g) Carcinogenicity of derivatives

N-Nitroso-*N*-methyl-*N*-acetoxymethylamine

(i) Oral administration

I.g. administration of 3.5 or 1.75 mg/kg bw to Sprague-Dawley rats twice-weekly resulted in squamous-cell carcinomas and papillomas of the forestomach in 13/16 and 18/20 animals, respectively (Wiessler & Schmähl, 1976).

(ii) Intraperitoneal administration

A single i.p. injection of 13 mg/kg bw *N*-nitroso-*N*-methyl-*N*-acetoxymethylamine to 4-5-week-old CD rats resulted in a high incidence (70-86%) of tumours, mostly in the intestine (Joshi *et al.*, 1977; Ward *et al.*, 1977).

(h) Factors that modify carcinogenicity in animals

Feeding of a protein-free diet for 1 week, then a single i.p. injection of 60 mg/kg bw NDMA, and a further week on protein-free diet induced 14/14 kidney tumours in Porton rats, compared with 0/9 in controls given the protein-free diet only (McLean & Magee, 1970). Similar results were obtained by Hilfrich *et al.* (1975).

In rats, the incidence of kidney tumours produced by feeding NDMA at a level of 500 mg/kg of diet for 2 weeks was markedly increased by subsequent treatment with 5000 mg/kg of diet of the nephrotoxin *N*-(3,5-dichlorophenyl)succinimide; pretreatment with this compound inhibited tumour induction (Ito *et al.*, 1974; Sugihara & Sugihara, 1976). A similar increase in the incidence of renal-cell tumours was produced by subsequent treatment with citrinin (Shinohara *et al.*, 1976).

Tumours of the kidney developed in 33% of male and 63% of female Wistar rats that received a single i.p. dose of 30 mg/kg bw NDMA. I.p. injections of 100, 200 or 300 mg/kg bw ethylmethanesulphonate 8 hours after NDMA injection increased kidney tumour rate, more in females than in males (Montesano *et al.*, 1974). In this experiment, 5/109 heart tumours of the left ventricle were observed in the combined treatment groups and diagnosed as either neurofibromas or neurinomas; 1/34 and 8/118 heart tumours were seen in the groups treated with NDMA or ethylmethanesulphonate, respectively (Haas *et al.*, 1974).

Actinomycin D, given before or after a single i.p. dose of NDMA, did not significantly modify kidney tumour incidence in Sprague-Dawley rats (Hilfrich *et al.*, 1975).

Gonadectomy abolished the kidney tumour response observed in male N20 mice after a single i.p. injection of 7.5 mg/kg bw (Noronha, 1975).

Combined gavage of 0.4 mg NDMA in 1 ml tap-water 5 times weekly for 24 weeks to rats together with 3-methylcholanthrene did not increase the incidence of liver tumours; however, tumours of the lung and skin were found (Hoch-Ligeti *et al.*, 1968). Hepatocarcinogenesis induced by 4 mg/kg bw/week NDMA was effectively suppressed by administration of 500 mg/kg bw/week disulfiram 2 hours before NDMA treatment but led to the an incidence of 59% of squamous-cell carcinomas in the paranasal sinus; this tumour type was not observed with NDMA or disulfiram alone (Schmähl *et al.*, 1976). Administration of a copper-deficient or excess-copper diet at the same time as treatment with 50 mg/l NDMA in the drinking-water did not change the incidence of liver or lung tumours; however, kidney neoplasms occurred in 57% of rats receiving the copper-deficient diet, as compared with 0% in the excess-copper groups (Carlton & Price, 1973). A diet high in fat and marginally deficient in lipotropes did not enhance hepatocarcinogenesis by NDMA, although this effect was seen for other nitrosamines (Rogers *et al.*, 1974).

Hepatocarcinogenesis in Sprague-Dawley rats after a single i.g. dose of 20 mg/kg bw NDMA was increased by pretreatment with carbon tetrachloride 42 or 60 hours before oral administration. A high incidence of papillary adenocarcinomas and nephroblastomas was observed in a group that received 40 mg/kg bw NDMA 42 hours after administration of carbon tetrachloride; no kidney tumours were seen in the group treated with NDMA only (Pound & Lawson, 1975; Pound *et al.*, 1973). A single i.p. injection of 12-15.6 mg/kg bw NDMA to female rats 24 hours after partial hepatectomy induced hepatocellular carcinomas; none developed in intact animals receiving NDMA (Craddock 1973, 1975). An increase in the incidence of NDMA-induced kidney tumours after partial hepatectomy was also seen (Craddock, 1971; Pound & Lawson, 1975).

Repeated i.p. injections of phorbol given after a single s.c. injection of 0.015 mg NDMA increased the incidences of lung and liver tumours in newborn AKR mice (Armuth & Berenblum, 1972). Cardesa *et al.* (1974b) described synergestic effects of i.p. injections of NDMA and *N*-nitrosodiethylamine; with NDMA alone, lung carcinomas and kidney tumours were seen, while with NDMA and *N*-nitrosodiethylamine lung adenomas and forestomach papillomas but no kidney tumours were seen.

Thyroidectomy significantly increased the tumour incidences in kidney and liver in NZR rats given single i.p. injections of 20 mg/kg bw NDMA; it reduced the sex difference in lung tumour incidence (male, 70%, female, 16%; compared with 54% and 39%, respectively) (Noronha & Goodall, 1976).

Treatment of Syrian golden hamsters with 15 mg/l NDMA in drinking-water and with a mixture of three antibiotics (gentamicin, nystatin and vancomycin) increased tumour incidence (liver carcinomas, cholangiocarcinomas, Kupffer-cell sarcomas) to 80% as compared with an incidence of 28% with NDMA alone in females, and to 21% compared to 4% in males (Love *et al.*, 1977).

Administration of aminoacetonitrile to rats decreased the carcinogenic effects of NDMA; the number of malignant liver tumours induced decreased by 80% (Hadjiolov, 1971).

3.2 Other relevant biological data

(a) Experimental systems

Toxic effects

In rats, the acute LD_{50} for NDMA was 40 mg/kg bw when given by oral administration, 37 mg/kg bw by inhalation (Druckrey *et al.*, 1967) and 43 mg/kg bw by i.p. administration (Heath, 1962). The i.p. LD_{50} in mice was 20 mg/kg bw (Frei, 1970). The s.c. LD_{50} was 30 mg/kg bw in Syrian golden hamsters (Haas *et al.*, 1973), 18 mg/kg bw in Chinese hamsters (Reznik, 1975), 43 mg/kg bw in female and 28 mg/kg bw in male European hamsters (Mohr *et al.*, 1974).

The major toxicity in a number of species arises from a severe centrilobular necrosis in the liver (Magee & Barnes, 1967; Magee & Swann, 1969). Inhibition of protein and nucleic acid synthesis in the liver by NDMA has been reviewed (Magee & Barnes, 1967; Magee & Swann, 1969; Pegg, 1977).

Embryotoxicity and teratogenicity

No teratogenic effects were observed in rats. A single dose of 30 mg/kg bw given intraperitoneally or orally, or 20 mg/kg bw injected intravenously, caused an increase in foetal mortality, particularly when given on days 3, 9, 10 or 12 of gestation (Napalkov & Alexandrov, 1968). After intraplacental injections of 0.1-0.3 mg NDMA into each embryonic sac on day 13 of gestation, all embryos died (Alexandrov, 1974).

Absorption, distribution and excretion

The uptake of NDMA from the gastrointestinal tract has been studied in rats. Uptake from the stomach was slow, but that from the upper part of the small intestine was very rapid ($t_{\frac{1}{2}}$: less than 5 min); absorption from the lower part of the small intestine and the caecum was slower but still much faster than from the stomach (Hashimoto *et al.*, 1976; Heading *et al.*, 1974). Comparisons of the relative methylation of liver and kidney DNA after small oral or i.v. doses of NDMA in rats have indicated that oral doses below 40 μg/kg bw were completely metabolized by the liver and did not enter the general circulation (Diaz Gomez *et al.*, 1977) [see also 'Metabolism'].

In goats, one hour after oral administration of 30 mg/kg bw, 12.2 mg/kg NDMA were found in milk and 10 mg/kg NDMA in blood. Only traces of NDMA were found in the milk after 24 hours (Juszkiewicz & Kowalski, 1974).

Metabolism

Available evidence suggests that NDMA requires metabolic activation to exert its toxic and carcinogenic effects. The rate of metabolism of NDMA *in vivo* has been examined by measuring the rate of loss of NDMA from the blood and exhalation of $^{14}CO_2$ following administration of ^{14}C-NDMA. In rats, a dose of 30 mg/kg administered by i.p. injection is metabolized within 6 hours (Heath, 1962; Magee *et al.*, 1976; Phillips *et al.*, 1975; Swann & McLean, 1971). The rate of metabolism of NDMA *in vitro* has been measured by the use of slices of liver and other organs (e.g., kidney, lung, small intestine, oesophagus) from rats, hamsters, monkeys, trout, goldfish and various amphibians. Labelled $^{14}CO_2$ was produced from ^{14}C-NDMA, and methylation of cellular macromolecules was observed (Den Engelse *et al.*, 1975; Montesano & Magee, 1974). These data, together with the distribution of methylated nucleic acids *in vivo* in rats, suggested that the liver is the principal site of NDMA metabolism (Swann & Magee, 1968). Oxidative *N*-demethylation to form formaldehyde has been demonstrated with liver microsomes from rats, mice and hamsters (Argus *et al.*, 1976; Czygan *et al.*, 1973a; Lake *et al.*, 1976; Lotlikar *et al.*, 1975; Mizrahi & Emmelot, 1962). Microsomal oxidation has been suggested to result in an unstable *N*-nitroso-*N*-methyl-*N*-hydroxymethylamine, which decomposes to yield a methylating species and formaldehyde (Druckrey *et al.*, 1967; Magee & Barnes, 1967). This mechanism is consistent with the observation that *N*-nitroso-*N*-methyl-*N*-acetoxymethylamine is hydrolysed to yield an alkylating intermediate (Roller *et al.*, 1975).

Microsome-mediated methylation of both protein and nucleic acid by NDMA has been demonstrated *in vitro* (Chin & Bosmann, 1976; Kim *et al.*, 1977). 7-Methylguanine derived from NDMA-d_6 has three deuterium atoms, indicating that it must be formed *via* a methyldiazonium ion or a methyl carbonium ion rather than from diazomethane (Lijinsky *et al.*, 1968).

NDMA treatment has been reported to induce methylation of cellular protein, including histones (Magee & Hultin, 1962; Turberville & Craddock, 1971).

Studies have been made of the alkylation of cellular nucleic acids after NDMA treatment *in vivo* or in tissue slices *in vitro*. The major product was 7-methylguanine, but a number of minor products have also been identified, including 1-methyl-, 3-methyl- and 7-methyladenine, O^6-methyl- and 3-methylguanine, 3-methylcytosine, 3-methyl- and O^4-methylthymine and methyl phospho esters (Lawley, 1974; Magee *et al.*, 1976; Montesano & Magee, 1974; O'Connor *et al.*, 1972, 1973, 1975; Pegg, 1977; Swann & Magee, 1968). Single s.c. injections of ^{14}C-NDMA into pregnant mice on day 12 of gestation produced no alkylation of DNA bases in embryonic tissues, but when given on day 18 of gestation, methylation of foetal liver and brain DNA bases was found. A similar extent of alkylation was obtained when 18-day-old foetuses were treated directly in the same manner (Bochert, 1975).

Studies have supported the hypothesis of Loveless (1969) that the formation of O^6-methylguanine may be of critical importance in carcinogenesis and mutagenesis, since this product is formed in much smaller amounts by other methylating agents which are less active as carcinogens or mutagens than NDMA (Lawley, 1974; Magee *et al.*, 1976; Pegg, 1977).

Distribution of methylated bases produced by NDMA may not be entirely random within DNA of the chromatin (Cooper *et al.*, 1975; Ramanathan *et al.*, 1976), and it has been demonstrated that hepatic mitochondrial DNA is alkylated more extensively than nuclear DNA (Wilkinson *et al.*, 1975; Wunderlich *et al.*, 1971/1972). Alteration in the velocity sedimentation rate of liver DNA in alkaline sucrose gradient, attributed to single-strand breaks, occurs in the DNA of rats treated with NDMA (Damjanov *et al.*, 1973). Repair of single-stranded regions in hepatic DNA following administration of NDMA, as determined by chromatography on benzoylated DEAE-cellulose, is more rapid than in kidney DNA (Huang & Stewart, 1977; Stewart & Huang, 1977).

Hepatic DNA damaged by alkylation after NDMA treatment is replicated (Rajalakshmi & Sarma, 1975). The persistence of O^6-methylguanine in DNA and the rate of cell division may be important factors in the tissue-specific induction of tumours by NDMA (Margison *et al.*, 1976; Nicoll *et al.*, 1975; Pegg, 1977). O^6-Methylguanine is removed from the DNA of liver and kidney by an enzyme system (Nicoll *et al.*, 1975; Pegg, 1977). There is evidence that NDMA-induced carcinogenic damage to the kidney can also be repaired (Swann *et al.*, 1976). Administration of NDMA induces selective proliferation of tubular epithelium and interstitial cells in rat kidney (Hard, 1975; Stewart & Magee, 1971).

Administration of aminoacetonitrile to rats reduced the metabolism of NDMA, the induction of hepatic DNA damage and the acute toxicity (Fiume *et al.*, 1970; Hadjiolov & Mundt, 1974; Stewart, 1974). Such pretreatment also reduced the production of a mutagenic metabolite from NDMA by rat liver microsomes (Bartsch *et al.*, 1975). Pretreatment of rats with pregnenolone-16α-carbonitrile (PCN) decreased the acute toxicity of NDMA (Somogyi *et al.*, 1972) but did not greatly reduce either conversion of ^{14}C-NDMA to exhaled $^{14}CO_2$ or methylation of nucleic acids (Grandjean & Somogyi, 1976). However, liver microsomes from PCN-pretreated rats showed an increased ability to convert NDMA to an intermediate mutagenic for *Salmonella typhimurium* G-46 (Bartsch *et al.*, 1975). The acute toxicity of NDMA in rats and mice and the *N*-7-methylation of guanine in liver DNA were reduced by simultaneous administration of disulfiram (Schmähl *et al.*, 1971). Microsomes from disulfiram-treated rats showed a decreased ability to convert NDMA into intermediates mutagenic for *S. typhimurium* G-46; mutagenicity was also reduced when disulfiram was added to the assay systems (Montesano & Bartsch, 1976).

Mutagenicity and other short-term tests

The mutagenic effects of NDMA have been reviewed by Montesano & Bartsch (1976). In the presence of a metabolic activation system, genetic activity has been demonstrated in *S. typhimurium* (reverse mutations), *Escherichia coli* (forward and reverse mutations), *Bacillus subtilis* (reverse mutations), *Saccharomyces cerevisiae* (back mutations, gene recombination and conversion), *Serratia marcescens* (reverse mutations) and *Neurospora crassa* (forward mutations) (Montesano & Bartsch, 1976). A mutagenic agent was produced from NDMA in the presence of mouse kidney microsomes, and there was a correlation between the ability to produce mutations in *S. typhimurium* G-46 and susceptibility for kidney tumours in different strains of mice (Weekes, 1975). NDMA was mutagenic in *S. typhimurium* G-46 in the presence of a microsomal fraction from human liver biopsies (Czygan *et al.*, 1973b).

NDMA has been tested in the host-mediated assay using mice or rats. Mutagenicity was shown in *S. typhimurium* strains G-46, C-207 and C-340 after their i.p. injection into Swiss albino mice that had received 3 i.m. injections of 0.1 ml of a 10% NDMA solution at 1-hour intervals (Gabridge & Legator, 1969). Fahrig (1975) observed mutagenicity in *S. cerevisiae* D-4 injected into the peritoneum, the testes or the tail vein of male Wistar rats injected subcutaneously with 740 mg/kg bw NDMA.

NDMA injected subcutaneously into mice at doses of 30 mg/kg bw or 300 mg/kg bw was mutagenic in a blood-mediated assay in which stationary cells of *E. coli* K-12 were injected intravenously (Mohn & Ellenberger, 1973).

NDMA and *N*-nitroso-*N*-methyl-*N*-acetoxymethylamine induced X-linked recessive lethal mutations in *Drosophila* (Fahmy *et al.*, 1975; Pasternak, 1962). *N*-Nitroso-*N*-methyl-*N*-acetoxymethylamine was also mutagenic in *S. typhimurium* TA 1530 and in bacteriophages R17 and T7 (Bartsch *et al.*, 1977; Shooter & Wiessler, 1976).

In the presence of a rat liver microsomal fraction from phenobarbital-treated rats, NDMA induced 8-azaguanine-resistant mutants in Chinese hamster V79 cells (Kuroki *et al.*, 1977). Concentrations from 8-135 mM induced chromosome aberrations and sister chromatid exchanges in Chinese hamster cells in the presence of liver microsomal preparations from rats (Natarajan *et al.*, 1976).

Chromosome aberrations, mainly dicentrics and deletions, were found in liver cells of Chinese hamsters injected intraperitoneally with 5 g/kg bw NDMA (Brooks & Cregger, 1973). In the dominant lethal test in mice, an i.p. dose of 9 mg/kg NDMA was ineffective (Epstein *et al.*, 1972), while 4.4 mg/kg administered subcutaneously produced a significant increase in dead implants (Propping *et al.*, 1972). Cultured lymphocytes taken from rats 6 hours after an i.p. injection of 30 mg/kg bw NDMA showed an increased frequency of chromosome aberrations (Lilly *et al.*, 1975).

Unscheduled DNA synthesis has been observed in isolated rat hepatocytes treated with NDMA (Williams, 1976, 1977) and in human fibroblasts in culture in the presence of NDMA and a mouse liver microsomal fraction (Laishes & Stich, 1973).

Rat liver epithelial-like cells maintained in culture were transformed by treatment with NDMA, and the transformed cells induced tumours at the site of injection in 32/42 newborn rats (Montesano *et al.*, 1973, 1975; Williams *et al.*, 1973). Cells cultured from kidneys of rats treated *in vivo* with a single i.p. dose of 60 mg/kg bw NDMA underwent transformation as determined by various *in vitro* criteria (Borland & Hard, 1974; Stewart & Hard, 1977). These transformed cells were described as morphologically similar to the putative precursors of NDMA-induced mesenchymal neoplasms (Hard & Butler, 1971b; Hard & Borland, 1977).

(b) Humans

In 4 men, laboratory exposure to NDMA gave rise to acute liver necrosis which later developed into cirrhosis; in one case, the acute liver injury proved to be fatal (Barnes & Magee, 1954; Freund, 1937).

Studies *in vitro* suggest that NDMA is metabolized by human liver and lung *via* the same metabolic pathway as in other mammalian species (Harris *et al.*, 1977; Montesano & Magee, 1970).

3.3 Case reports and epidemiological studies

No data were available to the Working Group.

4. Summary of Data Reported and Evaluation

4.1 Experimental data

N-Nitrosodimethylamine is carcinogenic in all animal species tested: mice, rats, Syrian golden, Chinese and European hamsters, guinea-pigs, rabbits, ducks, mastomys, various fish, newts and frogs. It induces benign and malignant tumours following its administration by various routes, including ingestion and inhalation, in various organs in various species. It produces tumours, mainly of the liver, kidney and respiratory tract. It is carcinogenic following its administration prenatally and in single doses. In several studies, dose-response relationships were established.

4.2 Human data

No case reports or epidemiological studies were available to the Working Group. Available information on occurrence suggests that the general population may be exposed to low levels of *N*-nitrosodimethylamine; however, no exposed group suitable for an epidemiological investigation has yet been identified. Reports of relatively high levels in certain pesticide formulations and of occupational exposures that may have occurred in the manufacture and use of rocket fuels may permit the identification of exposed groups.

4.3 Evaluation

There is *sufficient evidence* of a carcinogenic effect of *N*-nitrosodimethylamine in many experimental animal species. Similarities in its metabolism by human and rodent tissues have been demonstrated. Although no epidemiological data were available (and efforts should be directed toward this end), *N*-nitrosodimethylamine should be regarded for practical purposes as if it were carcinogenic to humans.

5. References

Alexandrov, V.A. (1968) Blastomogenic effect of dimethylnitrosamine on pregnant rats and their offspring. Nature (Lond.), 218, 280-281

Alexandrov, V.A. (1974) Embryotoxic and transplacental oncogenic action of symmetrical dialkylnitrosamines on the progeny of rats. Bull. exp. Biol. Med., 78, 1308-1310

Alliston, T.G., Cox, G.B. & Kirk, R.S. (1972) The determination of steam-volatile *N*-nitrosamines in foodstuffs by formation of electron-capturing derivatives from electrochemically derived amines. Analyst, 97, 915-920

Andersen, R.S. (1973) Carcinogenicity of phenols, alkylating agents, urethan, and a cigarette-smoke fraction in *Nicotiana* seedlings. Cancer Res., 33, 2450-2455

Anon. (1975) FMC decides to close NDMA plant in Baltimore. Chem. Marketing Reporter, 22 December, pp. 7-24

Argus, M.F. & Hoch-Ligeti, C. (1961) Comparative study of the carcinogenic activity of nitrosamines. J. nat. Cancer Inst., 27, 695-709

Argus, M.F., Arcos, J.C., Pastor, K.M., Wu, B.C. & Venkatesan, N. (1976) Dimethylnitrosamine-demethylase: absence of increased enzyme catabolism and multiplicity of effector sites in repression. Hemoprotein involvement. Chem.-biol. Interact., 13, 127-140

Armuth, V. & Berenblum, I. (1972) Systemic promoting action of phorbol in liver and lung carcinogenesis in AKR mice. Cancer Res., 32, 2259-2262

Ashley, L.M. & Halver, J.E. (1968) Dimethylnitrosamine-induced hepatic cell carcinoma in rainbow trout. J. nat. Cancer Inst., 41, 531-552

Barnes, J.M. & Magee, P.N. (1954) Some toxic properties of dimethylnitrosamine. Brit. J. industr. Med., 11, 167-174

Bartsch, H., Malaveille, C. & Montesano, R. (1975) Differential effect of phenobarbitone, pregnenolone-16α-carbonitrile and aminoacetonitrile on dialkylnitrosamine metabolism and mutagenicity *in vitro*. Chem.-biol. Interact., 10, 377-382

Bartsch, H., Margison, G.P., Malaveille, C., Camus, A.M., Brun, G. & Margison, J.M. (1977) Some aspects of metabolic activation of chemical carcinogens in relation to their organ specificity. Arch. Toxicol., 39, 51-63

Bochert, G. (1975) Comparative studies on the formation of methylated bases in DNA of adult and fetal mouse tissues by dimethylnitrosamine *in vivo*. In: Neubert, D. & Merker, H.-J., eds, New Approaches to the Evaluation of Abnormal Embryonic Development, Stuttgart, Georg Thieme, pp. 554-572

Borland, R. & Hard, G.C. (1974) Early appearance of 'transformed' cells from the kidneys of rats treated with a 'single' carcinogenic dose of dimethylnitrosamine (DMN) detected by culture *in vitro*. Europ. J. Cancer, 10, 177-184

Bretschneider, K. & Matz, J. (1974) Nitrosamine (NA) in der atmosphärischen und in der Luft am Arbeitsplatz. Arch. Geschwulstforsch., 43, 36-41

Bretschneider, K. & Matz, J. (1976) Occurrence and analysis of nitrosamines in air. In: Walker, E.A., Bogovski, P. & Griciute, L., eds, Environmental *N*-Nitroso Compounds Analysis and Formation, Lyon (IARC Scientific Publications No. 14), pp. 395-399

Brooks, A.L. & Cregger, V. (1973) Production of chromosome type aberrations in the liver cells of the Chinese hamster by dimethylnitrosamine (DMN) (Abstract No. 8). Mutation Res., 21, 214

Brooks, J.B., Cherry, W.B., Thacker, L. & Alley, C.C. (1972) Analysis by gas chromatography of amines and nitrosamines produced *in vivo* and *in vitro* by *Proteus mirabilis*. J. infect. Dis., 126, 143-153

Brunnemann, K.D. & Hoffmann, D. (1978) Chemical studies on tobacco smoke. LIX. Analysis of volatile nitrosamines in tobacco smoke and polluted indoor environments. In: Walker, E.A., Castegnaro, M., Griciute, L. & Lyle, R.E., eds, Environmental Aspects of *N*-Nitroso Compounds, Lyon (IARC Scientific Publications No. 19) (in press)

Brunnemann, K.D., Yu, L. & Hoffmann, D. (1977) Assessment of carcinogenic volatile *N*-nitrosamines in tobacco and in mainstream and sidestream smoke from cigarettes. Cancer Res., 37, 3218-3222

Campbell, J.S., Wiberg, G.S., Grice, H.C. & Lou, P. (1974) Stromal nephromas and renal cell tumors in suckling and weaned rats. Cancer Res., 34, 2399-2404

Cardesa, A., Pour, P., Althoff, J. & Mohr, U. (1973) Vascular tumors in female Swiss mice after intraperitoneal injection of dimethylnitrosamine. J. nat. Cancer Inst., 51, 201-208

Cardesa, A., Pour, P., Althoff, J. & Mohr, U. (1974a) Comparative studies of neoplastic response to a single dose of nitroso compounds. IV. The effect of dimethyl- and diethyl-nitrosamine in Swiss mice. Z. Krebsforsch., 81, 229-233

Cardesa, A., Pour, P., Althoff, J. & Mohr, U. (1974b) Effects of intraperitoneal injections of dimethyl- and diethylnitrosamine, alone or simultaneously on Swiss mice. Z. Krebsforsch., 82, 233-238

Carlton, W.W. & Price, P.S. (1973) Dietary copper and the induction of neoplasms in the rat by acetylaminofluorene and dimethylnitrosamine. Fd Cosmet. Toxicol., 11, 827-840

Chin, A.E. & Bosmann, H.B. (1976) Microsome-mediated methylation of DNA by *N,N*-dimethylnitrosamine *in vitro*. Biochem. Pharmacol., 25, 1921-1926

Clapp, N.K. (1973) Carcinogenicity of nitrosamines and methanesulphonate esters given intraperitoneally, in RF mice. Int. J. Cancer, 12, 728-733

Clapp, N.K. & Toya, R.E., Sr (1970) Effect of cumulative dose and dose rate on dimethylnitrosamine oncogenesis in RF mice. J. nat. Cancer Inst., 45, 495-498

Clapp, N.K., Craig, A.W. & Toya, R.E., Sr (1968) Pulmonary and hepatic oncogenesis during treatment of male RF mice with dimethylnitrosamine. J. nat. Cancer Inst., 41, 1213-1227

Clapp, N.K., Tyndall, R.L. & Otten, J.A. (1971) Differences in tumor types and organ susceptibility in BALB/c and RF mice following dimethylnitrosamine and diethylnitrosamine. Cancer Res., 31, 196-198

Cohen, J.B. & Bachman, J.D. (1978) Measurement of environmental nitrosamines. In: Walker, E.A., Castegnaro, M., Griciute, L. & Lyle, R.E., eds, Environmental Aspects of *N*-Nitroso Compounds, Lyon (IARC Scientific Publications No. 19) (in press)

Cohen, S.Z., Bontoyan, W.R. & Zweig, G. (1978) Analytical determination of *N*-nitroso compounds in pesticides by the United States Environmental Protection Agency. In: Walker, E.A., Castegnaro, M., Griciute, L. & Lyle, R.E., eds, Environmental Aspects of *N*-Nitroso Compounds, Lyon (IARC Scientific Publications No. 19) (in press)

Cooper, H.K., Margison, G.P., O'Connor, P.J. & Itzhaki, R.F. (1975) Heterogeneous distribution of DNA alkylation products in rat liver chromatin after *in vivo* administration of *N,N*-di[^{14}C]methylnitrosamine. Chem.-biol. Interact., 11, 483-492

Craddock, V.M. (1971) Liver carcinomas induced in rats by single administration of dimethylnitrosamine after partial hepatectomy. J. nat. Cancer Inst., 47, 889-907

Craddock, V.M. (1973) Induction of liver tumours in rats by a single treatment with nitroso compounds given after partial hepatectomy. Nature (Lond.), 245, 386-388

Craddock, V.M. (1975) Effect of a single treatment with the alkylating carcinogens dimethylnitrosamine, diethylnitrosamine and methyl methanesulphonate, on liver regenerating after partial hepatectomy. I. Test for induction of liver carcinomas. Chem.-biol. Interact., 10, 313-321

Crosby, N.T., Foreman, J.K., Palframan, J.F. & Sawyer, R. (1972) Estimation of steam-volatile *N*-nitrosamines in foods at the 1 μg/kg level. Nature (Lond.), 238, 342-343

Czygan, P., Greim, H., Garro, A.J., Hutterer, F., Schaffner, F., Popper, H., Rosenthal, O. & Cooper, D.Y. (1973a) Microsomal metabolism of dimethylnitrosamine and the cytochrome P-450 dependency of its activation to a mutagen. Cancer Res., 33, 2983-2986

Czygan, P., Greim, H., Garro, A.J., Hutterer, F., Rudick, J., Schaffner, F. & Popper, H. (1973b) Cytochrome P-450 content and the ability of liver microsomes from patients undergoing abdominal surgery to alter the mutagenicity of a primary and a secondary carcinogen. J. nat. Cancer Inst., 51, 1761-1764

Damjanov, I., Cox, R., Sarma, D.S.R. & Farber, E. (1973) Patterns of damage and repair of liver DNA induced by carcinogenic methylating agents *in vivo*. Cancer Res., 33, 2122-2128

Den Engelse, L., Bentvelzen, P.A.J. & Emmelot, P. (1969/70) Studies on lung tumours. I. Methylation of deoxyribonucleic acid and tumour formation following administration of dimethylnitrosamine to mice. Chem.-biol. Interact., 1, 394-406

Den Engelse, L., Hollander, C.F. & Misdorp, W. (1974) A sex-dependent difference in the type of tumours induced by dimethylnitrosamine in the livers of C3Hf mice. Europ. J. Cancer, 10, 129-135

Den Engelse, L., Gebbink, M. & Emmelot, P. (1975) Studies on lung tumours. III. Oxidative metabolism of dimethylnitrosamine by rodent and human lung tissue. Chem.-biol. Interact., 11, 535-544

Diaz Gomez, M.I., Swann, P.F. & Magee, P.N. (1977) The absorption and metabolism in rats of small oral doses of dimethylnitrosamine. Biochem. J., 164, 497-500

Druckrey, H., Preussmann, R., Ivankovic, S. & Schmähl, D. (1967) Organotrope carcinogene Wirkungen bei 65 verschiedenen *N*-Nitroso-Verbindungen an BD-ratten. Z. Krebsforsch., 69, 103-201

Du Plessis, L.S., Nunn, J.R. & Roach, W.A. (1969) Carcinogen in a Transkeian Bantu food additive. Nature (Lond.), 222, 1198-1199

Eisenbrand, G. & Preussmann, R. (1970) Eine neue Methode zur kolorimetrischen Bestimmung von Nitrosaminen nach Spaltung der *N*-Nitrosogruppe mit Bromwasserstoff in Eisessig. Arzneimittel-Forsch., 20, 1513-1517

Eisenbrand, G., Hodenberg, A. von & Preussmann, R. (1970) Trace analysis of *N*-nitroso compounds. II. Steam distillation at neutral, alkaline and acid pH under reduced and atmospheric pressure. Z. analyt. Chem., 251, 22-24

Eisenbrand, G., Rappardt, E. von, Zappe, R. & Preussmann, R. (1976) Trace analysis of volatile nitrosamines by a modified nitrogen-specific detector in pyrolytic mode and by ion-specific determination of heptafluorobutyramides in a gas chromatography-mass spectrometry system. In: Walker, E.A., Bogovski, P. & Griciute, L., eds, Environmental *N*-Nitroso Compounds Analysis and Formation, Lyon (IARC Scientific Publications No. 14), pp. 65-75

Eisenbrand, G., Janzowski, C. & Preussmann, R. (1977) Analysis, formation and occurrence of volatile and non-volatile *N*-nitroso compounds: recent results. In: Tinbergen, B.J. & Krol, B., eds, Proceedings of the Second International Symposium on Nitrite in Meat Products, Zeist, 1976, Wageningen, Centre for Agricultural Publishing and Documentation, pp. 155-169

Eisenbrand, G., Spiegelhalder, B., Janzowski, C., Kann, J. & Preussmann, R. (1978) Volatile and non-volatile *N*-nitroso compounds in foods and other environmental media. In: Walker, E.A., Castegnaro, M., Griciute, L. & Lyle, R.E., eds, Environmental Aspects of *N*-Nitroso Compounds, Lyon (IARC Scientific Publications No. 19) (in press)

Ender, F., Havre, G., Helgebostad, A., Koppang, N., Madsen, R., Ceh, L. & Björnson, O. (1964) Isolation and identification of a hepatotoxic factor in herring meal produced from sodium nitrite preserved herring. Naturwissenschaften, 51, 637-638

Epstein, S.S., Arnold, E., Andrea, J., Bass, W. & Bishop, Y. (1972) Detection of chemical mutagens by the dominant lethal assay in the mouse. Toxicol. appl. Pharmacol., 23, 288-325

Fahmy, O.G., Fahmy, M.J. & Wiessler, M. (1975) α-Acetoxy-dimethylnitrosamine: a proximate metabolite of the carcinogenic amine. Biochem. Pharmacol., 24, 1145-1148

Fahrig, R. (1975) Development of host-mediated mutagenicity tests - yeast systems. II. Recovery of yeast cells out of testes, liver, lung, and peritoneum of rats. Mutation Res., 31, 381-394

Fazio, T., Damico, J.N., Howard, J.W., White, R.H. & Watts, J.O. (1971a) Gas chromatographic determination and mass spectrometric confirmation of *N*-nitrosodimethylamine in smoke-processed marine fish. J. agric. Fd Chem., 19, 250-253

Fazio, T., White, R.H. & Howard, J.W. (1971b) Analysis of nitrite- and/or nitrate-processed meats for *N*-nitrosodimethylamine. J. Ass. off analyt. Chem., 54, 1157-1159

Fiddler, W., Feinberg, J.I., Pensabene, J.W., Williams, A.C. & Dooley, C.J. (1975) Dimethylnitrosamine in souse and similar jellied cured-meat products. Fd Cosmet. Toxicol., 13, 653-654

Fiddler, W., Pensabene, J.W., Doerr, R.C. & Dooley, C.J. (1977) The presence of dimethyl- and diethylnitrosamines in deionized water. Fd Cosmet. Toxicol., 15, 441-443

Fine, D.H. (1977) Human exposure to preformed nitrosamine compounds. In: Spengler, J.D., ed., Toxic Substances in the Air Environment, Pittsburgh, Air Pollution Control Association, pp. 168-181

Fine, D.H. (1978) An assessment of human exposure to *N*-nitroso compounds. In: Walker, E.A., Castegnaro, M., Griciute, L. & Lyle, R.E., eds, Environmental Aspects of *N*-Nitroso Compounds, Lyon (IARC Scientific Publications No. 19) (in press)

Fine D.H. & Rounbehler, D.P. (1976) *N*-Nitroso compounds in water. In: Keith, L.H., ed., Identification and Analysis of Organic Pollutants in Water, Ann Arbor, Michigan, Ann Arbor Science Press, pp. 255-264

Fine, D.H., Rounbehler, D.P., Belcher, N.M. & Epstein, S.S. (1976a) *N*-Nitroso compounds: detection in ambient air. Science, 192, 1328-1330

Fine, D.H., Rounbehler, D.P., Sawicki, E., Krost, K. & DeMarrais, G.A. (1976b) *N*-Nitroso compounds in the ambient community air of Baltimore, Maryland. Analyt. Lett., 9, 595-604

Fine, D.H., Rounbehler, D.P., Pellizzari, E.D., Bunch, J.E., Berkley, R.W., McCrae, J., Bursey, J.T., Sawicki, E., Krost, K. & DeMarrais, G.A. (1976c) *N*-Nitrosodimethylamine in air. Bull. environm. Contam. Toxicol., 15, 739-746

Fine, D.H., Rounbehler, D.P., Rounbehler, A., Silvergleid, A., Sawicki, E., Krost, K. & DeMarrais, G.A. (1977a) Determination of dimethylnitrosamine in air, water, and soil by thermal energy analysis: measurements in Baltimore, Md. Environm. Sci. Technol., 11, 581-584

Fine, D.H., Rounbehler, D.P., Fan, T. & Ross, R. (1977b) Human exposure to *N*-nitroso compounds in the environment. In: Hiatt, H.H., Watson, J.D. & Winsten, J.A., eds, Origins of Human Cancer, Book A, Cold Spring Harbor, N.Y., Cold Spring Harbor Laboratory, pp. 293-307

Fine, D.H., Ross, R., Rounbehler, D.P., Silvergleid, A. & Song, L. (1977c) Formation *in vivo* of volatile *N*-nitrosamines in man after ingestion of cooked bacon and spinach. Nature (Lond.), 265, 753-755

Fine, D.H., Ross, R., Fan, S., Rounbehler, D.P., Silvergleid, A., Song, L. & Morrison, J. (1978) Determination of *N*-nitroso pesticides in air, water and soil. In: Proceedings of the 172nd American Chemical Society National Meeting, San Francisco, 1976, Waltham, Mass., Thermo Electron Research Center (in press)

Fiume, L., Campadelli-Fiume, G., Magee, P.N. & Holsman, J. (1970) Cellular injury and carcinogenesis. Inhibition of metabolism of dimethylnitrosamine by aminoacetonitrile. Biochem. J., 120, 601-605

Fong, Y.Y. & Chan, W.C. (1973) Dimethylnitrosamine in Chinese marine salt fish. Fd Cosmet. Toxicol., 11, 841-845

Fong, Y.Y. & Chan, W.C. (1977) Nitrate, nitrite, dimethylnitrosamine and *N*-nitrosopyrrolidine in some Chinese food products. Fd Cosmet. Toxicol., 15, 143-145

Frei, J.V. (1970) Toxicity, tissue changes, and tumor induction in inbred Swiss mice by methylnitrosamine and -amide compounds. Cancer Res., 30, 11-17

Freund, H.A. (1937) Clinical manifestations and studies in parenchymatous hepatitis. Ann. int. Med., 10, 1144-1155

Fridman, A.L., Mukhametshin, F.M. & Novikov, S.S. (1971) Advances in the chemistry of aliphatic *N*-nitrosamines. Russ. chem. Rev., 40, 34-50

Fujii, K. & Sato, H. (1970) Response of adult mastomys (*Praomys natalensis*) to subcutaneous injection of *N*-nitrosodimethylamine. Gann, 61, 425-434

Gabridge, M.G. & Legator, M.S. (1969) A host-mediated microbial assay for the detection of mutagenic compounds. Proc. Soc. exp. Biol. (N.Y.), 130, 831-834

Gadbois, D.F., Ravesi, E.m. & Lundstrom, R.C. (1976) Occurrence of volatile *N*-nitrosamines in Japanese salmon roe. Fishery Bulletin, 74, 683-686

Geil, J.H., Stenger, R.J., Behki, R.M. & Morgan, W.S. (1968) Hepatotoxic and carcinogenic effects of dimethylnitrosamine in low dosage. Light and electron microscopic study. J. nat. Cancer Inst., 40, 713-730

Getz, J.W. (1960) Nitrosamines from secondary amines. US Patent 2,960,536, 15 November (to Food Machinery and Chemical Corp.) [Chem. Abstr., 55, 10317b]

Gough, T.A. (1978) An examination of some foodstuff for trace amounts of volatile nitrosamines using the thermal energy analyser. In: Walker, E.A., Castegnaro, M., Griciute, L. & Lyle, R.E., eds, Environmental Aspects of *N*-Nitroso Compounds, Lyon (IARC Scientific Publications No. 19) (in press)

Gough, T.A. & Walters, C.L. (1976) Volatile nitrosamines in fried bacon. In: Walker, E.A., Bogovski, P. & Griciute, L., eds, Environmental *N*-Nitroso Compounds Analysis and Formation, Lyon (IARC Scientific Publications No. 14), pp. 195-203

Gough, T.A., Goodhead, K. & Walters, C.L. (1976) Distribution of some volatile nitrosamines in cooked bacon. J. Sci. Fd Agric., 27, 181-185

Gough, T.A., McPhail, M.F., Webb, K.S., Wood, B.J. & Coleman, R.F. (1977) An examination of some foodstuffs for the presence of volatile nitrosamines. J. Sci. Fd Agric., 28, 345-351

Grandjean, C.J. & Somogyi, A. (1976) Effect of pregnenolone-16α-carbonitrile on the metabolism of dimethylnitrosamine and binding to rat liver macromolecules. Biochem. Pharmacol., 25, 2097-2098

Groenen, P.J., Jonk, R.J.G., van Ingen, C. & ten Noever de Brauw, M.C. (1976) Determination of eight volatile nitrosamines in thirty cured meat products with capillary gas chromatography-high-resolution mass spectrometry: the presence of nitrosodiethylamine and the absence of nitrosopyrrolidine. In: Walker, E.A., Bogovski, P. & Griciute, L., eds, Environmental *N*-Nitroso Compounds Analysis and Formation, Lyon (IARC Scientific Publications No. 14), pp. 321-331

Groenen, P.J., de Cock-Bethbeder, M.W., Jonk, R.J.G. & van Ingen, C. (1977) Further studies on the occurrence of volatile *N*-nitrosamines in meat products by combined gas chromatography and mass spectrometry. In: Tinbergen, B.J. & Krol, B., eds, Proceedings of the 2nd International Symposium on Nitrite in Meat Products, Zeist, 1976, Wageningen, Centre for Agricultural Publishing and Documentation, pp. 227-237

Haas, H., Mohr, U. & Krüger, F.W. (1973) Comparative studies with different doses of *N*-nitrosomorpholine, *N*-nitrosopiperidine, *N*-nitrosomethylurea, and dimethylnitrosamine in Syrian golden hamsters. J. nat. Cancer Inst., 51, 1295-1301

Haas, H., Hilfrich, J. & Mohr, U. (1974) Induction of heart tumours in Wistar rats after a single application of ethylmethanesulphonate and dimethylnitrosamine. Z. Krebsforsch., 81, 225-228

Hadjiolov, D. (1971) The inhibition of dimethylnitrosamine carcinogenesis in rat liver by aminoacetonitrile. Z. Krebsforsch., 76, 91-92

Hadjiolov, D. & Markow, D. (1973) Fine structure of hemangioendothelial sarcomas in the rat liver induced with *N*-nitrosodimethylamine. Arch. Geschwulstforsch., 42, 120-126

Hadjiolov, D. & Mundt, D. (1974) Effect of aminoacetonitrile on the metabolism of dimethylnitrosamine and methylation of RNA during liver carcinogenesis. J. nat. Cancer Inst., 52, 753-756

Hard, G.C. (1975) Autoradiographic analysis of proliferative activity in rat kidney epithelial and mesenchymal cell subpopulations following a carcinogenic dose of dimethylnitrosamine. Cancer Res., 35, 3762-3773

Hard, G.C. & Borland, R. (1977) Morphologic character of transforming renal cell cultures derived from Wistar rats given dimethylnitrosamine. J. nat. Cancer Inst., 58, 1377-1382

Hard, G.C. & Butler, W.H. (1971a) Morphogenesis of epithelial neoplasms induced in the rat kidney by dimethylnitrosamine. Cancer Res., 31, 1496-1505

Hard, G.C. & Butler, W.H. (1971b) Ultrastructural study of the development of interstitial lesions leading to mesenchymal neoplasia induced in the rat renal cortex by dimethylnitrosamine. Cancer Res., 31, 337-347

Hard, G.C., King, H., Borland, R., Stewart, B.W. & Dobrostanski, B. (1977) Length of *in vivo* exposure to a carcinogenic dose of dimethylnitrosamine necessary for subsequent expression of morphological transformation by rat kidney cells *in vitro*. Oncology, 34, 16-19

Harington, J.S., Nunn, J.R. & Irwig, L. (1973) Dimethylnitrosamine in the human vaginal vault. Nature (Lond.), 241, 49-50

Harris, C.C., Autrup, H., Stoner, G.D., McDowell, E.M., Trump, B.F. & Schafer, P. (1977) Metabolism of dimethylnitrosamine and 1,2-dimethylhydrazine in cultured human bronchi. Cancer Res., 37, 2309-2311

Hashimoto, S., Yokokura, T., Kawai, Y. & Mutai, M. (1976) Dimethylnitrosamine formation in the gastrointestinal tract of rats. Fd Cosmet. Toxicol., 14, 553-556

Havery, D.C. & Fazio, T. (1977) Survey of finfish and shellfish for volatile *N*-nitrosamines. J. Ass. off. analyt. Chem., 60, 517-519

Havery, D.C., Kline, D.A., Miletta, E.M., Joe, F.L., Jr & Fazio, T. (1976) Survey of food products for volatile *N*-nitrosamines. J. Ass. off. analyt. Chem., 59, 540-546

Havery, D.C., Fazio, T. & Howard, J.W. (1978) Survey of cured meat products for volatile *N*-nitrosamines: comparison of two analytical methods. In: Walker, E.A., Castegnaro, M., Griciute, L. & Lyle, R.E., eds, Environmental Aspects of *N*-Nitroso Compounds, Lyon (IARC Scientific Publications No. 19) (in press)

Heading, C.E., Phillips, J.C., Lake, B.G., Gangolli, S.D. & Lloyd, A.G. (1974) Some aspects of the metabolism of dimethylnitrosamine in the rat. Biochem. Soc. Trans., 2, 607-610

Heath, D.F. (1962) The decomposition and toxicity of dialkylnitrosamines in rats. Biochem. J., 85, 72-91

Hedler, L., Marquardt, P. & Schurr, C. (1976) The relation between the determinable quantities of volatile *N*-nitroso compounds and the peroxide number in soya bean oil. In: Walker, E.A., Bogovski, P. & Griciute, L., eds, Environmental *N*-Nitroso Compounds Analysis and Formation, Lyon (IARC Scientific Publications No. 14), pp. 361-374

Herrold, K.M. (1967) Histogenesis of malignant liver tumors induced by dimethylnitrosamine. An experimental study in Syrian hamsters. J. nat. Cancer Inst., 39, 1099-1111

Hicks, R.M., Gough, T.A. & Walters, C.L. (1978) Demonstration of the presence of nitrosamines in human urine. Preliminary observations on a possible aetiology for bladder cancer in association with chronic urinary tract infection. In: Walker, E.A., Castegnaro, M., Griciute, L. & Lyle, R.E., eds, Environmental Aspects of *N*-Nitroso Compounds, Lyon (IARC Scientific Publications No. 19) (in press)

Hilfrich, J., Haas, H., Kmoch, N., Montesano, R., Mohr, U. & Magee, P.N. (1975) The modification of the renal carcinogenicity of dimethylnitrosamine by actinomycin D and a protein deficient diet. Brit. J. Cancer, 32, 578-587

Hoch-Ligeti, C., Argus, M.F. & Arcos, J.C. (1968) Combined carcinogenic effects of dimethylnitrosamine and 3-methylcholanthrene in the rat. J. nat. Cancer Inst., 40, 535-549

Homburger, F., Handler, A.H., Soto, E., Hsueh, S.-S., Van Dongen, C.G. & Russfield, A.B. (1976) Adenocarcinoma of the glandular stomach following 3-methylcholanthrene, *N*-nitrosodiethylamine, or *N*-nitrosodimethylamine feeding in carcinogen-susceptible inbred Syrian hamsters. J. nat. Cancer Inst., 57, 141-144

Huang, D.P., Gough, T.A., Webb, K.S. & Ho, J.H.C. (1978a) Volatile nitrosamines in some traditional Southern Chinese food products. J. Fd Safety, 1 (in press)

Huang, D.P., Gough, T.A. & Ho, J.H.C. (1978b) Analysis for volatile nitrosamines of salt-preserved foodstuffs traditionally consumed by Southern Chinese. In: Blaudin de-Thé, G. & Ito, Y., eds, Nasopharyngeal Carcinoma: Etiology and Control, Lyon (IARC Scientific Publications No. 20) (in press)

Huang, P.H.T. & Stewart, B.W. (1977) Differences in patterns of structural change by rat liver DNA following administration of dimethylnitrosamine and methyl methanesulfonate. Cancer Res., 37, 3796-3801

Hurst, R.E. (1976) Dimethylnitrosamine levels in untreated herring meals. J. Sci. Fd Agric., 27, 600-602

IARC (1972) IARC Monographs on the Evaluation of Carcinogenic Risk of Chemicals to Man, 1, Lyon, pp. 95-106

IARC (1974) IARC Monographs on the Evaluation of Carcinogenic Risk of Chemicals to Man, 4, Some Aromatic Amines, Hydrazine and Related Substances, *N*-Nitroso Compounds and Miscellaneous Alkylating Agents, Lyon, pp. 137-143

IARC (1975) Annual Report 1975, Lyon, International Agency for Research on Cancer, p. 120

IARC (1976) Annual Report 1976, Lyon, International Agency for Research on Cancer, p. 53

IARC (1977a) Annual Report 1977, Lyon, International Agency for Research on Cancer, p. 63

IARC (1977b) Annual Report 1977, Lyon, International Agency for Research on Cancer, p. 57

IARC (1977c) Annual Report 1977, Lyon, International Agency for Research on Cancer, p. 64

Ii, Y., Cardesa, A., Patil, K., Althoff, J. & Pour, P. (1976) Comparative studies of neoplastic response to a single dose of nitroso compounds. Z. Krebsforsch., 86, 165-170

Ingram, A.J. (1972) The lethal and hepatocarcinogenic effects of dimethylnitrosamine injection in the newt *Triturus helveticus*. Brit. J. Cancer, 26, 206-215

Ireton, H.J.C., McGiven, A.R. & Davies, D.J. (1972) Renal mesenchymal tumours induced in rats by dimethylnitrosamine: light- and electron-microscope studies. J. Path., 108, 181-185

Issenberg, P. & Sornson, H. (1976) A monitoring method for volatile nitrosamine levels in laboratory atmospheres. In: Walker, E.A., Bogovski, P. & Griciute, L., eds, Environmental *N*-Nitroso Compounds Analysis and Formation, Lyon (IARC Scientific Publications No. 14), pp. 97-108

Ito, N. (1973) Experimental studies on tumors of the urinary system of rats induced by chemical carcinogens. Acta path. jap., 23, 87-109

Ito, N., Hiasa, Y., Kamamoto, Y., Makiura, S., Sugihara, S., Marugami, M. & Okajima, E. (1971) Histopathological analysis of kidney tumors in rats induced by chemical carcinogens. Gann, 62, 435-4444

Ito, N., Sugihara, S., Makiura, S., Arai, M., Hirao, K., Denda, A. & Nishio, O. (1974) Effect of *N*-(3,5-dichlorophenyl)succinimide on the histological pattern and incidence of kidney tumors in rats induced by dimethylnitrosoamine. Gann, 65, 131-138

Iyengar, J.R., Panalaks, T., Miles, W.F. & Sen, N.P. (1976) A survey of fish products for volatile *N*-nitrosamines. J. Sci. Fd Agric., 27, 527-530

Jasmin, G. & Cha, J.W. (1969) Renal adenomas induced in rats by dimethylnitrosamine. An electron microscopic study. Arch. Path., 87, 267-278

Jasmin, G. & Riopelle, J.L. (1968) Renal adenomas induced by dimethylnitrosamine. Enzyme histochemistry in the rat. Arch. Path., 85, 298-305

Jasmin, G. & Riopelle, J.L. (1969) Transplantation de trois tumeurs rénales induites chez le rat par la diméthylnitrosamine. Int. J. Cancer, 4, 299-311

Johnson, D.E. & Rhoades, J.W. (1972) *N*-Nitrosamines in smoke condensate from several varieties of tobacco. J. nat. Cancer Inst., 48, 1845-1847

Joint Iran-International Agency for Research on Cancer Study Group (1977) Esophageal cancer studies in the Caspian littoral of Iran: results of population studies - a prodrome. J. nat. Cancer Inst., 59, 1127-1138

Joshi, S.R., Rice, J.M., Wenk, M.L., Roller, P.P. & Keefer, L.K. (1977) Selective induction of intestinal tumors in rats by methyl(acetoxymethyl)nitrosamine, an ester of the presumed reactive metabolite of dimethylnitrosamine. J. nat. Cancer Inst., 58, 1531-1535

Juszkiewicz, T. & Kowalski, B. (1974) Passage of nitrosamines from rumen into milk in goats. In: Bogovski, P. & Walker, E.A., eds, *N*-Nitroso Compounds in the Environment, Lyon (IARC Scientific Publications No. 9), pp. 173-176

Juszkiewicz, T. & Kowalski, B. (1976) An investigation of the possible presence or formation of nitrosamines in animal feeds. In: Walker, E.A., Bogovski, P. & Griciute, L., eds, Environmental *N*-Nitroso Compounds Analysis and Formation, Lyon (IARC Scientific Publications No. 14), pp. 375-383

Kann, J., Tauts, O., Raja, K. & Kalve, R. (1976) Nitrosamines and their precursors in some Estonian foodstuffs. In: Walker, E.A., Bogovski, P. & Griciute, L., eds, Environmental *N*-Nitroso Compounds Analysis and Formation, Lyon (IARC Scientific Publications No. 14), pp. 385-394

Kann, J., Spiegelhalder, B., Eisenbrand, G. & Preussmann, R. (1978) Occurrence of volatile *N*-nitrosamines in animal diets. Z. Krebsforsch. (in press)

Keefer, L.K., Lijinsky, W. & Garcia, H. (1973) Deuterium isotope effect on the carcinogenicity of dimethylnitrosamine in rat liver. J. nat. Cancer Inst., 51, 299-302

Khudoley, V.V. (1973) Morphological changes in the liver of fish (*Lebistes reticulatus*) under the action of diethyl- and dimethylnitrosamines. Vop. Onkol., 19, 88-94

Khudoley, V.V. (1977) The induction of tumors in *Rana temporaria* with nitrosamines. Neoplasma, 24, 249-251

Kim, S., Lotlikar, P.D., Chin, W. & Magee, P. (1977) Protein bound carboxylmethyl ester as a precursor of methanol formation during oxidation of dimethylnitrosamine *in vitro* (Abstract No. 189). Proc. Amer. Ass. Cancer Res., 18, 48

Klimsch, H.-J., Stadler, L. & Brahm, S. (1976) Quantitative Bestimmung flüchtiger Nitrosamine in Zigarettenrauchkondensat. Z. Lebensmittel-Untersuch., 162, 131-138

Kowalewski, K. & Todd, E.F. (1971) Carcinoma of the gallbladder induced in hamsters by insertion of cholesterol pellets and feeding dimethyl-nitrosamine. Proc. Soc. exp. Biol. (N.Y.), 136, 482-486

Kuroki, T., Drevon, C. & Montesano, R. (1977) Microsome-mediated mutagenesis in V79 Chinese hamster cells by various nitrosamines. Cancer Res., 37, 1044-1050

Kuwahara, A., Otsuka, H. & Nagamatsu, A. (1972) Induction of hemangiomatous lesions with dimethylnitrosoamine: influence of route of administration and strain of mice. Gann, 63, 499-502

Laishes, B.A. & Stich, H.F. (1973) Repair synthesis and sedimentation analysis of DNA of human cells exposed to dimethylnitrosamine and activated dimethylnitrosamine. Biochem. biophys. Res. Commun., 52, 827-833

Lake, B.G., Phillips, J.C., Heading, C.E. & Gangolli, S.D. (1976) Studies on the *in vitro* metabolism of dimethylnitrosamine by rat liver. Toxicology, 5, 297-309

Lakritz, L., Wasserman, A.E., Gates, R. & Spinelli, A.M. (1978) Preliminary observations on amines and nitrosamines in non-normal human gastric contents. In: Walker, E.A., Castegnaro, M., Griciute, L. & Lyle, R.E., eds, Environmental Aspects of *N*-Nitroso Compounds, Lyon (IARC Scientific Publications No. 19) (in press)

Lawley, P.D. (1974) Some chemical aspects of dose-response relationships in alkylation mutagenesis. Mutation Res., 23, 283-295

Le Page, R.N. & Christie, G.S. (1969a) Induction of liver tumours in the guinea pig by feeding dimethylnitrosamine. Pathology, 1, 49-56

Le Page, R.N. & Christie, G.S. (1969b) Induction of liver tumours in the rabbit by feeding dimethylnitrosamine. Brit. J. Cancer, 23, 125-131

Lijinsky, W. & Greenblatt, M. (1972) Carcinogen dimethylnitrosamine produced *in vivo* from nitrite and aminopyrine. Nature New Biol., 236, 177-178

Lijinsky, W., Loo, J. & Ross, A.E. (1968) Mechanism of alkylation of nucleic acids by nitrosodimethylamine. Nature (Lond.), 218, 1174-1175

Lilly, L.J., Bahner, B. & Magee, P.N. (1975) Chromosome aberrations induced in rat lymphocytes by *N*-nitroso compounds as a possible basis for carcinogen screening. Nature (Lond.), 258, 611-612

Lotlikar, P.D., Baldy, W.J., Jr & Dwyer, E.N. (1975) Dimethylnitrosamine demethylation by reconstituted liver microsomal cytochrome P-450 enzyme system. Biochem. J., 152, 705-708

Love, L.A., Pelfrene, A. & Garcia, H. (1977) Effect of intestinal microflora suppression on liver carcinogenicity of dimethylnitrosamine in Syrian hamsters. J. nat. Cancer Inst., 58, 1835-1836

Loveless, A. (1969) Possible relevance of *O*-6 alkylation of deoxyguanosine to the mutagenicity and carcinogenicity of nitrosamines and nitrosamides. Nature (Lond.), 223, 206-207

Magee, P.N. & Barnes, J.M. (1956) The production of malignant primary hepatic tumours in the rat by feeding dimethylnitrosamine. Brit. J. Cancer, 10, 114-122

Magee, P.N. & Barnes, J.M. (1959) The experimental production of tumours in the rat by dimethylnitrosamine (*N*-nitroso dimethylamine). Acta un. int. cancr., 15, 187-190

Magee, P.N. & Barnes, J.M. (1962) Induction of kidney tumours in the rat with dimethylnitrosamine (*N*-nitrosodimethylamine). J. Path. Bact., 84, 19-31

Magee, P.N. & Barnes, J.M. (1967) Carcinogenic nitroso compounds. Adv. Cancer Res., 10, 163-246

Magee, P.N. & Hultin, T. (1962) Toxic liver injury and carcinogenesis. Methylation of proteins of rat-liver slices by dimethylnitrosamine *in vitro*. Biochem. J., 83, 106-114

Magee, P.N. & Swann, P.F. (1969) Nitroso compounds. Brit. med. Bull., 25, 240-244

Magee, P.N., Montesano, R. & Preussmann, R. (1976) *N*-Nitroso compounds and related carcinogens. In: Searle, C.E., ed., Chemical Carcinogens (ACS Monograph 173), Washington DC, American Chemical Society, pp. 491-625

Margison, G.P., Margison, J.M. & Montesano, R. (1976) Methylated purines in the deoxyribonucleic acid of various Syrian-golden-hamster tissues after administration of a hepatocarcinogenic dose of dimethylnitrosamine. Biochem. J., 157, 627-634

McCormick, A., Nicholson, M.J., Baylis, M.A. & Underwood, J.G. (1973) Nitrosamines in cigarette smoke condensate. Nature (Lond.), 244, 237-238

McCracken, M.D., Bottoms, G.D. & Carlton, W.W. (1973) Tumorigenesis of dimethylnitrosamine in the Pekin duck (Abstract No. 23). Toxicol. appl. Pharmacol., 25, 447-448

McGiven, A.R. & Ireton, H.J.C. (1972) Renal epithelial dysplasia and neoplasia in rats given dimethylnitrosamine. J. Path., 108, 187-190

McLean, A.E.M. & Magee, P.N. (1970) Increased renal carcinogenesis by dimethyl nitrosamine in protein deficient rats. Brit. J. exp. Path., 51, 587-590

Mirna, A., Harada, K., Rapp, U. & Kaufmann, H. (1976) *N*-Nitrosamine in Futtermitteln. Fleischwirtschaft, 56, 1014

Mizrahi, I.J. & Emmelot, P. (1962) The effect of cysteine on the metabolic changes produced by two carcinogenic *N*-nitrosodialkylamines in rat liver. Cancer Res., 22, 339-351

Mohn, G. & Ellenberger, J. (1973) Mammalian blood-mediated mutagenicity tests using a multipurpose strain of *Escherichia coli* K-12. Mutation Res., 19, 257-260

Mohr, U., Haas, H. & Hilfrich, J. (1974) The carcinogenic effects of dimethylnitrosamine and nitrosomethylurea in European hamsters (*Cricetus cricetus* L.). Brit. J. Cancer, 29, 359-364

Moiseev, G.E. & Benemansky, V.V. (1975) On carcinogenic activity of low concentrates of nitrosodimethylamine in inhalation. Vop. Onkol., 21, 107-109

Montesano, R. & Bartsch, H. (1976) Mutagenic and carcinogenic *N*-nitroso compounds: possible environmental hazards. Mutation Res., 32, 179-228

Montesano, R. & Magee, P.N. (1970) Metabolism of dimethylnitrosamine by human liver slices *in vitro*. Nature (Lond.), 228, 173-174

Montesano, R. & Magee, P.N. (1974) Comparative metabolism *in vitro* of nitrosamines in various animal species including man. In: Montesano, R. & Tomatis, L., eds, Chemical Carcinogenesis Essays, Lyon (IARC Scientific Publications No. 10), pp. 39-56

Montesano, R., Saint Vincent, L. & Tomatis, L. (1973) Malignant transformation *in vitro* of rat liver cells by dimethylnitrosamine and *N*-methyl-*N*'-nitro-*N*-nitrosoguanidine. Brit. J. Cancer, 28, 215-220

Montesano, R., Mohr, U., Magee, P.N., Hilfrich, H. & Haas, H. (1974) Additive effect in the induction of kidney tumours in rats treated with dimethylnitrosamine and ethylmethanesulphonate. Brit. J. Cancer, 29, 50-58

Montesano, R., Saint Vincent, L., Drevon, C. & Tomatis, L. (1975) Production of epithelial and mesenchymal tumours with rat liver cells transformed *in vitro*. Int. J. Cancer, 16, 550-558

Murphy, G.P., Mirand, E.A., Johnston, G.S., Schmidt, J.D. & Scott, W.W. (1966) Renal tumors induced by a single dose of dimethylnitrosamine: morphologic, functional, enzymatic, and hormonal characterization. Invest. Urol., 4, 39-56

Napalkov, N.P. & Alexandrov, V.A. (1968) On the effects of blastomogenic substances on the organism during embryogenesis. Z. Krebsforsch., 71, 32-50

Natarajan, A.T., Tates, A.D., Van Buul, P.P.W., Meijers, M. & De Vogel, N. (1976) Cytogenetic effects of mutagens/carcinogens after activation in a microsomal system *in vitro*. I. Induction of chromosome aberrations and sister chromatid exchanges by diethylnitrosamine (DEN) and dimethylnitrosamine (DMN) in CHO cells in the presence of rat-liver microsomes. Mutation Res., 37, 83-90

Nicoll, J.W., Swann, P.F. & Pegg, A.E. (1975) Effect of dimethylnitrosamine on persistence of methylated guanines in rat liver and kidney DNA. Nature (Lond.), 254, 261-262

Noronha, R.F.X. (1975) The inhibition of dimethylnitrosamine-induced renal tumorigenesis in NZO/Bl mice by orchiectomy. Invest. Urol., 13, 136-141

Noronha, R.F.X. & Goodall, C.M. (1972) Nasal tumours in starved rats injected once with dimethylnitrosamine. N.Z. med. J., 75, 374-375

Noronha, R.F.X. & Goodall, C.M. (1976) Enhancement of hepatic and renal tumorigenesis in thyroidectomized NZR/Gd rats treated with dimethylnitrosamine. J. surg. Oncol., 8, 539-550

O'Connor, P.J., Capps, M.J., Craig, A.W., Lawley, P.D. & Shah, S.A. (1972) Differences in the patterns of methylation in rat liver ribosomal ribonucleic acid after reaction *in vivo* with methyl methanesulphonate and *NN*-dimethylnitrosamine. Biochem. J., 129, 519-528

O'Connor, P.J., Capps, M.J. & Craig, A.W. (1973) Comparative studies of the hepatocarcinogen *N,N*-dimethylnitrosamine *in vivo*: reaction sites in rat liver DNA and the significance of their relative stabilities. Brit. J. Cancer, 27, 153-166

O'Connor, P.J., Margison, G.P. & Craig, A.W. (1975) Phosphotriesters in rat liver deoxyribonucleic acid after the administration of the carcinogen *NN*-dimethylnitrosamine *in vivo*. Biochem. J., 145, 475-482

Otsuka, H. & Kuwahara, A. (1971) Hemangiomatous lesions of mice treated with nitrosodimethylamine. Gann, 62, 147-156

Panalaks, T., Iyengar, J.R. & Sen, N.P. (1973) Nitrate, nitrite, and dimethylnitrosamine in cured meat products. J. Ass. off. analyt. Chem., 56, 621-625

Panalaks, T., Iyengar, J.R., Donaldson, B.A., Miles, W.F. & Sen, N.P. (1974) Further survey of cured meat products for volatile *N*-nitrosamines. J. Ass. off. analyt. Chem., 57, 806-812

Pasternak, L. (1962) Mutagene Wirkung von Dimethylnitrosamin bei *Drosophila melanogaster*. Naturwissenschaften, 49, 381

Pegg, A.E. (1977) Formation and metabolism of alkylated nucleosides: possible role in carcinogenesis by nitroso compounds and alkylating agents. Adv. Cancer Res., 25, 195-269

Pellizzari, E.D., Bunch, J.E., Bursey, J.T., Berkley, R.E., Sawicki, E. & Krost, K. (1976) Estimation of *N*-nitrosodimethylamine levels in ambient air by capillary gas-liquid chromatography/mass spectrometry. Analyt. Lett., 9, 579-594

Pensabene, J.W., Fiddler, W., Dooley, C.J., Doerr, R.C. & Wasserman, A.E. (1972) Spectral and gas chromatographic characteristics of some *N*-nitrosamines. J. agric. Fd Chem., 20, 274-277

Phillips, J.C., Lake, B.G., Heading, C.E., Gangolli, S.D. & Lloyd, A.G. (1975) Studies on the metabolism of dimethylnitrosamine in the rat. I. Effect of dose, route of administration and sex. Fd Cosmet. Toxicol., 13, 203-209

Pliss, G.B. & Khudoley, V.V. (1975) Tumor induction by carcinogenic agents in aquarium fish. J. nat. Cancer Inst., 55, 129-136

Pound, A.W. & Lawson, T.A. (1975) Partial hepatectomy and toxicity of dimethylnitrosamine and carbon tetrachloride, in relation to the carcinogenic action of dimethylnitrosamine. Brit. J. Cancer, 32, 596-603

Pound, A.W., Lawson, T.A. & Horn, L. (1973) Increased carcinogenic action of dimethylnitrosamine after prior administration of carbon tetrachloride. Brit. J. Cancer, 27, 451-459

Prager, B., Jacobson, P., Schmidt, P. & Stern, D., eds (1922) Beilsteins Handbuch der Organischen Chemie, 4th ed., Vol. 4, Syst. No. 335, Berlin, Springer, p. 84

Preussmann, R., Walker, E.A., Wasserman, A.E. & Castegnaro, M., eds (1978) Environmental Carcinogens - Selected Methods of Analysis, Vol. 1, Nitrosamines, Lyon (IARC Scientific Publications No. 18) (in press)

Propping, P., Röhrborn, G. & Buselmaier, W. (1972) Comparative investigations on the chemical induction of point mutations and dominant lethal mutations in mice. Mol. gen. Genet., 117, 197-209

Radomski, J.L. & Hearn, W.L. (1976) Nitrates, nitrites and the induction of bladder cancer from nitrosamines (Abstract No. 18). Proc. Amer. Ass. Cancer Res., 17, 5

Rainey, W.T., Christie, W.H. & Lijinsky, W. (1978) Mass spectrometry of *N*-nitrosamines. Biomed. Mass Spectrom. (in press)

Rajalakshmi, S. & Sarma, D.S.R. (1975) Replication of hepatic DNA in rats treated with dimethylnitrosamine. Chem.-biol. Interact., 11, 245-252

Ramanathan, R., Rajalakshmi, S., Sarma, D.S.R. & Farber, E. (1976) Non-random nature of *in vivo* methylation by dimethylnitrosamine and the subsequent removal of methylated products from rat liver chromatin DNA. Cancer Res., 36, 2073-2079

Reznik, G. (1975) The carcinogenic effect of dimethylnitrosamine on the Chinese hamster (*Cricetulus griseus*). Cancer Lett., 1, 25-28

Reznik, G., Mohr, U. & Kmoch, N. (1976) Carcinogenic effects of different nitroso-compounds in Chinese hamsters. I. Dimethylnitrosamine and *N*-diethylnitrosamine. Brit. J. Cancer, 33, 411-418

Rhoades, J.W. & Johnson, D.E. (1972) *N*-Dimethylnitrosamine in tobacco smoke condensate. Nature (Lond.), 236, 307-308

Riopelle, J.L. & Jasmin, G. (1969) Nature, classification, and nomenclature of kidney tumors induced in the rat by dimethylnitrosamine. J. nat. Cancer Inst., 42, 643-662

Rogers, A.E., Sanchez, O., Feinsod, F.M. & Newberne, P.M. (1974) Dietary enhancement of nitrosamine carcinogenesis. Cancer Res., 34, 96-99

Roller, P.P., Shimp, D.R. & Keefer, L.K. (1975) Synthesis and solvolysis of methyl(acetoxymethyl)nitrosamine. Solution chemistry of the presumed carcinogenic metabolite of dimethylnitrosamine. Tetrahedron Lett., 25, 2065-2068

Rounbehler, D.P., Ross, R., Fine, D.H., Iqbal, Z.M. & Epstein, S.S. (1977) Quantitation of dimethylnitrosamine in the whole mouse after biosynthesis *in vivo* from trace levels of precursors. Science, 197, 917-918

Sakshaug, J., Sögnen, E., Hansen, M.A. & Koppang, N. (1965) Dimethylnitrosamine: its hepatotoxic effect in sheep and its occurrence in toxic batches of herring meal. Nature (Lond.), 206, 1261-1262

Sato, S., Matsushima, T., Tanaka, N., Sugimura, T. & Takashima, F. (1973) Hepatic tumors in the guppy (*Lebistes reticulatus*) induced by aflatoxin B_1, dimethylnitrosamine and 2-acetylaminofluorene. J. nat. Cancer Inst., 50, 765-778

Schmähl, D. & Preussmann, R. (1959) Cancerogene Wirkung von Nitrosodimethylamin bei Ratten. Naturwissenschaften, 46, 175

Schmähl, D., Krüger, F.W., Ivankovic, S. & Preissler, P. (1971) Verminderung der Toxizität von Dimethylnitrosamin bei Ratten und Mäusen nach Behandlung mit Disulfiram. Arzneimittel-Forsch., 21, 1560-1562

Schmähl, D., Krüger, F.W., Habs, M. & Diehl, B. (1976) Influence of disulfiram on the organotropy of the carcinogenic effect of dimethylnitrosamine and diethylnitrosamine in rats. Z. Krebsforsch., 85, 271-276

Sen, N.P. (1972) The evidence for the presence of dimethylnitrosamine in meat products. Fd Cosmet. Toxicol., 10, 219-223

Sen, N.P., Donaldson, B., Iyengar, J.R. & Panalaks, T. (1973) Nitrosopyrrolidine and dimethylnitrosamine in bacon. Nature (Lond.), 241, 473-474

Sen, N.P., Donaldson, B., Charbonneau, C. & Miles, W.F. (1974) Effect of additives on the formation of nitrosamines in meat curing mixtures containing spices and nitrite. J. agric. Fd Chem., 22, 1125-1130

Sen, N.P., Seaman, S. & Miles, W.F. (1976a) Dimethylnitrosamine and nitrosopyrrolidine in fumes produced during the frying of bacon. Fd Cosmet. Toxicol., 14, 167-170

Sen, N.P., Iyengar, J.R., Miles, W.F. & Panalaks, T. (1976b) Nitrosamines in cured meat products. In: Walker, E.A., Bogovski, P. & Griciute, L., eds, Environmental *N*-Nitroso Compounds Analysis and Formation, Lyon (IARC Scientific Publications No. 14), pp. 333-342

Sen, N.P., Donaldson, B.A., Seaman, S., Iyengar, J.R. & Miles, W.F. (1978) Recent studies in Canada on the analysis and occurrence of volatile and non-volatile *N*-nitroso compounds in foods. In: Walker, E.A., Castegnaro, M., Griciute, L. & Lyle, R.E., eds, Environmental Aspects of *N*-Nitroso Compounds, Lyon (IARC Scientific Publications No. 19) (in press)

Shabad, L.M. & Savluchinskaya, L.A. (1971) Some results of studying the blastomogenic action of nitrosamines on mice. Biull. eksp. Biol. Med., 71, 76-80

Shinohara, Y., Arai, M., Hirao, K., Sugihara, S., Nakanishi, K., Tsunoda, H. & Ito, N. (1976) Combination effect of citrinin and other chemicals on rat kidney tumorigenesis. Gann, 67, 147-155

Shooter, K.V. & Wiessler, M. (1976) The interaction of acetoxy-dimethylnitrosamine, a proximate metabolite of the carcinogenic amine, and bacteriophages R17 and T7. Chem. biol.-Interact., 14, 1-11

Skaare, J.U. & Dahle, H.K. (1975) Gas chromatographic determination and mass spectrometric confirmation of *N*-nitrosodimethylamine in fish meal. J. Chromat., 111, 426-429

Smetanin, E.E. (1971) On transplacental blastomogenic effect of dimethylnitrosamine and nitrosomethylurea. Vop. Onkol., 17, 75-81

Somogyi, A., Conney, A.H., Kuntzman, R. & Solymoss, B. (1972) Protection against dimethylnitrosamine toxicity by pregnenolone-16α-carbonitrile. Nature (Lond.), 237, 61-63

Stenback, F., Ferrero, A., Montesano, R. & Shubik, P. (1973) Synergistic effect of ferric oxide on dimethylnitrosamine carcinogenesis in the Syrian golden hamster. Z. Krebsforsch., 79, 31-38

Stephany, R.W. & Schuller, P.L. (1978) Some new data on the intake of nitrate, nitrite and volatile *N*-nitrosamines and on the occurrence of volatile *N*-nitrosamines in human urine and veal calves. In: Walker, E.A., Castegnaro, M., Griciute, L. & Lyle, R.E., eds, Environmental Aspects of *N*-Nitroso Compounds, Lyon (IARC Scientific Publications No. 19) (in press)

Stephany, R.W., Freudenthal, J. & Schuller, P.L. (1976) Quantitative and qualitative determination of some volatile nitrosamines in various meat products. In: Walker, E.A., Bogovski, P. & Griciute, L., eds, Environmental *N*-Nitroso Compounds Analysis and Formation, Lyon (IARC Scientific Publications No. 14), pp. 343-354

Stewart, B.W. (1974) Inhibition of dimethylnitrosamine-induced strand breakage in rat liver DNA by aminoacetonitrile. Biochim. biophys. acta, 366, 261-263

Stewart, B.W. & Hard, G.C. (1977) Distinctive patterns of proliferative activity in kidney cell cultures derived from normal, dimethylnitrosamine-treated, and renal tumour-bearing rats. J. nat. Cancer Inst., 58, 1615-1619

Stewart, B.W. & Huang, P.H.T. (1977) Analysis by benzoylated-DEAE-cellulose of carcinogen-induced DNA damage *in vivo* (Abstract No. 91). Proc. Amer. Ass. Cancer Res., 18, 23

Stewart, B.W. & Magee, P.N. (1971) Effect of a single dose of dimethylnitrosamine on biosynthesis of nucleic acid and protein in rat liver and kidney. Biochem. J., 125, 943-952

Sugihara, R. & Sugihara, S., Jr (1976) Electron microscopic observations on the morphogenesis of renal cell carcinoma induced in rat kidney by dimethylnitrosamine and *N*-(3,5-dichlorophenyl)succinimide. Cancer Res., 36, 533-550

Swann, P.F. & Magee, P.N. (1968) Nitrosamine-induced carcinogenesis. The alkylation of nucleic acids of the rat by *N*-methyl-*N*-nitrosourea, dimethylnitrosamine, dimethyl sulphate and methyl methanesulphonate. Biochem. J., 110, 39-47

Swann, P.F. & McLean, A.E.M. (1971) Cellular injury and carcinogenesis. The effect of a protein-free high-carbohydrate diet on the metabolism of dimethylnitrosamine in the rat. Biochem. J., 124, 283-288

Swann, P.F., Magee, P.N., Mohr, U., Reznik, G., Green, U. & Kaufman, D.G. (1976) Possible repair of carcinogenic damage caused by dimethylnitrosamine in rat kidney. Nature (Lond.), 263, 134-136

Takayama, S. & Oota, K. (1963) Malignant tumors induced in mice fed with *N*-nitrosodimethylamine. Gann, 54, 465-472

Takayama, S. & Oota, K. (1965) Induction of malignant tumors in various strains of mice by oral administration of *N*-nitrosodimethylamine and *N*-nitrosodiethylamine. Gann, 56, 189-199

Taylor, H.W. & Lijinsky, W. (1975) Tumor induction in rats by feeding aminopyrine or oxytetracycline with nitrite. Int. J. Cancer, 16, 211-215

Taylor, H.W., Lijinsky, W., Nettesheim, P. & Snyder, C.M. (1974) Alteration of tumor response in rat liver by carbon tetrachloride. Cancer Res., 34, 3391-3395

Telling, G.M., Bryce, T.A., Hoar, D., Osborne, D. & Welti, D. (1974) Progress in the analysis of volatile *N*-nitroso compounds. In: Bogovski, P. & Walker, E.A., eds, *N*-Nitroso Compounds in the Environment, Lyon (IARC Scientific Publications No. 9), pp. 12-17

Terracini, B. & Magee, P.N. (1964) Renal tumours in rats following injection of dimethylnitrosamine at birth. Nature (Lond.), 202, 502-503

Terracini, B., Palestro, G., Ramella Gigliardi, M. & Montesano, R. (1966) Carcinogenicity of dimethylnitrosamine in Swiss mice. Brit. J. Cancer, 20, 871-876

Terracini, B., Magee, P.N. & Barnes, J.M. (1967) Hepatic pathology in rats on low dietary levels of dimethylnitrosamine. Brit. J. Cancer, 21, 559-565

Terracini, B., Palestro, G., Ruà, S. & Revisio, A. (1969) Studio sul ruolo dell'iperplasia compensatoria nella cancerogenesi renale da dimetilnitrosamina nel ratto. Tumori, 55, 357-370

Tomatis, L. & Cefis, F. (1967) The effects of multiple and single administration of dimethylnitrosamine to hamsters. Tumori, 53, 447-452

Tomatis, L., Magee, P.N. & Shubik, P. (1964) Induction of liver tumors in the Syrian golden hamster by feeding dimethylnitrosamine. J. nat. Cancer Inst., 33, 341-345

Toth, B. & Shubik, P. (1967) Carcinogenesis in AKR mice injected at birth with benzo[*a*]pyrene and dimethylnitrosamine. Cancer Res., 27, 43-51

Toth, B., Magee, P.N. & Shubik, P. (1964) Carcinogenesis study with dimethylnitrosamine administered orally to adult and subcutaneously to newborn BALB/c mice. Cancer Res., 24, 1712-1721

Turberville, C. & Craddock, V.M. (1971) Methylation of nuclear proteins by dimethylnitrosamine and by methionine in the rat *in vivo*. Biochem. J., 124, 725-739

US Environmental Protection Agency (1977) Requirement for certain pesticide registrants and applicants for registration to submit analyses of pesticides for *N*-nitroso contaminants. Fed. Regist., 42, 51640-51641

US Occupational Safety & Health Administration (1976) Toxic and hazardous substances. US Code of Federal Regulations, Title 29, part 1910.1016, pp. 56-59

Vesselinovitch, S.D. (1969) The sex-dependent difference in the development of liver tumors in mice administered dimethylnitrosamine. Cancer Res., 29, 1024-1027

Ward, J.M., Rice, J.M., Roller, P.P. & Wenk, M.L. (1977) Natural history of intestinal neoplasms induced in rats by a single injection of methyl(acetoxymethyl)nitrosamine. Cancer Res., 37, 3046-3052

Wasserman, A.E., Fiddler, W., Doerr, R.C., Osman, S.F. & Dooley, C.J. (1972) Dimethylnitrosamine in frankfurters. Fd Cosmet. Toxicol., 10, 681-684

Weekes, U.Y. (1975) Metabolism of dimethylnitrosamine to mutagenic intermediates by kidney microsomal enzymes and correlation with reported host susceptibility to kidney tumors. J. nat. Cancer Inst., 55, 1199-1201

Wiessler, M. & Schmähl, D. (1976) Zur carcinogenen Wirkung von *N*-Nitroso-Verbindungen. V. Acetoxymethyl-Methyl-Nitrosamin. Z. Krebsforsch., 85, 47-49

Wilkinson, R., Hawks, A. & Pegg, A.E. (1975) Methylation of rat liver mitochondrial deoxyribonucleic acid by chemical carcinogens and associated alterations in physical properties. Chem.-biol. Interact., 9, 157-167

Williams, G.M. (1976) The use of liver epithelial cultures for the study of chemical carcinogenesis. Amer. J. Path., 85, 739-754

Williams, G.M. (1977) Detection of chemical carcinogens by unscheduled DNA synthesis in rat liver primary cell cultures. Cancer Res., 37, 1845-1851

Williams, G.M., Elliott, J.M. & Weisburger, J.H. (1973) Carcinoma after malignant conversion *in vitro* of epithelial-like cells from rat liver following exposure to chemical carcinogens. Cancer Res., 33, 606-612

Wunderlich, V., Tetzlaff, I. & Graffi, A. (1971/72) Studies on nitrosodimethylamine: preferential methylation of mitochondrial DNA in rats and hamsters. Chem.-biol. Interact., 4, 81-89

Zak, F.G., Holzner, J.H., Singer, E.J. & Popper, H. (1960) Renal and pulmonary tumors in rats fed dimethylnitrosamine. Cancer Res., 20, 96-99

Zwicker, G.M., Carlton, W.W. & Tuite, J. (1972) Carcinogenic activity of toxigenic penicillia (Abstract). Lab. Invest., 26, 497

N-NITROSODI-*n*-PROPYLAMINE

1. Chemical and Physical Data

1.1 Synonyms and trade names

Chem. Abstr. Services Reg. No.: 621-64-7

Chem. Abstr. Name: *N*-Nitroso-*N*-propyl-1-propanamine

N,*N*-Di-*n*-propylnitrosamine; di-*n*-propylnitrosamine; DPNA; NDPA; *N*-nitrosodipropylamine

1.2 Structural and molecular formulae and weight

$$O{=}N{-}N\begin{cases}CH_2{-}CH_2{-}CH_3\\CH_2{-}CH_2{-}CH_3\end{cases}$$

$C_6H_{14}N_2O$ Mol. wt: 130.2

1.3 Chemical and physical properties of the pure substance

(a) Description: Yellow liquid

(b) Boiling-point: 81°C (5 mm) (Druckrey *et al.*, 1967)

(c) Density: d_4^{20} 0.9160

(d) Refractive index: n_D^{20} 1.4437

(e) Spectroscopy data: λ_{max} 233 and 339 nm (E_1^1 = 583.5 and 6.5) in water (Druckrey *et al.*, 1967); mass spectroscopy data are given by Pensabene *et al.* (1972) and Rainey *et al.* (1978).

(f) Solubility: Soluble in water (approximately 1%), in organic solvents and in lipids

(g) Volatility: Can be steam-distilled quantitatively (Eisenbrand *et al.*, 1970)

(h) Stability: Stable at room temperature for more than 14 days in neutral or alkaline aqueous solutions in the dark (Druckrey *et al.*, 1967); slightly less stable in acidic solutions; light-sensitive, especially to ultra-violet light

(i) Reactivity: Strong oxidants (peracids) oxidize it to the corresponding nitramine; can be reduced to the corresponding hydrazine and/or amine; relatively resistant to hydrolysis but can be split by hydrogen bromide in acetic acid (Eisenbrand *et al.*, 1970). Photochemically reactive (Fridman *et al.*, 1971)

1.4 Technical products and impurities

No data were available to the Working Group.

2. Production, Use, Occurrence and Analysis

2.1 Production and use

(a) Production

N-Nitrosodi-*n*-propylamine (NDPA) was first prepared by Vincent in 1886 from di-*n*-propylamine and nitrous acid (Prager *et al.*, 1922). No evidence was found that NDPA has been produced commercially.

(b) Use

No data were available to the Working Group.

2.2 Occurrence

(a) Waste-water

NDPA was reported to occur in the waste-water from 3/18 chemical factories at levels of 0.12 and 2.8 μg/l[1] (Cohen & Bachman, 1978).

(b) Food

NDPA has been detected at levels of 20-30 μg/kg[1] in cheese (Cerutti *et al.*, 1975).

---

[1]These results were not confirmed by mass spectroscopy (see also 'General Remarks on the Substances Considered', p. 40).

(c) Alcoholic beverages

NDPA has been shown to be present in a high proportion of samples of apple brandy at levels of 0-3.6 μg/kg. Its presence has also been demonstrated in a number of samples of cognac, rum and whiskey at levels of 0-0.2 μg/kg (IARC, 1977).

(d) Pesticides

Fine *et al.* (1977) reported 154,000 μg/l NDPA in the herbicide Treflan (trifluralin, emulsified concentrate of α,α,α-trifluoro-2,6-dinitro-*N*,*N*-dipropyl-*para*-toluidine); Cohen *et al.* (1978) found levels varying from 190,000-17,000 μg/l. The lower level reflects an effort by the manufacturer to reduce the nitrosamine contamination (US Environmental Protection Agency, 1977). NDPA has also been found in isopropalin (4-isopropyl-2,6-dinitro-*N*,*N*-dipropylaniline) at a level of 86,000 μg/l (Cohen *et al.*, 1978).

2.3 Analysis

An IARC Manual gives selected methods for the analysis of volatile *N*-nitrosamines, including NDPA (Preussmann *et al.*, 1978).

On 29 September 1977, the US Environmental Protection Agency issued a notice requiring all registrants of pesticide products that are potentially contaminated with *N*-nitroso compounds to analyse commercial samples which have been stored for at least 18 days to determine the extent of contamination. This notice prescribes in general terms the types of analytical methods to be used for volatile *N*-nitroso compounds (e.g., gas chromatography plus mass spectrometry or thermal energy analysis and others) as well as for non-volatile *N*-nitroso compounds (e.g., high-pressure liquid chromatography plus ultra-violet spectroscopy). Confirmation of positive results by gas chromatography and mass spectrometry or by valid independent methods is required when possible (US Environmental Protection Agency, 1977).

3. Biological Data Relevant to the Evaluation of Carcinogenic Risk to Man

3.1 Carcinogenicity and related studies in animals

(a) Oral administration[1]

Rat: Groups of BD rats were given *N*-nitrosodi-*n*-propylamine (NDPA) in the drinking-water at doses of 4, 8, 15 or 30 mg/kg bw/day. Of 48 animals, 45 developed liver carcinomas after average induction times of 300, 202, 155 or 120 days, respectively (average total dose to induce tumours in 50% of animals, 1.15-3.2 g/kg bw). In addition, 8 animals which received doses of 8 or 15 mg/kg bw/day showed papillomas or carcinomas of the oesophagus and 6, carcinomas of the tongue (Druckrey *et al.*, 1967).

(b) Subcutaneous and/or intramuscular administration

Rat: Groups of 10 male and 10 female 12-week-old Sprague-Dawley rats were injected subcutaneously with 1/5, 1/10 or 1/20 the LD_{50} NDPA (LD_{50}: 487 mg/kg bw) once weekly for life. Twenty male and 20 female untreated Sprague-Dawley rats served as controls. The average total dose ranged between 0.93 and 2.7 g/kg bw. A high incidence of neoplasms was observed in the apical parts of the nasal cavities (35) and in the endoturbinals of the nasal cavities (13). Of a total of 58 effective animals, 45 developed 48 tumours of the nasal and/or paranasal cavities, 19 of which were malignant. In addition, 13 liver tumours (mainly liver-cell carcinomas), 11 adenomas or carcinomas of the lung and 11 squamous-cell papillomas of the oesophagus were seen. Tumours of the kidney (2 adenomas, 1 adenocarcinoma) developed in 3 animals treated with 48 mg/kg bw (1/10 LD_{50}) (Althoff *et al.*, 1973a; Reznik *et al.*, 1975).

---

[1] The Working Group was aware of a study in monkeys, reported in an abstract, in which liver tumours were found following i.p. and/or oral administration of NDPA; however, the results of this study have not been fully reported (Adamson *et al.*, 1974).

Hamster: Groups of 20 male and 20 female Syrian golden hamsters were treated with 1.2% NDPA in olive oil subcutaneously once weekly for life at 5 dose levels, 3.75, 7.5, 15, 30 or 60 mg/kg bw. Of 185 effective animals, 134 had 591 tumours of the nasal and paranasal cavities, 163 had 1224 tumours of the laryngobronchial tract, and 56 had 112 tumours of the lung; a few tumours occurred in a variety of other organs. The first neoplasms were seen after 16 weeks. Among 20 male and 20 female controls, 2 thyroid adenomas, 1 cortical adenoma of the adrenal gland and 1 papilloma of the vagina were observed (Althoff *et al.*, 1973b; Pour *et al.*, 1973).

(c) Carcinogenicity of metabolites and derivatives (see also section 3.2a)

N-Nitroso-2-hydroxy-*n*-propyl-*n*-propylamine

Subcutaneous and/or intramuscular administration

Groups of 10 male and 10 female Sprague-Dawley rats were injected subcutaneously once weekly for life with 255, 127 or 64 mg/kg bw (1/5, 1/10 or 1/20 LD_{50}; LD_{50}: 1273 mg/kg bw); 53/59 animals developed benign and malignant tumours, mainly in the nasal cavity (47 squamous-cell papillomas and carcinomas) and the liver (25 hepatocellular carcinomas, haemangioendotheliomas, hepatomas). Other tumour sites were the lung (7) and oesophagus (10) (Reznik *et al.*, 1975).

Groups of 10 male and 10 female Syrian golden hamsters received weekly s.c. injections of *N*-nitroso-2-hydroxypropyl-*n*-propylamine in olive oil for life at 3 dose levels (1/10, 1/20 or 1/40 of the LD_{50}; LD_{50}: 1500 mg/kg bw). The effective number of animals was 43; the average survival time ranged from 39-46 weeks. Tumours of the nasal cavities were seen in 33-69% of treated animals; 33-54% had laryngotracheal tumours; and 7-40% had liver tumours described as cholangiomas and haemangioendotheliomas. A few tumours occurred at a variety of other sites (Pour *et al.*, 1974a,c).

Results obtained on the carcinogenicity of derivatives are summarized in Table 1.

Table 1

Carcinogenicity of derivatives of *N*-nitrosodi-*n*-propylamine

Compound	Species tested	Main tumour sites	References
N-Nitroso-bis(2-hydroxy-*n*-propyl)amine	Wistar rats	Respiratory tract, liver, thyroid, kidney, urinary bladder and pancreas	Konishi *et al.*, 1976
	Sprague-Dawley rats	Kidney, nasal cavities, respiratory tract, thyroid, oesophagus and liver	Reznik & Mohr, 1976
	Syrian golden hamsters	Pancreas, nasal cavities, respiratory tract, liver, gall bladder, kidney, lip and vaginal epithelium	Althoff *et al.*, 1976; Krüger *et al.*, 1974; LeVitt *et al.*, 1977; Pour *et al.*, 1974b, 1975a,b, 1977a
	Guinea-pigs	Liver	Rao & Reddy, 1977
N-Nitroso-2-oxo-*n*-propyl-*n*-propylamine	Sprague-Dawley rats	Liver	Althoff *et al.*, 1974
	Syrian golden hamsters	Nasal cavities, respiratory tract, liver and kidney	Pour *et al.*, 1974c,d
N-nitroso-bis(2-oxo-*n*-propyl)-amine	Syrian golden hamsters	Pancreas, lung, liver and gall bladder	Pour *et al.*, 1975c, 1977b
N-Nitroso-bis(2-acetoxy-*n*-propyl)amine	Syrian golden hamsters	Respiratory tract, liver, pancreas, nasal cavities, gall bladder, lip and vaginal epithelium	Pour *et al.*, 1976a,b, 1977a
N-Nitroso-2,2'-dimethyldi-*n*-propylamine	Syrian golden hamsters	Nasal cavities and respiratory tract	Althoff *et al.*, 1975

3.2 Other relevant biological data

(a) Experimental systems

Toxic effects

The acute LD_{50} of NDPA was 480 mg/kg bw after oral administration to BD rats (Druckrey *et al.*, 1967); the s.c. LD_{50} was 487 mg/kg bw in rats and 600 mg/kg bw in Syrian golden hamsters (Pour *et al.*, 1973; Reznik *et al.*, 1975).

No data on the embryotoxicity or teratogenicity of NDPA were available to the Working Group.

Absorption, distribution and excretion

In goats, one hour after oral administration of 30 mg/kg bw NDPA, 4.9 mg/kg NDPA were found in milk and 1.6 mg/kg in blood. Only traces were found in the milk after 24 hours (Juszkiewicz & Kowalski, 1974).

Metabolism

Urine collected during 48 hours after administration of an oral LD_{50} dose to rats contained the following compounds: *N*-nitroso-3-hydroxy-*n*-propyl-*n*-propylamine, *N*-nitroso-2-carboxyethyl-*n*-propylamine and, to a lesser extent, *N*-nitroso-2-hydroxy-*n*-propyl-*n*-propylamine and *N*-nitroso-carboxymethyl-*n*-propylamine (Blattmann & Preussmann, 1973) [see also, section 3.1 (c)].

Administration of [1-^{14}C]-NDPA to rats produced 7-[^{14}C]-*n*-propyl-guanine together with 7-[^{14}C]-methylguanine in the liver RNA. In contrast, administration of [2-^{14}C]-NDPA led to production of only 7-[^{14}C]-*n*-propyl-guanine in rat liver RNA (Krüger, 1971).

NDPA incubated in the presence of a rat-liver microsomal system and 3,4-dichlorothiophenol as a trapping agent yields the corresponding methyl and propyl thioethers (Preussman *et al.*, 1976).

Mutagenicity and other short-term tests

NDPA produced reverse mutations in *Salmonella typhimurium* TA 1530, TA 1535 and TA 100 in the presence of microsomal fractions from rat and hamster liver and hamster lung (Bartsch *et al.*, 1976; Camus *et al.*, 1976; Olajos & Cornish, 1976; Sugimura *et al.*, 1976). NDPA also produced reverse mutations in *Escherichia coli* in the presence of rat liver microsomal fractions (Nakajima *et al.*, 1974).

In the presence of a liver microsomal system from phenobarbital-treated rats, NDPA induced 8-azaguanine-resistant mutants in Chinese hamster V79 cells (Kuroki *et al.*, 1977).

A study was made of the abilities of liver, kidney and lung fractions from untreated or phenobarbital-treated rats and hamsters to convert β-oxidized metabolites or synthetic putative intermediates, including *N*-nitroso(2-hydroxy-*n*-propyl)-*n*-propylamine, *N*-nitroso-bis(2-hydroxy-*n*-propyl)amine, *N*-nitroso-bis(2-acetoxy-*n*-propyl)amine, *N*-nitroso(2-oxo-*n*-propyl)amine and *N*-nitrosomethyl-*N*-*n*-propylamine into intermediates mutagenic for *S. typhimurium* TA 1530 (Camus *et al.*, 1976).

(b) Humans

No data were available to the Working Group.

3.3 Case reports and epidemiological studies

No data were available to the Working Group.

4. Summary of Data Reported and Evaluation

4.1 Experimental data

N-Nitrosodi-*n*-propylamine is carcinogenic in rats after its oral administration and in rats and hamsters after its subcutaneous injection. It produces benign and malignant tumours of the liver, kidney, oesophagus and respiratory tract. The metabolite *N*-nitroso-*N*-(2-hydroxy-*n*-propyl)-*n*-propylamine is also carcinogenic in rats and hamsters: it produces benign and malignant tumours of the respiratory tract and liver after its subcutaneous injection.

4.2 Human data

No case reports or epidemiological studies were available to the Working Group. Available information on occurrence suggests that the general population may be exposed sporadically to low levels of *N*-nitrosodi-*n*-propylamine; however, no exposed group suitable for an epidemiological investigation has yet been identifed. The report of relatively high levels in one pesticide formulation may permit the identification of exposed groups.

4.3 Evaluation

There is *sufficient evidence* of a carcinogenic effect of *N*-nitrosodi-*n*-propylamine in two experimental animal species. Although no epidemiological data were available (and efforts should be directed toward this end), *N*-nitrosodi-*n*-propylamine should be regarded for practical purposes as if it were carcinogenic to humans.

5. References

Adamson, R.H., Correa, P. & Dalgard, D.W. (1974) Induction of tumors in non-human primates with various chemical carcinogens (Abstract No. 45). Toxicol. appl. Pharmacol., 29, 93

Althoff, J., Krüger, F.W., Hilfrich, J., Schmähl, D. & Mohr, U. (1973a) Carcinogenicity of β-hydroxylated dipropylnitrosamine. Naturwissenschaften, 60, 55

Althoff, J., Krüger, F.W. & Mohr, U. (1973b) Carcinogenic effect of dipropylnitrosamine and compounds related by β-oxidation. J. nat. Cancer Inst., 51, 287-288

Althoff, J., Hilfrich, J., Krüger, F.W. & Bertram, B. (1974) The carcinogenic effect of 2-oxo-propyl-propylnitrosamine in Sprague-Dawley rats. Z. Krebsforsch., 81, 23-28

Althoff, J., Eagen, M. & Grandjean, C. (1975) Carcinogenic effect of 2,2'-dimethyldipropylnitrosamine in Syrian hamsters. J. nat. Cancer Inst., 55, 1209-1211

Althoff, J., Pour, P., Malick, L. & Wilson, R.B. (1976) Pancreatic neoplasms induced in Syrian golden hamsters. Amer. J. Path., 83, 517-530

Bartsch, H., Malaveille, C. & Montesano, R. (1976) The predictive value of tissue-mediated mutagenicity assays to assess the carcinogenic risk of chemicals. In: Montesano, R., Bartsch, H. & Tomatis, L., eds, Screening Tests in Chemical Carcinogenesis, Lyon (IARC Scientific Publications No. 12), pp. 467-491

Blattmann, L. & Preussmann, R. (1973) Struktur von Metaboliten carcinogener Dialkylnitrosamine im Rattenurin. Z. Krebsforsch., 79, 3-5

Camus, A., Bertram, B., Krüger, F.W., Malaveille, C. & Bartsch, H. (1976) Mutagenicity of β-oxidized *N*,*N*-di-*n*-propylnitrosamine derivatives in *S. typhimurium* mediated by rat and hamster tissues. Z. Krebsforsch., 86, 293-302

Cerutti, G., Zappavigna, R. & Santini, P.L. (1975) *N*-Alkylnitrosamines in domestic and imported cheeses. Latte, 3, 224-227 [Chem. Abstr., 83, 130147c]

Cohen, J.B. & Bachman, J.D. (1978) Measurement of environmental nitrosamines. In: Walker, E.A., Castegnaro, M., Griciute, L. & Lyle, R.E., eds, Environmental Aspects of *N*-Nitroso Compounds, Lyon (IARC Scientific Publications No. 19) (in press)

Cohen, S.Z., Bontoyan, W.R. & Zweig, G. (1978) Analytical determination of *N*-nitroso compounds in pesticides by the United States Environmental Protection Agency. In: Walker, E.A., Castegnaro, M., Griciute, L. & Lyle, R.E., eds, Environmental Aspects of *N*-Nitroso Compounds, Lyon (IARC Scientific Publications No. 19) (in press)

Druckrey, H., Preussmann, R., Ivankovic, S. & Schmähl, D. (1967) Organotrope carcinogene Wirkungen bei 65 verschiedenen *N*-Nitroso-Verbindungen an BD-Ratten. Z. Krebsforsch., 69, 103-201

Eisenbrand, G., Hodenberg, A. von & Preussmann, R. (1970) Trace analysis of *N*-nitroso compounds. II. Steam distillation at neutral, alkaline and acid pH under reduced and atmospheric pressure. Z. analyt. Chem., 251, 22-24

Fine, D.H., Rounbehler, D.P., Fan, T. & Ross, R. (1977) Human exposure to *N*-nitroso compounds in the environment. In: Hiatt, H.H., Watson, J.D. & Winsten, J.A., eds, Origins of Human Cancer, Book A, Cold Spring Harbor, N.Y., Cold Spring Harbor Laboratory, pp. 293-307

Fridman, A.L., Mukhametshin, F.M. & Novikov, S.S. (1971) Advances in the chemistry of aliphatic *N*-nitrosamines. Russ. chem. Rev., 40, 34-50

IARC (1977) Annual Report 1977, Lyon, International Agency for Research on Cancer, p. 57

Juszkiewicz, T. & Kowalski, B. (1974) Passage of nitrosamines from rumen into milk in goats. In: Bogovski, P. & Walker, E.A., eds, *N*-Nitroso Compounds in the Environment, Lyon (IARC Scientific Publications No. 9), pp. 173-176

Konishi, Y., Denda, A., Kondo, H. & Takahashi, S. (1976) Lung carcinomas induced by oral administration of *N*-bis(2-hydroxypropyl)nitrosamine in rats. Gann, 67, 773-780

Krüger, F.W. (1971) Metabolismus von Nitrosaminen *in vivo*. I. Über die β-Oxidation aliphatischer Di-*n*-alkylnitrosamine: die Bildung von 7-Methylguanin neben 7-Propyl- bzw. 7-Butylguanin nach Applikation von Di-*n*-propyl- oder Di-*n*-butylnitrosamin. Z. Krebsforsch., 76, 145-154

Krüger, F.W., Pour, P. & Althoff, J. (1974) Induction of pancreas tumours by di-isopropanolnitrosamine. Naturwissenschaften, 61, 328

Kuroki, T., Drevon, C. & Montesano, R. (1977) Microsome-mediated mutagenesis in V79 Chinese hamster cells by various nitrosamines. Cancer Res., 37, 1044-1050

Levitt, M.H., Harris, C.C., Squire, R., Springer, S., Wenk, M., Mollelo, C., Thomas, D., Kingsbury, E. & Newkirk, C. (1977) Experimental pancreatic carcinogenesis. I. Morphogenesis of pancreatic adenocarcinoma in the Syrian golden hamster induced by *N*-nitroso-bis(2-hydroxypropyl)amine. Amer. J. Path., 88, 5-28

Nakajima, T., Tanaka, A. & Tojyo, K.-I. (1974) The effect of metabolic activation with rat liver preparations on the mutagenicity of several *N*-nitrosamines on a streptomycin-dependent strain of *Escherichia coli*. Mutation Res., 26, 361-366

Olajos, E.J. & Cornish, H.H. (1976) Mutagenicity of dialkylnitrosamines: metabolites and derivatives (Abstract No. 43). Toxicol. appl. Pharmacol., 37, 109-110

Pensabene, J.W., Fiddler, W., Dooley, C.J., Doerr, R.C. & Wasserman, A.E. (1972) Spectral and gas chromatographic characteristics of some *N*-nitrosamines. J. agric. Fd Chem., 20, 274-277

Pour, P., Krüger, F.W., Cardesa, A., Althoff, J. & Mohr, U. (1973) Carcinogenic effect of di-*n*-propylnitrosamine in Syrian golden hamsters. J. nat. Cancer Inst., 51, 1019-1027

Pour, P., Krüger, F.W., Althoff, J., Cardesa, A. & Mohr, U. (1974a) Effect of *beta*-oxidized nitrosamines on Syrian golden hamsters. I. 2-Hydroxypropyl-*n*-propylnitrosamine. J. nat. Cancer Inst., 52, 1245-1249

Pour, P., Krüger, F.W., Althoff, J., Cardesa, A. & Mohr, U. (1974b) Cancer of the pancreas induced in the Syrian golden hamster. Amer. J. Path., 76, 349-358

Pour, P., Althoff, J., Cardesa, A., Krüger, F.W. & Mohr, U. (1974c) Effect of *beta*-oxidized nitrosamines on Syrian golden hamsters. II. 2-Oxo-propyl-*n*-propylnitrosamine. J. nat. Cancer Inst., 52, 1869-1874

Pour, P., Cardesa, A., Althoff, J. & Mohr, U. (1974d) Tumorigenesis in the nasal olfactory region of Syrian golden hamsters as a result of di-*n*-propylnitrosamine and related compounds. Cancer Res., 34, 16-26

Pour, P., Krüger, F.W., Althoff, J., Cardesa, A. & Mohr, U. (1975a) A new approach for induction of pancreatic neoplasms. Cancer Res., 35, 2259-2268

Pour, P., Krüger, F.W., Althoff, J., Cardesa, A. & Mohr, U. (1975b) Effect of *beta*-oxidized nitrosamines on Syrian hamsters. III. 2,2'-Dihydroxy-di-*n*-propylnitrosamine. J. nat. Cancer Inst., 54, 141-146

Pour, P., Althoff, J., Krüger, F., Schmähl, D. & Mohr, U. (1975c) Induction of pancreatic neoplasms by 2,2'-dioxopropyl-*N*-propylnitrosamine. Cancer Lett., 1, 3-6

Pour, P., Althoff, J., Gingell, R., Kupper, R., Krüger, F. & Mohr, U. (1976a) *N*-Nitroso-bis(2-acetoxypropyl)amine as a further pancreatic carcinogen in Syrian golden hamsters. Cancer Res., 36, 2877-2884

Pour, P., Althoff, J., Gingell, R., Kupper, R., Krüger, F.W. & Mohr, U. (1976b) A further pancreatic carcinogen in Syrian golden hamsters: *N*-nitroso-bis(2-acetoxypropyl)amine. Cancer Lett., 1, 197-202

Pour, P., Althoff, J. & Nagel, D. (1977a) Induction of epithelial neoplasms by local application of *N*-nitroso-bis(2-hydroxypropyl)amine and *N*-nitroso-bis(2-acetoxypropyl)amine. Cancer Lett., 3, 109-113

Pour, P., Althoff, J., Krüger, F.W. & Mohr, U. (1977b) A potent pancreatic carcinogen in Syrian hamsters: *N*-nitroso-bis(2-oxopropyl)amine. J. nat. Cancer Inst., 58, 1449-1453

Prager, B., Jacobson, P., Schmidt, P. & Stern, D., eds (1922) Beilsteins Handbuch der Organischen Chemie, 4th ed., Vol. 4, Syst. No. 337, Berlin, Springer, p. 146

Preussmann, R., Arjungi, K.N. & Ebers, G. (1976) *In vitro* detection of nitrosamines and other indirect alkylating agents by reaction with 3,4-dichlorothiophenol in the presence of rat liver microsomes. Cancer Res., 36, 2459-2462

Preussmann, R., Walker, E.A., Wasserman, A.E. & Castegnaro, M., eds (1978) Environmental Carcinogens - Selected Methods of Analysis, Vol. 1, Nitrosamines, Lyon (IARC Scientific Publications No. 18) (in press)

Rainey, W.T., Christie, W.H. & Lijinsky, W. (1978) Mass spectrometry of *N*-nitrosamines. Biomed. Mass Spectrom. (in press)

Rao, M.S. & Reddy, J.K. (1977) Induction of malignant vascular tumors of the liver in guinea pigs treated with 2,2'-dihydroxy-di-*n*-propylnitrosamine. J. nat. Cancer Inst., 58, 387-392

Reznik, G. & Mohr, U. (1976) Induction of renal pelvic tumours in Sprague-Dawley rats by di-isopropanolnitrosamine. Cancer Lett., 2, 87-92

Reznik, G., Mohr, U. & Krüger, F.W. (1975) Carcinogenic effects of di-*n*-propylnitrosamine, β-hydroxypropyl-*n*-propylnitrosamine, and methyl-*n*-propylnitrosamine on Sprague-Dawley rats. J. nat. Cancer Inst., 54, 937-943

Sugimura, T., Yahagi, T., Nagao, M., Takeuchi, M., Kawachi, T., Hara, K., Yamasaki, E., Matsushima, T., Hashimoto, Y. & Okada, M. (1976) Validity of mutagenicity tests using microbes as a rapid screening method for environmental carcinogens. In: Montesano, R., Bartsch, H. & Tomatis, L., eds, Screening Tests in Chemical Carcinogenesis, Lyon (IARC Scientific Publications No. 12), pp. 81-101

US Environmental Protection Agency (1977) Requirement for certain pesticide registrants and applicants for registration to submit analyses of pesticides for *N*-nitroso contaminants. Fed. Regist., 42, 51640-51641

N-NITROSO-*N*-ETHYLUREA

This substance was considered previously by an IARC Working Group, in December 1971 (IARC, 1972). Since that time new data have become available, and these have been incorporated into the monograph and taken into account in the present evaluation.

1. Chemical and Physical Data

1.1 Synonyms and trade names

Chem. Abstr. Services Reg. No.: 759-73-9

Chem. Abstr. Name: *N*-Ethyl-*N*-nitrosourea

ANH; ENU; 1-ethyl-1-nitrosourea; NEU; nitrosoethylurea; NSC 45403

1.2 Structural and molecular formulae and weight

$$O{=}N{-}N(CH_2{-}CH_3){-}C({=}O){-}NH_2$$

$C_3H_7N_3O_2$ Mol. wt: 117.1

1.3 Chemical and physical properties of the pure substance

(a) Description: Yellow-pink crystals

(b) Melting-point: 103-104°C (decomposition) (Druckrey *et al.*, 1967)

(c) Spectroscopy data: λ_{max} 233 nm (E^1_1 = 469) in water (Druckrey *et al.*, 1967)

(d) Solubility: Soluble in water (approximately 1.3%) and in polar organic solvents; insoluble in non-polar organic solvents

(e) Stability: Decomposes to diazoethane in alkaline solutions; stability in aqueous solutions is pH-dependent (20°C) (Druckrey *et al.*, 1967):

pH	4.0	6.0	7.0	8.0	9.0
half-life (hrs)	190	31	1.5	0.1	0.05

Sensitive to humidity and light and should be refrigerated for storage

(f) Reactivity: Highly reactive (Garrett *et al.*, 1965; McCalla *et al.*, 1968). Reaction rates with various biologically important nucleophiles have been determined (Veleminský *et al.*, 1970).

1.4 Technical products and impurities

No data were available to the Working Group.

2. Production, Use, Occurrence and Analysis

2.1 Production and use

For background information on this section, see preamble, p. 22.

(a) Production

N-Nitroso-*N*-ethylurea (NEU) was first prepared in 1919 by the reaction of *N*-ethylurea with nitrous acid (Werner, 1919). Although NEU is available in small quantities for research purposes, no evidence was found that it has been produced commercially.

(b) Use

NEU has been used in the laboratory synthesis of diazoethane. Its mutagenic effect has been studied for promoting the growth of various plants (Ezhakova, 1973; Nikiforova, 1973; Samoshkin & Rodyankov, 1973). No evidence was found that it has been used commercially for these purposes.

2.2 Occurrence

No data were available to the Working Group.

2.3 Analysis

NEU is labile, and this complicates its analysis. High-pressure liquid chromatographic conditions for *N*-nitrosoureas have been reviewed by Montgomery *et al.* (1977). Selective detectors used for analysis of this compound include those of Fine *et al.* (1977) and Singer *et al.* (1977). A method for the analysis of alkylureas in fish has been developed (Mirvish *et al.*, 1978).

3. Biological Data Relevant to the Evaluation of Carcinogenic Risk to Man

3.1 Carcinogenicity and related studies in animals

(a) Oral administration

Rat: Ten-day-old BD-IX rats were given single oral doses of 10, 20, 40 or 80 mg/kg bw *N*-nitroso-*N*-ethylurea (NEU), and malignant neurogenic tumours were induced in the brain, spinal cord and peripheral nervous system in 75/80 animals. Even at the lowest dose, 23/26 animals died with neurogenic tumours (21 with brain tumours). At the highest dose, 9/16 rats had nephroblastomas (Druckrey *et al.*, 1970a).

Single oral administrations of 10 mg/kg bw NEU to 10-day-old BD-IX rats induced tumours in 8/19 animals. Tumours of the central and of the peripheral nervous systems were seen in 4 and 4 animals, respectively (Cravioto *et al.*, 1974).

It was reported in an abstract that among 39 MRC rats given 60 mg NEU/l of drinking-water on 5 days/week for 52 weeks, 7 tumours of the stomach (3 papillomas, 1 squamous-cell carcinoma and 3 sarcomas, all in males), 9 tumours of the large intestine (6 adenocarcinomas and 3 sarcomas, all in males), 9 adenocarcinomas of the mammary gland (8 in females and 1 in a male) and 12 myelocytic leukaemias were observed (Pelfrene *et al.*, 1975).

Of 104 female Donryu rats given NEU at dose levels of 100-400 mg/l of drinking-water, 87 developed leukaemias (Ogiu *et al.*, 1974, 1976).

Opossum: A variety of epithelial and mesenchymal embryonal neoplasms of the eye, liver, brain, kidney, muscle and jaw (including neuroectodermal tumours of the eye and nephroblastomas), closely analogous to tumours of human infancy, were found in opossums (*Didelphis virginiana* Kerr) treated orally from birth to 16 weeks of age with 100 mg/kg bw NEU in either single or split doses (Jurgelski *et al.*, 1974, 1976).

(b) Subcutaneous and/or intramuscular administration

Newborn mouse: One-day-old A, C57BL, DBAf and IF mice given single s.c. injections of NEU at dose levels ranging from 10-160 mg/kg bw developed a high incidence of tumours. Liver tumours ranging from hepatomas to hepatocellular carcinomas occurred most frequently in C57BL (28/44) and DBAf (20/75) mice, lung adenomas and adenocarcinomas in A mice (38/80) and lymphomas in A (16/80) and DBAf (20/75) mice. C57BL, DBAf and IF mice developed several tumours of the nervous system (1/44, 8/75 and 5/57, respectively) (Searle & Jones, 1976).

Newborn and suckling rat: Rats were injected subcutaneously with single doses of 5, 10, 20, 40 or 80 mg/kg bw NEU at birth, and 10-day-old rats received single doses of 10, 20 or 40 mg/kg bw. Mainly tumours of the central and peripheral nervous system were produced. At the lowest dose (5 mg/kg bw), 9/28 rats had tumours of the nervous system; at 10 mg/kg bw, 70% of the animals had tumours of the nervous system; at higher doses, all animals except one had tumours of the nervous system. No difference in response was observed between the newborn and the 10-day-old animals (Druckrey *et al.*, 1970a).

Single s.c. injections of 10 mg/kg bw NEU to newborn (approximately 24-hr-old) Wistar-derived albino rats and Lister hooded rats resulted in tumours of the nervous system in 33/34 animals: 53 brain tumours, 9 spinal-cord tumours and 9 peripheral nervous system tumours were found. No strain differences in response to the carcinogen were observed (Jones *et al.*, 1973; Searle *et al.*, 1972).

(c) Intraperitoneal administration

Newborn, suckling and adult mouse: It was reported in an abstract that doses of 60 or 120 mg/kg bw NEU injected into $C3HxAF_1$ mice less than 24 hours, 15 days or 6 weeks old, produced multiple types of tumours, including intracranial neurogenic and renal epithelial neoplasms. The multiplicity and frequency of tumour types were dependent upon age at the time of treatment (more than 20 different types in the two younger groups, only 4 types of primary tumours in the 6-week-old mice) (Lombard & Vesselinovitch, 1971; Vesselinovitch & Lombard, 1971).

First generation hybrids of C57BL/6JxC3Heb/FeJ ($B6C3F_1$) and C3HeB/FeJxA/J ($C3AF_1$) mice were given single i.p. injections of 60 or 120 mg/kg bw NEU at 1, 15 or 42 days of age. By the 90th week of age, most animals had died due to the development of benign and malignant tumours at multiple sites. Newborn animals were more susceptible to liver, kidney and ovarian tumours, and young adults to lung, Harderian gland, stomach, and lymphoreticular system tumours. The sex of the animals influenced the development of tumours of the liver (males), Harderian gland (males) and lymphoreticular system (females). $C3AF_1$ mice were more susceptible to lung tumours than $B6C3AF_1$ mice; the latter more readily developed tumours of the liver, Harderian gland, lymphoreticular system, ovaries and mammary gland (Vesselinovitch *et al.*, 1974). Most of the renal epithelial tumours resembled the corresponding human renal adenomas (Lombard *et al.*, 1974).

Rat: Monthly i.p. injections of 10 mg/animal NEU for 3 months caused thymic lymphomas in 3/10 adult Wistar rats. Monthly treatment with 10 mg/animal for 5 months produced thymic lymphomas in 9/20 treated rats and myeloid leukaemias in 5 others (Hadjiolov, 1972).

(d) Intravenous administration

Rat: Weekly i.v. doses of 10 mg/kg bw NEU to BD rats for 25 weeks produced leukaemias in 9/16 animals and 4 gliomas of the brain, 1 glioma of the spinal cord and 1 adenocarcinoma of the small intestine in 4 rats (Druckrey *et al.*, 1967). Treatment of 30-day-old rats with a single dose of 20, 40 or 80 mg/kg bw produced tumours predominantly of the brain and peripheral nervous system. With 20 mg/kg bw, 18/29 rats had tumours of the nervous system. More tumours outside the nervous system (ovary, uterus and, especially, kidney) were seen in animals given the highest dose (Druckrey *et al.*, 1970a).

Rats treated during pregnancy with single i.v. injections of 60-150 mg/kg bw NEU developed predominantly malignant tumours in the uterus and vagina late in life; these tumours were not produced by treatment in non-pregnant females (Alexandrov, 1969; Ivankovic, 1969).

Monkey: In a study reported in an abstract, malignant tumours (mainly of the ovary, uterus, vascular endothelium, bone, bone marrow and skin) were observed in 2/4 male and 5/9 female young patas monkeys (*Erythrocebus patas*) 700-900 days after the start of treatment with i.v. injections of 12 mg/kg bw NEU every 2 weeks for 2 years (Rice *et al.*, 1977).

(e) Other experimental systems

Prenatal exposure: Since the first reports of Druckrey *et al.* (1966) and Ivankovic *et al.* (1966) in rats, NEU has been investigated extensively for transplacental carcinogenicity.

The offspring of female A/J, A/He, C3Hf/He, C57BL/6 and GP mice given single i.p. injections of NEU at doses ranging from 29-117 mg/kg bw between the 12th and 19th day of gestation were found to have pulmonary adenomas and, occasionally, lymphocytic leukaemias at 12 weeks of age. Hepatomas were seen in A and C3Hf mice after 40 weeks (Rice, 1969).

Single i.p. injections of 59 mg/kg bw NEU on day 12, 14, 16 or 18 of gestation were given to AKR/J, SWR/J, DBA/2J, C57BL/6J and C57L/J mice. The incidence, type and latency of tumours depended on both the strain and the day of gestation on which NEU was given. The most common tumours were single or multiple pulmonary adenomas and leukaemias, which appeared after NEU treatment on days 16 and 18, respectively. Hepatomas, Harderian gland adenomas, tumours of endocrine glands and neurogenic tumours were also found, to a lesser extent. Hepatomas occurred preferentially in males (Diwan & Meier, 1974).

Mice were given i.p. injections of 59 mg/kg bw NEU on the 16th day of gestation. A lower incidence of pulmonary adenomas (18/36) and a longer latent period (16-20 weeks) were observed in (AKR/J females x SWR/J males) F_1 offspring than in (SWR/J females x AKR/J males) F_1 offspring, in which the incidence of lung tumours was 36/39, with a latent period of 10 weeks or less (Diwan *et al.*, 1974).

Differences in the susceptibilities of different strains of mice to NEU were also described by Denlinger *et al.* (1974). Ten of the 31 offspring of 5 C3HeB/FeJ mice which had been injected intravenously with a single dose of 20 mg/kg bw NEU on the 19th day of pregnancy, developed neurogenic tumours. This is a relatively high rate compared with results of earlier studies performed with other mouse strains.

It was reported in an abstract that perinatal treatment of 4555 DBA/2, C3H, C57BL/6, NZW, A, (C3HxC57BL/6) F_1 and (C3HxA) F_1 mice with NEU caused tumours of the peripheral nervous system in 74 animals and of the central nervous system in 43. The latent period ranged from 150-1000 days. In 1903 controls, only 1 primary neurinoma was seen (Wechsler *et al.*, 1974).

Ivankovic & Druckrey (1968) gave single i.v. injections of NEU to female BD-IX rats, varying the dose and the day of application during pregnancy. On the 15th day of gestation, 7 different single doses of between 5 and 80 mg/kg bw were injected. Of 222 offspring, 193 (87%) died with malignant neurogenic tumours. At the lowest dosage (5 mg/kg bw, approximately 2% of LD_{50}), 63% of the offspring developed neurogenic tumours (see Table 1). The yield of neurogenic tumours in the progeny was highest when the compound was administered during the last week of pregnancy; no tumours were observed in the offspring when the mothers were treated before the 12th day of gestation. Similar results were obtained in the same and other strains of rats and by the same and other routes of administration (Cravioto *et al.*, 1973, 1974; Druckrey *et al.*, 1970b; Graw *et al.*, 1974; Koestner *et al.*, 1971; Koyama *et al.*, 1972).

Table 1[a]

Dose, mg/kg bw i.v. on day 15 of pregnancy	Incidence of neurogenic tumours in offspring	Induction period (days)
80	5/5	160-230
70	21/22	120-490
60	51/51	not given
40	41/42	not given
20	18/21	120-600
10	32/41	132-640
5	25/40	190-700

[a]From Ivankovic & Druckrey, 1968

A single oral application of 30 mg/kg bw to Sprague-Dawley rats on day 19 of gestation caused a total of 1847 malignant tumours in about 90% of the 1068 offspring. The tumours were located mainly in the brain, the spinal cord and the trigeminal nerve. Medium induction time was 240 days. Various additional treatments did not affect the tumour incidence (Schmähl *et al.*, 1974).

Single i.v. injections of 1, 5, 20 or 50 mg/kg bw NEU to 2-4 Sprague-Dawley (CD) rats and single injections of 50 mg/kg bw NEU to 3 Fischer (CDF) rats, both on the 20th day of gestation, caused neuroectodermal tumours in offspring of rats at all dose levels. A directly proportional relationship was observed between dose levels and tumour incidences, while mean survival times were inversely related to exposure (see Table 2). A strain difference was also noted: at the 50 mg/kg bw level 69% of the Fischer rats and only 27% of the Sprague-Dawley rats died of brain tumours (Swenberg *et al.*, 1972).

Table 2[a]

Tumour incidence and survival of rats receiving NEU transplacentally

Dose to mother mg/kg bw	Strain	Number of rats with neuroectodermal tumours/total number of rats	Mean survival time (days)
1	SD	5/41	655
5	SD	19/24	477
20	SD	17/17	288
50	SD	25/25	211
50	Fischer	26/26	258

[a]From Swenberg *et al.*, 1972

The possibility was investigated that an increased cancer risk may persist for several generations in otherwise untreated descendants of NEU-treated mothers. A single i.p. dose of 40 mg/kg bw NEU given to 11 female BDVI rats on the 16th day of pregnancy caused tumours in 10 rats of the parental generation: 5 had tumours of the nervous tissue, and 7 had tumours at other sites. In the F_1 generation, mainly nervous system tumours were found (48/55); only 6/55 animals had tumours at other sites. In the F_2 generation, bred by brother-to-sister mating from F_1, no nervous tumours were observed, but 6/25 animals had tumours at other sites. In the F_3 generation, 3/38 animals had nervous system neoplasms, and 11/38 had tumours at other sites (Tomatis *et al.*, 1977).

Alexandrov & Napalkov (1976) demonstrated in rats that both a teratogenic and a carcinogenic effect can occur in the same target organ. The induction of microcephaly by i.p. administration of 5 mg/kg bw *N*-nitroso-*N*-methylurea (NMU) on the 15th day of pregnancy did not preclude the induction of brain tumours by the administration of 20 mg/kg bw NEU on the 17th day of pregnancy. Similarly, the induction of brain tumours by the administration of 20 mg/kg bw NEU on the 17th day of pregnancy was not influenced by the administration of 20 mg/kg bw NMU on the 21st day of pregnancy.

The morphology and growth of tumours of the nervous system have been described by Grossi-Paoletti *et al.* (1970), Kleihues *et al.* (1968), Thomas & Kersting (1968) and Wechsler *et al.* (1969).

When 30 mg/kg bw NEU were given by i.v. injection to Syrian golden hamsters on day 15 of pregnancy, 14/22 offspring developed tumours, mainly of the nervous system (5 tumours of the trigeminal nerve and 11 tumours of the peripheral nerves). No tumours of the brain or spinal cord were observed (Mennel & Zülch, 1972). The morphology and growth of such nervous system tumours have been described by Wechsler *et al.* (1969).

Three rabbits received 1 or 2 i.v. injections of 40 mg/kg bw NEU between days 23 and 28 of gestation. Eight of the 10 offspring that survived longer than 90 days developed adenosarcomas of the kidney within a mean latent period of 600 days (in 3 animals, the tumours were bilateral). Metastases to the lung, parietal pleura and para-aortic lymph nodes were observed in 3 animals. No tumours were observed in the mothers (Güthert *et al.*, 1973). Kidney tumours, including adenomas, adenocarcinomas and adenocarcinosarcomas were also found in the offspring of rabbits which had received i.v. or i.p. injections of NEU between days 18-32 of gestation (Fox *et al.*, 1975; Stavrou & Lübbe, 1975; Stavrou *et al.*, 1975).

Neurogenic tumours of the peripheral nervous system were observed in offspring of rabbits treated on day 8 or 10 of gestation with single i.v. doses of 50 mg/kg bw (Stavrou *et al.*, 1977).

Adenomas of the sweat glands (hidradenomas) and papillomas of the skin were produced in litters of pigs whose mothers were given 6 i.v. injections of 20 mg/kg bw NEU between the 20th and the 31st day of gestation (Kupfer *et al.*, 1969).

In a study reported in an abstract, female patas monkeys (*Erythrocebus patas*) received i.v. injections of 21 mg/kg bw NEU weekly or every two weeks, commencing at 30 or 60 days of pregnancy and continuing until parturition. One male infant whose mother had received 18 weekly injections starting at 30 days of pregnancy died 78 days post parturition with a hepatoma and an intracerebral haemangiosarcoma. No tumours had been observed in 33 other infants two years post parturition (Rice *et al.*, 1977).

Results of a study still in progress indicate that following treatment of 6 female monkeys (*Macaca mulatta*) with single i.v. injections of 25-70 mg/kg bw NEU 3-70 days before parturition, or treatment of 2 monkeys with 2 i.v. injections of 15-25 mg/kg bw NEU at 71 and 2 days or 63 and 15 days before parturition, no tumours occurred in the surviving offspring, aged 5-6 years; one infant whose mother had received 70 mg/kg bw was delivered stillborn (Jänisch *et al.*, 1977).

Intracerebral injection: A single intracerebral injection of 0.01-0.05 mg/animal (1.25-6.25 mg/kg bw) NEU to 1-, 3- and 10-day-old BD-IX rats resulted in 70 neurogenic tumours, mostly of the brain (37), in 85 animals. A clear dependency of tumour yield and length of latent period on both dose and age of rats at treatment could be established. Malignant neurinomas of the trigeminal nerve appeared only as a result of treatment on the first day of life (Druckrey *et al.*, 1973).

Single intracerebral administration of 10 mg/kg bw NEU to 1-day-old Long Evans rats induced neurogenic tumours, mostly in the central nervous system, in 9/11 animals (Cravioto *et al.*, 1974).

Intra-arterial administration: The injection of 0.04 mg NEU (1 mg/kg bw) into the left carotid of 25-day-old BDVI rats under nembutal anaesthesia (30 mg/kg bw) produced only 1 malignant neurinoma in 21 treated rats (Druckrey *et al.*, 1973).

Various routes of administration: Long Evans rats were treated intracerebrally or subcutaneously with 10 or 50 mg/kg bw when newborn, or were treated transplacentally with i.v. injections of 10 mg/kg bw on the 17th day of gestation. No differences in incidences of neurogenic tumours (80-86%) could be established for the various routes of administration (Cravioto *et al.*, 1974; Fornatto & Schiffer, 1972; Grossi-Paoletti *et al.*, 1972a,b).

(f) Carcinogenicity of precursors

Neurogenic tumours were found in 4/20 and non-neurogenic tumours in 11/20 Sprague-Dawley rats after administration of 0.03% ethylurea in the drinking-water and 0.3% sodium nitrite in the diet. When the concentration of ethylurea was decreased to 0.01%, and the nitrite concentration kept constant, 18/20 animals developed non-neurogenic tumours, and none developed neurogenic tumours (Koestner & Wechsler, 1974; Koestner *et al.*, 1975).

The typical transplacental neurocarcinogenic effect of NEU has been observed after oral administration of ethylurea and sodium nitrite to pregnant BD-IX rats (Ivankovic & Preussmann, 1970; Ramadan & Wechsler, 1975). These results were confirmed in inbred E rats (Osske *et al.*, 1972).

None of 38 offspring of 6 Wistar rats treated twice orally with 150 mg/kg bw ethylurea, 100 mg/kg bw sodium nitrite and 200 mg/kg bw ascorbic acid on the 22nd day of gestation died of malignant tumours within 295 days after birth. However, administration of ascorbic acid had no influence on the carcinogenic activity of already formed NEU (Ivankovic *et al.*, 1973). An inhibitory effect of sodium ascorbate on transplacental carcinogenesis by ethylurea and sodium nitrite was also found in Syrian golden hamsters (Rustia, 1975).

Daily intragastric administration of 100 mg/kg bw ethylurea and 50 mg/kg bw sodium nitrite to adult Syrian golden hamsters for 40 days resulted in benign and malignant tumours in a broad spectrum of organs, including the forestomach, vagina, ovaries and peripheral nervous system, in 55/64 treated animals. Multiple neoplasms (average, more than 3/animal) were seen in 85% of the hamsters; the tumours had an average latency of 46 weeks (Rustia, 1974).

Four consecutive daily i.g. doses of 100 mg/kg bw ethylurea and 50 mg/kg bw sodium nitrite administered from day 12-15 of gestation to 8 Syrian golden hamsters induced neurogenic tumours in the peripheral nervous system of the offspring. Females had a higher tumour incidence, a greater multiplicity of neurogenic tumours and shorter latencies than the males (Rustia & Schenken, 1976; Rustia & Shubik, 1974).

Feeding ethylurea and sodium nitrite to pregnant rabbits on days 17, 18 and 19 of gestation resulted in the induction of kidney tumours in the progeny (Fox *et al.*, 1977).

(g) Factors that modify carcinogenicity in animals

BD rats were given simultaneous s.c. administrations of 10 mg/kg bw NEU and 1 mg/kg bw anhydrous cobalt chloride or anhydrous cupric sulphate once weekly; all of 24 rats treated with cobalt and NEU developed local sarcomas at the injection site, and, in addition, 2 malignant neurinomas were seen. Of those treated with copper and NEU, 4 animals developed local sarcomas. A single i.p. injection of 25-90 mg/kg bw NEU with 5-10 mg/kg bw anhydrous cupric sulphate or anhydrous cobalt chloride caused local sarcomas in the abdominal cavity in 6/20 animals. Rats treated with NEU or with cobalt or copper salts alone did not develop local sarcomas (Ivankovic *et al.*, 1972).

When the offspring of Sprague-Dawley rats given a single oral dose of 30 mg/kg bw NEU on day 19 of gestation were treated postnatally with cyclophosphamide or Freunds' adjuvant an increased incidence of mammary tumours was observed (Schmähl *et al.*, 1974).

A reduction in the incidence of neurogenic tumours was observed in the offspring of Sprague-Dawley rats given X-irradiation (200 rads) on day 15 or 16 of gestation and injected i.p. with 10 mg/kg bw NEU 1-4 days later. Most of the 60 offspring of irradiated and NEU-treated mothers exhibited microcephaly and other malformations, and 10 (16.7%) developed neurogenic tumours by 15 months of age, in comparison with a tumour rate of 46/74 (62.2%) in the offspring of mothers treated with NEU alone (Warkany *et al.*, 1976).

3.2 Other relevant biological data

(a) Experimental systems

Toxic effects

The acute LD_{50} of NEU in rats was 240 mg/kg bw after administration by s.c. or i.v. injection, and 300 mg/kg bw after oral administration (Druckrey, 1972; Druckrey *et al.*, 1967, 1970a).

The major toxic effects result from severe damage to haematopoietic, lymphoid and other tissues with a rapid rate of cell turnover (Magee & Barnes, 1967; Magee & Swann, 1969).

Embryotoxicity and teratogenicity

Female rats were given a single i.v. dose of 20, 40, 60, 70 or 80 mg/kg bw NEU on day 15 of gestation; 80 mg/kg bw caused the death of 50% of the foetuses, and all surviving foetuses showed malformed extremities. With 20 mg/kg bw, no malformations could be detected; doses of 40-70 mg/kg bw induced distinct dose-related abnormalities of the paws (Druckrey *et al.*, 1966; Ivankovic & Druckrey, 1968).

I.v. doses of 20 mg/kg bw NEU to rats on day 17 of gestation resulted in microcephaly (Alexandrov & Napalkov, 1976).

When rats were treated with a single dose of 20 mg/kg bw NEU by i.v. injection during pregnancy, peaks of embryonic mortality were noted on days 4 (40%) and 9 (25%) of gestation. Teratogenic effects, such as hydrocephaly and exencephaly, were observed in about 60% of the surviving foetuses that had been exposed to NEU on days 9 and 10 of gestation (Alexandrov, 1973).

In 15 mice treated on day 8 of gestation with i.p. doses of 60 mg/kg bw NEU and examined on day 14 of gestation, embryolethality was 57% in

C57L/J mice and 20% in DBA/2J mice; most of the surviving embryos had mainly eye defects, hydrocephaly, exencephaly, spina bifida and some skeletal abnormalities. When exposed on day 12 of gestation, 76% of C57BL/6J and 59% of C57L/J foetuses had skeletal malformations after birth (Diwan, 1974).

In Syrian golden hamsters, i.p. injections of 60 mg/kg bw NEU on day 8 of gestation resulted in 53% resorptions and 94% malformations in the live embryos on day 15 of gestation (Givelber & DiPaolo, 1969).

Absorption, distribution and excretion

NEU was rapidly lost from the blood after its i.v. injection, with a half-life of 5-6 minutes (Swann & Magee, 1971). The high chemical reactivity of NEU renders it unlikely that enzymic catalysis is involved in its decomposition.

Metabolism

NEU is a direct alkylating agent and has been shown to ethylate nucleic acids both *in vitro* and *in vivo* (Goth & Rajewsky, 1974a,b; Lawley, 1974; Pegg, 1977; Singer, 1975; Swann & Magee, 1971). 7-Ethylguanine, O^6-ethylguanine, 3-ethyladenine and 7-ethyladenine and ethylphosphate triesters have been detected in rat tissues after administration of NEU *in vivo* (Goth & Rajewsky, 1974a,b; Singer & Fraenkel-Conrat, 1975; Swann & Magee, 1971). O^6-Ethylguanine was lost from DNA of brain (a target organ) much more slowly than from liver DNA, whereas no such difference was observed for the rate of loss of the other ethylated products (Goth & Rajewsky, 1974a,b).

Administration of NEU led to an altered sedimentation pattern in alkaline sucrose gradients of DNA from brain (Hadjiolov & Venkov, 1975) and liver (Cox *et al.*, 1973).

Decomposition of NEU yields cyanate, which reacts with proteins. This carbamoylation has been found to be important in the toxicity of NEU to cells in culture (Knox, 1976).

Mutagenicity and other short-term tests

NEU induces mutations in *Salmonella typhimurium*, *Escherichia coli*, lower and higher plants, in *Drosophila melanogaster* and in other organisms (for reviews, see Montesano & Bartsch, 1976; Neale, 1976). A mutation yield of 85% X-linked recessive lethal and visible mutations was seen in *Drosophila* exposed to 4-5 mg NEU (Rapoport, 1962).

Treatment of cultured human fibroblasts with NEU induced both chromatid and chromosome aberrations (Sanger & Eisen, 1976). The effect of NEU on human chromosomes from cultured blood lymphocytes and on rat and mouse bone-marrow chromosomes *in vivo* was studied. The incidence of single chromatid and isochromatid breaks, exchanges and multiple breaks in human lymphocytes *in vitro* was dose-dependent at doses ranging from 25-200 μg/ml. Treatment of mice and rats with i.p. injections of 100 or 200 mg/kg bw produced similar lesions, the incidence of which was dependent on the dose and on the time of sampling after injection (Soukup & Au, 1975). I.p. doses of 50 and 100 mg/kg bw to mice produced chromosome aberrations in germ cells (Ramaiya, 1969).

Primary cell cultures derived from the brains of rats treated transplacentally with NEU *in vivo* were maintained for 200 days, and after long-term culture showed characteristics of transformation. These transformed cells, which were not present in cultures from control rats, induced tumours when transplanted back into newborn rats (Laerum & Rajewsky, 1975; Laerum *et al*., 1977).

(b) Humans

No data were available to the Working Group.

3.3 Case reports and epidemiological studies

No data were available to the Working Group.

4. Summary of Data Reported and Evaluation

4.1 Experimental data

N-Nitroso-*N*-ethylurea is carcinogenic in all animal species tested: mice, rats, Syrian golden hamsters, rabbits, opossums, pigs and monkeys. It produces benign and malignant tumours following its administration by different routes, including single oral doses; the main target organ appears to vary with the route of administration. Prenatal exposure to the substance has been shown to be particularly effective in producing tumours of the nervous system. In several studies, dose-response relationships were established.

4.2 Human data

No case reports or epidemiological studies were available to the Working Group. No information on the occurrence or use of *N*-nitroso-*N*-ethylurea was available.

4.3 Evaluation

There is *sufficient evidence* of a carcinogenic effect of *N*-nitroso-*N*-ethylurea in several experimental animal species. Although no epidemiological data or information on occurrence were available, *N*-nitroso-*N*-ethylurea should be regarded for practical purposes as if it were carcinogenic to humans.

5. References

Alexandrov, V.A. (1969) Uterine, vaginal and mammary tumours induced by nitrosoureas in pregnant rats. Nature (Lond.), 224, 1064-1065

Alexandrov, V.A. (1973) Embryotoxic and teratogenic effects of chemical carcinogens. In: Tomatis, L. & Mohr, U., eds, Transplacental Carcinogenesis, Lyon (IARC Scientific Publications No. 4), pp. 112-126

Alexandrov, V.A. & Napalkov, N.P. (1976) Experimental study of relationship between teratogenesis and carcinogenesis in the brain of the rat. Cancer Lett., 1, 345-350

Cox, R., Damjanov, I. & Irving, C.C. (1973) Damage and repair of hepatic DNA by ethylating carcinogens (Abstract No. 111). Proc. Amer. Ass. Cancer Res., 14, 28

Cravioto, H., Weiss, J.F., Weiss, E. de C., Goebel, H.H. & Ransohoff, J. (1973) Biological characteristics of peripheral nerve tumors induced with ethylnitrosourea. Acta neuropath. (Berl.), 23, 265-280

Cravioto, H.M., Weiss, J.F., Goebel, H.H., Weiss, E. de C. & Ransohoff, J.F. (1974) Preferential induction of central or peripheral nervous system tumors in rats by nitrosourea derivatives. J. Neuropath. exp. Neurol., 33, 595-615

Denlinger, R.H., Koestner, A. & Wechsler, W. (1974) Induction of neurogenic tumors in C3HeB/FeJ mice by nitrosourea derivatives: observations by light microscopy, tissue culture, and electron microscopy. Int. J. Cancer, 13, 559-571

Diwan, B.A. (1974) Strain-dependent teratogenic effects of 1-ethyl-1-nitrosourea in inbred strains of mice. Cancer Res., 34, 151-157

Diwan, B.A. & Meier, H. (1974) Strain- and age-dependent transplacental carcinogenesis by 1-ethyl-1-nitrosourea in inbred strains of mice. Cancer Res., 34, 764-770

Diwan, B.A., Meier, H. & Huebner, R.J. (1974) Transplacental effects of 1-ethyl-1-nitrosourea in inbred strains of mice. IV. Rapid tumor induction in strain crosses. J. nat. Cancer Inst., 52, 893-895

Druckrey, H. (1972) Organospecific carcinogenesis in the digestive tract. In: Nakahara, W., Takayama, S., Sugimura, T. & Odashima, S., eds, Topics in Chemical Carcinogenesis, Tokyo, University of Tokyo Press, pp. 73-103

Druckrey, H., Ivankovic, S. & Preussmann, R. (1966) Teratogenic and carcinogenic effects in the offspring after single injection of ethylnitrosourea to pregnant rats. Nature (Lond.), 210, 1378-1379

Druckrey, H., Preussmann, R., Ivankovic, S. & Schmähl, D. (1967) Organotrope carcinogene Wirkungen bei 65 verschiedenen *N*-Nitroso-Verbindungen an BD-Ratten. Z. Krebsforsch., 69, 103-201

Druckrey, H., Schagen, B. & Ivankovic, S. (1970a) Erzeugung neurogener Malignome durch einmalige Gabe von Äthyl- nitrosoharnstoff (ÄNH) an neugeborene und junge BD IX-Ratten. Z. Krebsforsch., 74, 141-161

Druckrey, H., Landschütz, C. & Ivankovic, S. (1970b) Transplacentare Erzeugung maligner Tumoren des Nervensystems. II. Äthyl-nitrosoharnstoff an 10 genetisch definierten Rattenstämmen. Z. Krebsforsch., 73, 371-386

Druckrey, H., Ivankovic, S. & Gimmy, J. (1973) Cancerogene Wirkung von Methyl- und Äthylnitrosoharnstoff (MNH und ÄNH) nach einmaliger intracerebraler bzw. intracarotidaler Injektion bei neugeborenen und jungen BD-Ratten. Z. Krebsforsch., 79, 282-297

Ezhakova, O.F. (1973) Effect of chemical mutagens on self-compatibility of white clover. In: Rapoport, I.A., ed., Proceedings of the All Union Conference on Chemical Mutagens, Utilization of Chemical Mutagens in Agriculture and Medicine, 1972, Moscow, Nauka, pp. 262-264 [Chem. Abstr., 80, 56080v]

Fine, D.H., Rounbehler, D.P., Silvergleid, A. & Ross, R. (1977) Trace analysis of polar and apolar *N*-nitroso compounds by combined high-performance liquid chromatography and thermal energy analysis. In: Tinbergen, B.J. & Krol, B., eds, Proceedings of the Second International Symposium on Nitrite in Meat Products, Zeist, 1976, Wageningen, Centre for Agricultural Publishing and Documentation, pp. 191-199

Fornatto, L. & Schiffer, D. (1972) *In vitro* culture observations on neurinoma induced experimentally in the rat by ethylnitrosourea. Acta neuropath. (Berl.), 20, 199-206

Fox, R.R., Diwan, B.A. & Meier, H. (1975) Transplacental induction of primary renal tumors in rabbits treated with 1-ethyl-1-nitrosourea. J. nat. Cancer Inst., 54, 1439-1448

Fox, R.R., Diwan, B.A. & Meier, H. (1977) Transplacental carcinogenic effects of combined treatment of ethylurea and sodium nitrite in rabbits. J. nat. Cancer Inst., 59, 427-429

Garrett, E.R., Goto, S. & Stubbins, J.F. (1965) Kinetics of solvolyses of various *N*-alkyl-*N*-nitrosoureas in neutral and alkaline solutions. J. pharm. Sci., 54, 119-123

Givelber, H.M. & DiPaolo, J.A. (1969) Teratogenic effects of *N*-ethyl-*N*-nitrosourea in the Syrian hamster. Cancer Res., 29, 1151-1155

Goth, R. & Rajewsky, M.F. (1974a) Persistence of *O*6-ethylguanine in rat-brain DNA: correlation with nervous system-specific carcinogenesis by ethylnitrosourea (elimination rates of ethylated bases/DNA repair/DNA replication/determinants of neoplastic transformation). Proc. nat. Acad. Sci. (Wash.), 71, 639-643

Goth, R. & Rajewsky, M.F. (1974b) Molecular and cellular mechanisms associated with pulse-carcinogenesis in the rat nervous system by ethylnitrosourea: ethylation of nucleic acids and elimination rates of ethylated bases from the DNA of different tissues. Z. Krebsforsch., 82, 37-64

Graw, J., Zeller, W.J. & Ivankovic, S. (1974) Entstehung von neurogenen Malignomen bei den Nachkommen von Sprague-Dawley Ratten nach perkutaner Applikation von Äthylnitrosoharnstoff (ÄNH) während der Tragzeit. Z. Krebsforsch., 81, 169-172

Grossi-Paoletti, E., Paoletti, P., Schiffer, D. & Fabiani, A. (1970) Experimental brain tumours induced in rats by nitrosourea derivatives. II. Morphological aspects of nitrosoethylurea tumours obtained by transplacental induction. J. neurol. Sci., 11, 573-581

Grossi-Paoletti, E., Paoletti, P., Pezzotta, S., Schiffer, D. & Fabiani, A. (1972a) Tumors of the nervous system induced by ethylnitrosourea administered either intracerebrally or subcutaneously to newborn rats. Morphological and biochemical characteristics. J. Neurosurg., 37, 580-590

Grossi-Paoletti, E., Pezzotta, S. & Paoletti, P. (1972b) Tumors of the nervous system induced in rats by intracerebral administration of ethylnitrosourea. Pharmacol. Res. Commun., 4, 201-212

Güthert, H., Jäckel, E.M. & Warzok, R. (1973) Zur karzinogenen Wirkung von *N*-Äthyl-*N*-nitrosoharnstoff (ÄNH) bei Kaninchen. Zbl. allg. Path., 117, 461-471

Hadjiolov, D. (1972) Thymic lymphoma and myeloid leukemia in the rat induced with ethylnitrosourea. Z. Krebsforsch., 77, 98-100

Hadjiolov, D. & Venkov, L. (1975) Strand breakage in rat brain DNA and its repair induced by ethylnitrosourea *in vivo*. Z. Krebsforsch., 84, 223-225

IARC (1972) IARC Monographs on the Evaluation of Carcinogenic Risk of Chemicals to Man, 1, Lyon, pp. 135-140

Ivankovic, S. (1969) Erzeugung von Genitalkrebs bei trächtigen Ratten. Arzneimittel-Forsch., 19, 1040-1041

Ivankovic, S. & Druckrey, H. (1968) Transplacentare Erzeugung maligner Tumoren des Nervensystems. I. Äthyl-nitroso-harnstoff (ÄNH) an BD IX-Ratten. Z. Krebsforsch., 71, 320-360

Ivankovic, S. & Preussmann, R. (1970) Transplazentare Erzeugung maligner Tumoren nach oraler Gabe von Äthylharnstoff und Nitrit an Ratten. Naturwissenschaften, 57, 460

Ivankovic, S., Druckrey, H. & Preussmann, R. (1966) Erzeugung neurogener Tumoren bei den Nachkommen nach einmaliger Injektion von Äthylnitrosoharnstoff an schwangere Ratten. Naturwissenschaften, 53, 410

Ivankovic, S., Zeller, W.J. & Schmähl, D. (1972) Steigerung der carcinogenen Wirkung von Äthyl-nitrosoharnstoff durch Schwermetalle. Naturwissenschaften, 59, 369

Ivankovic, S., Zeller, W.J., Schmähl, D. & Preussmann, R. (1973) Verhinderung der pränatal carcinogenen Wirkung von Äthylharnstoff und Nitrit durch Ascorbinsäure. Naturwissenschaften, 60, 525

Jänisch, W., Schreiber, D., Warzok, R. & Scholtze, P. (1977) Versuche mit den Kanzerogenen Methyl- und Äthylnitrosoharnstoff bei *Macaca mulatta*. Arch. Geschwulstforsch., 47, 123-126

Jones, E.L., Searle, C.E. & Smith, W.T. (1973) Tumours of the nervous system induced in rats by the neonatal administration of *N*-ethyl-*N*-nitrosourea. J. Path., 109, 123-139

Jurgelski, W., Jr, Hudson, P., Zimmerman, L.E., Falk, H.L. & Kotin, P. (1974) Induction of malignant intraocular medulloepitheliomas in opossums orally exposed to a chemical carcinogen (ethyl nitrosourea) early in postnatal life (Abstract No. 90). Amer. J. Path., 74, 40a

Jurgelski, W., Jr, Hudson, P.M., Falk, H.L. & Kotin, P. (1976) Embryonal neoplasms in the opossum: a new model for solid tumors of infancy and childhood. Science, 193, 328-332

Kleihues, P., Matsumoto, S., Wechsler, W. & Zülch, K.J. (1968) Morphologie und Wachstum der mit Äthylnitrosoharnstoff transplazentar erzeugten Tumoren des Nervensystems. Verh. dtsch. Ges. Path., 52, 372-380

Knox, P. (1976) Carcinogenic nitrosamides and cell cultures. Nature (Lond.), 259, 671-673

Koestner, A. & Wechsler, W. (1974) Induction of neurogenic- and non-neurogenic neoplasms by feeding precursors of methyl- and ethylnitrosourea to adult rats (Abstract No. 39). J. Neuropath. exp. Neurol., 33, 178

Koestner, A., Swenberg, J.A. & Wechsler, W. (1971) Transplacental production with ethylnitrosourea of neoplasms of the nervous system in Sprague-Dawley rats. Amer. J. Path., 63, 37-50

Koestner, A., Denlinger, R.H. & Wechsler, W. (1975) Induction of neurogenic and lymphoid neoplasms by the feeding of threshold levels of methyl- and ethylnitrosourea precursors to adult rats. Fd Cosmet. Toxicol., 13, 605-609

Koyama, T., Handa, J., Handa, H. & Matsumoto, S. (1972) Ethylnitrosourea-induced brain tumor in SD-JCL rats (Abstract No. 2290). Clin. Neurol. (Tokyo), 12, 95-104

Kupfer, M., Kupfer, G., Zintzsch, I., Juhls, H. & Ehrentraut, W. (1969) Hautmissbildungstumoren bei Ferkeln nach transplazentarer Einwirkung von Äthylnitrosoharnstoff. Beitrag zur Genese der Schweissdrüsen-adenome. Arch. Geschwulstforsch., 34, 25-33

Laerum, O.D. & Rajewsky, M.F. (1975) Neoplastic transformation of fetal rat brains cells in culture after exposure to ethylnitrosourea *in vivo*. J. nat. Cancer Inst., 55, 1177-1187

Laerum, O.D., Rajewsky, M.F., Schachner, M., Stavrou, D., Haglid, K.G. & Haugen, A. (1977) Phenotypic properties of neoplastic cell lines developed from fetal rat brain cells in culture after exposure to ethylnitrosourea *in vivo*. Z. Krebsforsch., 89, 273-295

Lawley, P.D. (1974) Some chemical aspects of dose-response relationships in alkylation mutagenesis. Mutation Res., 23, 283-295

Lombard, L.S. & Vesselinovitch, S.D. (1971) Pathogenesis of renal tumors in mice treated with ethylnitrosourea (Abstract No. 220). Proc. Amer. Ass. Cancer Res., 12, 55

Lombard, L.S., Rice, J.M. & Vesselinovitch, S.D. (1974) Renal tumors in mice: light microscopic observations of epithelial tumors induced by ethylnitrosourea. J. nat. Cancer Inst., 53, 1677-1685

Magee, P.N. & Barnes, J.M. (1967) Carcinogenic nitroso compounds. Adv. Cancer Res., 10, 163-246

Magee, P.N. & Swann, P.F. (1969) Nitroso compounds. Brit. med. Bull., 25, 240-244

McCalla, D.R., Reuvers, A. & Kitai, R. (1968) Inactivation of biologically active *N*-methyl-*N*-nitroso compounds in aqueous solution: effect of various conditions of pH and illumination. Canad. J. Biochem., 46, 807-811

Mennel, H.D. & Zülch, K.J. (1972) Zur Morphologie transplacentar erzeugter neurogener Tumoren beim Goldhamsters. Acta neuropath. (Berl.), 21, 194-203

Mirvish, S.S., Karlowski, K., Sams, J.P. & Arnold, S.D. (1978) Studies related to nitrosamide formation: nitrosation in solvent:water and solvent systems, nitrosomethylurea formation in the rat stomach, and analysis of a fish product for ureas. In: Walker, E.A., Castegnaro, M., Griciute, L. & Lyle, R.E., eds, Environmental Aspects of *N*-Nitroso Compounds, Lyon (IARC Scientific Publications No. 19) (in press)

Montesano, R. & Bartsch, H. (1976) Mutagenic and carcinogenic *N*-nitroso compounds: possible environmental hazards. Mutation Res., 32, 179-228

Montgomery, J.A., Johnston, T.P., Thomas, H.J., Piper, J.R. & Temple, C., Jr (1977) The use of microparticulate reversed-phase packing in high pressure liquid chromatography of compounds of biological interest. Adv. Chromatogr., 15, 169-195

Neale, S. (1976) Mutagenicity of nitrosamides and nitrosamidines in micro-organisms and plants. Mutation Res., 32, 229-266

Nikiforova, I.L. (1973) Use of chemical mutagens in the breeding of fast-ripening forms of barley under the conditions of the Karelian ASSR. In: Rapoport, I.A., ed., Proceedings of the All Union Conference on Chemical Mutagens, Utilization of Chemical Mutagens in Agriculture and Medicine, 1972, Moscow, Nauka, pp. 210-214 [Chem. Abstr., 80, 56078a]

Ogiu, T., Nakadate, M. & Odashima, S. (1974) Rapid and selective induction of erythroleukemia in female Donryu rats by 1-ethyl-1-nitrosourea. Gann, 65, 377

Ogiu, T., Nakadate, M. & Odashima, S. (1976) Rapid and selective induction of erythroleukemia in female Donryu rats by continuous oral administration of 1-ethyl-1-nitrosourea. Cancer Res., 36, 3043-3046

Osske, G., Warzok, R. & Schneider, J. (1972) Diaplazentare Tumorinduktion durch endogen gebildeten *N*-Äthyl-*N*-nitrosoharnstoff bei Ratten. Arch. Geschwulstforsch., 40, 244-247

Pegg, A.E. (1977) Formation and metabolism of alkylated nucleosides: possible role in carcinogenesis by nitroso compounds and alkylating agents. Adv. Cancer Res., 25, 195-269

Pelfrene, A., Mirvish, S.S. & Garcia, H. (1975) Carcinogenic action of ethylnitroso cyanamide (ENC), 1-nitrosohydantoin (NH), and ethyl-nitrosourea (ENU) in the rat (Abstract No. 466). Proc. Amer. Ass. Cancer Res., 16, 117

Ramadan, M.A. & Wechsler, W. (1975) Tansplacental induction of neurogenic tumors in BD IX rats by intragastric administration of ethylnitrosourea precursors. Z. Krebsforsch., 84, 177-187

Ramaiya, L.K. (1969) The cytogenetic effect of *N*-nitrosoethylurea, hydroxylamine and X-rays on the germ-cells of male mice. Genetika, 5, 74-86

Rapoport, I.A. (1962) 85% Mutation in the sex chromosome under the influence of nitrosoethylurea. Dokl. Biol. Sci., 146, 1044-1046

Rice, J.M. (1969) Transplacental carcinogenesis in mice by 1-ethyl-1-nitrosourea. Ann. N.Y. Acad. Sci., 163, 813-827

Rice, J.M., London, W.T., Palmer, A.E., Sly, D.L. & Williams, G.M. (1977) Direct and transplacental carcinogenesis by ethylnitrosourea in the patas monkey (*Erythrocebus patas*) (Abstract No. 210). Proc. Amer. Ass. Cancer Res., 18, 53

Rustia, M. (1974) Multiple carcinogenic effects of the ethylnitrosourea precursors ethylurea and sodium nitrite in hamsters. Cancer Res., 34, 3232-3244

Rustia, M. (1975) Inhibitory effect of sodium ascorbate on ethylurea and sodium nitrite carcinogenesis and negative findings in progeny after intestinal inoculation of precursors into pregnant hamsters. J. nat. Cancer Inst., 55, 1389-1394

Rustia, M. & Schenken, J. (1976) Transplacental effects of ethylnitrosourea precursors ethylurea and sodium nitrite in hamsters. Z. Krebsforsch., 85, 201-217

Rustia, M. & Shubik, P. (1974) Prenatal induction of neurogenic tumors in hamsters by precursors ethylurea and sodium nitrite. J. nat. Cancer Inst., 52, 605-608

Samoshkin, E.N. & Rodyankov, E.P. (1973) Effect of some chemical mutagens on the growth of red-leafed ash seedlings. Izv. Vyssh. Ucheb. Zaved., Les. Zh., 16, 14-16 [Chem. Abstr., 80, 23096b]

Sanger, W.G. & Eisen, J.D. (1976) Clastogenic effects of methylnitrosourea and ethylnitrosourea on chromosomes from human fibroblast cell lines. Mutation Res., 34, 415-426

Schmähl, D., Mundt, D. & Schmidt, K.G. (1974) Experimental investigations on the influence upon the chemical carcinogenesis. 1st communication: studies with ethylnitroso-urea. Z. Krebsforsch., 82, 91-100

Searle, C.E. & Jones, E.L. (1976) The multipotential carcinogenic action of *N*-ethyl-*N*-nitrosourea administered neonatally to mice. Brit. J. Cancer, 33, 612-625

Searle, C.E., Jones, E.L. & Smith, W.T. (1972) Induction of brain tumours in high yield by administration of *N*-ethyl-*N*-nitrosourea to newborn rats. Experientia, 28, 1452-1453

Singer, B. (1975) The chemical effects of nucleic acid alkylation and their relation to mutagenesis and carcinogenesis. Prog. Nucleic Acid Res. mol. Biol., 15, 219-284

Singer, B. & Fraenkel-Conrat, H. (1975) The specificity of different classes of ethylating agents toward various sites in RNA. Biochemistry, 14, 772-782

Singer, G.M., Singer, S.S. & Schmidt, D.G. (1977) A nitrosamide-specific detector for use with high-pressure liquid chromatography. J. Chromat., 133, 59-66

Soukup, S.W. & Au, W. (1975) The effect of ethylnitrosourea on chromosome aberrations *in vitro* and *in vivo*. Humangenetik, 29, 319-328

Stavrou, D. & Lübbe, I. (1975) Transplazentare Induktion von Nierentumoren beim Kaninchen durch Äthylnitrosoharnstoff (Abstract No. 12). Zbl. alg. Path., 119, 320

Stavrou, D., Hänichen, T. & Wriedt-Lübbe, I. (1975) Oncogene Wirkung von Äthylnitrosoharnstoff beim Kaninchen während der pränatalen Periode. Z. Krebsforsch., 84, 207-215

Stavrou, D., Dahme, E. & Schröder, B. (1977) Transplacentare neuroonkogene Wirkung von Äthylnitrosoharnstoff beim Kaninchen während der frühen Graviditätsphase. Z. Krebsforsch., 89, 331-339

Swann, P.F. & Magee, P.N. (1971) Nitrosamine-induced carcinogenesis. The alkylation of *N*-7 of guanine of nucleic acids of the rat by diethylnitrosamine, *N*-ethyl-*N*-nitrosourea and ethyl methanesulphonate. Biochem. J., 125, 841-847

Swenberg, J.A., Koestner, A., Wechsler, W. & Denlinger, R.H. (1972) Quantitative aspects of transplacental tumor induction with ethylnitrosourea in rats. Cancer Res., 32, 2656-2660

Thomas, C. & Kersting, G. (1968) Pathomorphologische Vergleichsuntersuchungen diaplazentar und postnatal erzeugter Hirntumoren. Verh. dtsch. Ges. Path., 52, 384-388

Tomatis, L., Ponomarkov, V. & Turusov, V. (1977) Effects of ethylnitrosourea administration during pregnancy on three subsequent generations of BDVI rats. Int. J. Cancer, 19, 240-248

Veleminský, J., Osterman-Golkar, S. & Ehrenberg, L. (1970) Reaction rates and biological action of *N*-methyl- and *N*-ethyl-*N*-nitrosourea. Mutation Res., 10, 169-174

Vesselinovitch, S.D. & Lombard, L.S. (1971) Broad spectrum carcinogenicity of ethylnitrosourea in the newborn and infant mice (Abstract No. 221). Proc. Amer. Ass. Cancer Res., 12, 56

Vesselinovitch, S.D., Rao, K.V.N., Mihailovich, N., Rice, J.M. & Lombard, L.S. (1974) Development of broad spectrum of tumors by ethylnitrosourea in mice and the modifying role of age, sex and strain. Cancer Res., 34, 2530-2538

Warkany, J., Mandybur, T.I. & Kalter, H. (1976) Oncogenic response of rats with X-ray-induced microcephaly to transplacental ethylnitrosourea. J. nat. Cancer Inst., 56, 59-64

Wechsler, W., Kleihues, P., Matsumoto, S., Zülch, K.J., Ivankovic, S., Preussmann, R. & Druckrey, H. (1969) Pathology of experimental neurogenic tumors chemically induced during prenatal and postnatal life. Ann. N.Y. Acad. Sci., 159, 360-408

Wechsler, W., Rice, J.M., Vesselinovitch, S.D. & Arai, T. (1974) Perinatale Tumorinduktion mit Äthylnitrosoharnstoff: Ein Beitrag zur Frage der Organotropie alkylierender Resorptivkanzerogene bei verschiedenen Mäusestämmen (Abstract No. 13). Verh. dtsch. Ges. Path., 58, 546

Werner, E.A. (1919) XCIV. The constitution of carbamides. IX. The interaction of nitrous acid and mono-substituted ureas. The preparation of diazomethane, diazoethane, diazo-*n*-butane, and diazoisopentane from the respective nitrosoureas. J. chem. Soc., 115, 1093-1102

N-NITROSOFOLIC ACID

1. Chemical and Physical Data

1.1 Synonyms and trade names

Chem. Abstr. Services Reg. No.: 29291-35-8

Chem. Abstr. Name: *N*-{4-[(2-Amino-3,4-dihydro-4-oxo-6-pteridinyl)methyl]amino}benzoyl-*N*-nitroso-L-glutamic acid

N-Nitroso-*N*-pteroyl-L-glutamic acid

1.2 Structural and molecular formulae and weight

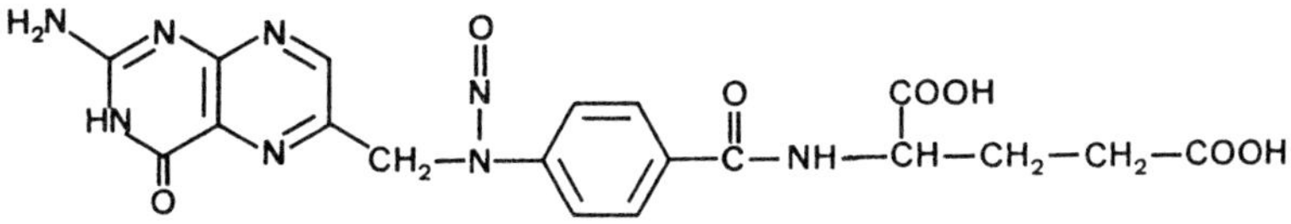

$C_{19}H_{18}N_8O_7$ Mol. wt: 470

1.3 Chemical and physical properties of the pure substance

(a) Description: White crystals

(b) Solubility: Slightly soluble in water and in polar organic solvents; very soluble in aqueous alkalis

1.4 Technical products and impurities

No data were available to the Working Group.

2. Production, Use, Occurrence and Analysis

2.1 Production and use

(a) Production

N-Nitrosofolic acid has been prepared for laboratory use by the reaction of sodium nitrite with a solution of folic acid in hydrochloric acid (Cosulich, 1951; Cosulich & Smith, 1949).

No evidence was found that *N*-nitrosofolic acid has been produced commercially.

(b) Use

No data were available to the Working Group.

2.2 Occurrence

No data were available to the Working Group.

2.3 Analysis

No data were available to the Working Group.

3. Biological Data Relevant to the Evaluation of Carcinogenic Risk to Man

3.1 Carcinogenicity and related studies in animals

Intraperitoneal injection

Newborn mouse: A group of (C57Bl/6JxC3HeB/FeJ)F_1 mice received 125 mg/kg bw *N*-nitrosofolic acid suspended in trioctanoin intraperitoneally on days 1, 4 and 7 after birth; the experiment was terminated at 85 weeks. Of 14 male animals that lived 50 or more weeks (12 survivors at 79 weeks), 3 developed lung adenocarcinomas (first tumour at 79 weeks), 1 a liver-cell carcinoma (85 weeks), and 1 a neurofibrosarcoma (79 weeks). Of 15 females that lived 50 or more weeks (13 survivors at 79 weeks), 1 had a lung adenocarcinoma (84 weeks), and 1 had lesions described as 'liver-cell hyperplasia'. In the control group, which received 3 x 5 ml/kg bw trioctanoin intraperitoneally, 1/12 females had a liver-cell carcinoma and 2/14 males exhibited 'liver-cell hyperplasia'; no lung tumours were observed (Wogan *et al.*, 1975) [The increased incidence of tumours is not statistically significant ($P>0.05$)].

3.2 Other relevant biological data

(a) Experimental systems

Toxic effects

The LD_{50} of single i.p. injections of *N*-nitrosofolic acid given to mice 24 hours after birth was estimated to be 330 mg/kg bw (Wogan *et al.*, 1975).

No data on the embryotoxicity, teratogenicity or metabolism of this compound were available to the Working Group.

Mutagenicity and other short-term tests

N-Nitrosofolic acid was mutagenic in *Salmonella typhimurium* TA 1535, TA 1538, TA 98 and TA 100 in the presence of a rat liver microsomal fraction (Purchase *et al.*, 1976) [Full details of the procedure were not given].

(b) Humans

No data were available to the Working Group.

3.3 Case reports and epidemiological studies

No data were available to the Working Group.

4. Comments on Data Reported and Evaluation

4.1 Experimental data

N-Nitrosofolic acid has been tested only in newborn mice by intraperitoneal injection, with inconclusive results.

4.2 Human data

No case reports or epidemiological studies were available to the Working Group. No data on the occurrence or use of this material were available which would permit the identification of exposed groups.

4.3 Evaluation

No evaluation of the carcinogenicity of *N*-nitrosofolic acid could be made on the basis of the available data.

5. References

Cosulich, D.B. (1951) Nitroso derivatives of substituted pteridines. US Patent 2,537,006, 9 January (to American Cyanamid Co.) [Chem. Abstr., 45, 5194]

Cosulich, D.B. & Smith, J.M., Jr (1949) N^{10}-Nitrosopteroylglutamic acid. J. Amer. chem. Soc., 71, 3574

Purchase, I.F.H., Longstaff, E., Ashby, J., Styles, J.A., Anderson, D., Lefevre, P.A. & Westwood, F.R. (1976) Evaluation of six short term tests for detecting organic chemical carcinogens and recommendations for their use. Nature (Lond.), 264, 624-627

Wogan, G.N., Paglialunga, S., Archer, M.C. & Tannenbaum, S.R. (1975) Carcinogenicity of nitrosation products of ephedrine, sarcosine, folic acid, and creatinine. Cancer Res., 35, 1981-1984

N-NITROSOMETHYLETHYLAMINE

1. Chemical and Physical Data

1.1 Synonyms and trade names

Chem. Abstr. Services Reg. No.: 10595-95-6

Chem. Abstr. Name: *N*-Methyl-*N*-nitroso-ethamine

N,N-Methylethylnitrosamine; NEMA; NMEA

1.2 Structural and molecular formulae and weight

$$O{=}N{-}N(CH_3){-}CH_2{-}CH_3$$

$C_3H_8N_2O$ Mol. wt: 88.1

1.3 Chemical and physical properties of the pure substance

(a) Description: Yellow liquid

(b) Boiling-point: 163°C (747 mm); 70°C (35 mm); 57-58°C (12 mm)

(c) Density: d_4^{18} 0.9448

(d) Spectroscopy data: λ_{max} 230 and 335 nm (E_1^1 = 886 and 9) in water (Druckrey *et al.*, 1967); mass spectroscopy data are given by Pensabene *et al.* (1972) and Rainey *et al.* (1978).

(e) Solubility: Soluble in water (30%) and in organic solvents and lipids

(f) Volatility: Can be steam-distilled

(g) Stability: Stable at room temperature for more than 14 days in neutral or alkaline aqueous solutions in the dark (Druckrey *et al.*, 1967); slightly less stable in acidic solutions; light sensitive, especially to ultra-violet light

(h) Reactivity: Strong oxidants (peracids) oxidize it to the corresponding nitramine; can be reduced to the corresponding hydrazine and/or amine; relatively resistant to hydrolysis but can be split by hydrogen bromide in acetic acid (Eisenbrand & Preussmann, 1970). Photochemically reactive (Fridman *et al.*, 1971)

1.4 Technical products and impurities

No data were available to the Working Group.

2. Production, Use, Occurrence and Analysis

2.1 Production and use

(a) Production

N-Nitrosomethylethylamine (NMEA) has been prepared by the reaction of sodium nitrite with a solution of *N,N'*-dimethyl-*N,N'*-diethyl methylenediamine in concentrated hydrochloric acid (Graymore, 1938). It can also be prepared by the reaction of sodium nitrite with methylethylamine at 60°C (Druckrey *et al.*, 1967).

No evidence was found that NMEA has been produced commercially.

(b) Use

No data were available to the Working Group.

2.2 Occurrence

(a) Tobacco smoke condensate

McCormick *et al.* (1973) reported the presence of NMEA in 7/11 samples of tobacco smoke condensate at levels of 1-40 ng/cigarette. Klimsch *et al.* (1976) reported levels of up to 25 ng/cigarette.

Hoffmann *et al.* (1974) found up to 35 ng/cigarette in mainstream smoke, and Brunnemann & Hoffmann (1978) and Brunnemann *et al.* (1977) up to 30 ng/cigarette and 75 ng/cigar in sidestream smoke.

(b) Food

NMEA was found at levels of 1.1 μg/kg[1] in 1/6 samples of smoked horsemeat and at levels of 0.2 μg/kg in 1/5 luncheon meats (Groenen *et al.*, 1977). Gough (1978) reported 0.2 μg/kg[1] NMEA in bacon and chicken and in complete meals containing mushrooms, and 0.1 μg/kg[1] in cured meats. Using procedures which would have detected levels above 1 μg/kg, no evidence was found that this compound occurs in other foodstuffs (Groenen *et al.*, 1976).

2.3 Analysis

An IARC manual gives selected methods for the analysis of volatile *N*-nitrosamines, including *N*-nitrosomethylethylamine (Preussmann *et al.*, 1978).

3. Biological Data Relevant to the Evaluation of Carcinogenic Risk to Man

3.1 Carcinogenicity and related studies in animals

Oral administration

Rat: A group of 15 female BD rats was given *N*-nitrosomethylethylamine (NMEA) in the drinking-water at doses of 1 or 2 mg/kg bw/day. Nine of 15 animals developed hepatocellular carcinomas, and 1 animal a fibrosarcoma of the vagina. The average induction time was 500 or 360 days, respectively; the average total dose to induce tumours in 50% of animals was 0.42 or 0.75 g/kg bw, respectively (Druckrey *et al.*, 1967).

3.2 Other relevant biological data

(a) Experimental systems

Toxic effects

The oral LD_{50} of NMEA in BD rats was 90 mg/kg bw (Druckrey *et al.*, 1967).

---

[1]These results were not confirmed by mass spectroscopy (see also 'General Remarks on the Substances Considered', p. 40).

No data on the embryotoxicity, teratogenicity, metabolism or mutagenicity of this compound were available to the Working Group.

(b) Humans

No data were available to the Working Group.

3.3 Case reports and epidemiological studies

No data were available to the Working Group.

4. Summary of Data Reported and Evaluation

4.1 Experimental data

N-Nitrosomethylethylamine is carcinogenic in rats after its oral administration, the only species and route tested: it produces hepatocellular carcinomas.

4.2 Human data

No case reports or epidemiological studies were available to the Working Group. Available information on occurrence suggests that the general population may be exposed sporadically to low levels of *N*-nitrosomethylethylamine; however, no exposed group suitable for an epidemiological investigation has yet been identified. Reports suggest that tobacco smokers may be exposed to *N*-nitrosomethylethylamine together with other *N*-nitroso compounds.

4.3 Evaluation

There is *sufficient evidence* of a carcinogenic effect of *N*-nitrosomethylethylamine in one experimental animal species. No epidemiological data were available.

5. References

Brunnemann, K.D. & Hoffmann, D. (1978) Chemical studies on tobacco smoke. LIX. Analysis of volatile nitrosamines in tobacco smoke and polluted indoor environments. In: Walker, E.A., Castegnaro, M., Griciute, L. & Lyle, R.E., eds, Environmental Aspects of *N*-Nitroso Compounds, Lyon (IARC Scientific Publications No. 19) (in press)

Brunnemann, K.D., Yu, L. & Hoffmann, D. (1977) Assessment of carcinogenic volatile *N*-nitrosamines in tobacco and in mainstream and sidestream smoke from cigarettes. Cancer Res., 37, 3218-3222

Druckrey, H., Preussmann, R., Ivankovic, S. & Schmähl, D. (1967) Organotrope carcinogene Wirkungen bei 65 verschiedenen *N*-Nitroso-Verbindungen an BD-Ratten. Z. Krebsforsch., 69, 103-201

Eisenbrand, G. & Preussmann, R. (1970) Eine neue Methode zur kolorimetrischen Bestimmung von Nitrosaminen nach Spaltung der *N*-Nitrosogruppe mit Bromwasserstoff in Eisessig. Arzneimittel-Forsch., 20, 1513-1517

Fridman, A.L., Mukhametshin, F.M. & Novikov, S.S. (1971) Advances in the chemistry of aliphatic *N*-nitrosamines. Russ. chem. Rev., 40, 34-50

Gough, T.A. (1978) An examination of some foodstuff for trace amounts of volatile nitrosamines using the thermal energy analyser. In: Walker, E.A., Castegnaro, M., Griciute, L. & Lyle, R.E., eds, Environmental Aspects of *N*-Nitroso Compounds, Lyon (IARC Scientific Publications No. 19) (in press)

Graymore, J. (1938) The cyclic methyleneamines. Hydrolysis of quaternary compounds. Preparation of aliphatic secondary amines. I. J. chem. Soc., Part II, 1311-1313

Groenen, P.J., Jonk, R.J.G., van Ingen, C. & ten Noever de Brauw, M.C. (1976) Determination of eight volatile nitrosamines in thirty cured meat products with capillary gas chromatography-high-resolution mass spectrometry: the presence of nitrosodiethylamine and the absence of nitrosopyrrolidine. In: Walker, E.A., Bogovski, P. & Griciute, L., eds, Environmental *N*-Nitroso Compounds Analysis and Formation, Lyon (IARC Scientific Publications No. 14), pp. 321-331

Groenen, P.J., de Cock-Bethbeder, M.W., Jonk, R.J.G. & van Ingen, C. (1977) Further studies on the occurrence of volatile *N*-nitrosamines in meat products by combined gas chromatography and mass spectrometry. In: Tinbergen, B.J. & Krol, B., eds, Proceedings of the 2nd International Symposium on Nitrite in Meat Products, Zeist, 1976, Wageningen, Centre for Agricultural Publishing and Documentation, pp. 227-237

Hoffmann, D., Rathkamp, G. & Liu, Y.Y. (1974) Chemical studies on tobacco smoke. XXVI. On the isolation and identification of volatile and non-volatile *N*-nitrosamines and hydrazines in cigarette smoke. In: Bogovski, P. & Walker, E.A., eds, *N*-Nitroso Compounds in the Environment, Lyon (IARC Scientific Publications No. 9), pp. 159-165

Klimsch, H.-J., Stadler, L. & Brahm, S. (1976) Quantitative Bestimmung flüchtiger Nitrosamine in Zigarettenrauchkondensat. Z. Lebensmittel-Untersuch., 162, 131-138

McCormick, A., Nicholson, M.J., Baylis, M.A. & Underwood, J.G. (1973) Nitrosamines in cigarette smoke condensate. Nature (Lond.), 244, 237-238

Pensabene, J.W., Fiddler, W., Dooley, C.J., Doerr, R.C. & Wasserman, A.E. (1972) Spectral and gas chromatographic characteristics of some *N*-nitrosamines. J. agric. Fd Chem., 20, 274-277

Preussmann, R., Walker, E.A., Wasserman, A.E. & Castegnaro, M., eds (1978) Environmental Carcinogens - Selected Methods of Analysis, Vol. 1, Nitrosamines, Lyon (IARC Scientific Publications No. 18) (in press)

Rainey, W.T., Christie, W.H. & Lijinsky, W. (1978) Mass spectrometry of *N*-nitrosamines. Biomed. Mass Spectrom. (in press)

N-NITROSO-*N*-METHYLUREA

This substance was considered previously by an IARC Working Group, in December 1971 (IARC, 1972). Since that time new data have become available, and these have been incorporated into the monograph and taken into account in the present evaluation.

1. Chemical and Physical Data

1.1 Synonyms and trade names

Chem. Abstr. Services Reg. No.: 684-93-5

Chem. Abstr. Name: *N*-Methyl-*N*-nitrosourea

Methyl nitrosourea; 1-methyl-1-nitrosourea; MNU; NMH; NMU; *N*-nitroso-*N*-methylcarbamide; nitrosomethylurea; NSC 23909

1.2 Structural and molecular formulae and weight

$O=N-N(CH_3)-C(=O)-NH_2$

$C_2H_5N_3O_2$ Mol. wt: 103.1

1.3 Chemical and physical properties of the pure substance

(a) Description: Pale-yellow crystals

(b) Melting-point: 124°C (decomposition) (Druckrey *et al.*, 1967)

(c) Spectroscopy data: λ_{max} 231 nm (E^1_1 = 571) in water (Druckrey *et al.*, 1967)

(d) Solubility: Soluble in water (approximately 1.4%) and in polar organic solvents; insoluble in non-polar organic solvents

(e) Stability: Decomposes to diazomethane in alkaline solutions; stability in aqueous solutions is pH-dependent (20°C) (Druckrey *et al.*, 1967):

pH	4.0	6.0	7.0	8.0	9.0
half-life (hrs)	125	24	1.2	0.1	0.03

The pure compound is sensitive to humidity and light and should be refrigerated for storage.

(f) Reactivity: The compound is highly reactive (Garrett *et al.*, 1965; McCalla *et al.*, 1968). Reaction rates with various biologically important nucleophiles have been measured (Veleminský *et al.*, 1970).

1.4 Technical products and impurities

No data were available to the Working Group.

2. Production, Use, Occurrence and Analysis

2.1 Production and use

For background information on this section, see preamble, p. 22.

(a) Production

N-Nitroso-*N*-methylurea (NMU) was first prepared by Brüning in 1889 by the reaction of sodium nitrite with an aqueous solution of methylurea nitrate (Prager *et al.*, 1922). Although NMU is available in small quantities for research purposes, no evidence was found that it has been produced in significant commercial quantities.

(b) Use

NMU has commonly been used for the laboratory synthesis of diazomethane, but it has been largely replaced by other reagents such as *N*-nitroso-*N*-methyl-*para*-toluenesulphonamide.

NMU has been studied for use as a cancer chemotherapy agent by a number of investigators. A review was recently published in connection with a clinical study of its use in combination with cyclophosphamide

Kolarič, 1977). It has also been studied for its mutagenic effects on various plants (Kerkadze *et al.*, 1974; Nikiforova, 1972; Zhuravel & Shlyapunov, 1972).

2.2 Occurrence

No data were available to the Working Group.

2.3 Analysis

NMU is labile, and this complicates its analysis. High-pressure liquid chromatography conditions for *N*-nitrosoureas have been reviewed by Montgomery *et al.* (1977). Selective detectors used for analysis of this compound include those of Fine *et al.* (1977) and Singer *et al.* (1977). A method for the analysis of alkylureas in fish has been developed (Mirvish *et al.*, 1978).

3. Biological Data Relevant to the Evaluation of Carcinogenic Risk to Man

3.1 Carcinogenicity and related studies in animals

(a) Oral administration

Rat: In a lifetime feeding study, doses of 8 and 4 mg/kg bw/day *N*-nitroso-*N*-methylurea (NMU) produced squamous-cell carcinomas of the forestomach at cumulative doses of 700-1400 mg/kg bw (Druckrey *et al.*, 1961, 1967). Carcinomas of the forestomach were seen at doses of 10 mg/kg bw given once every 2 weeks and 20 mg/kg bw given once every 4 weeks over a period of 9 months; malignant tumours of the brain (sarcomas, gliomas) and the peripheral nervous system (described as neurosarcomas) were also observed (Schreiber & Jänisch, 1967). Continuous administration of NMU in the drinking-water produced tumours of the brain, mainly gliomas, and one neurinoma of the spinal cord, but no tumours of the forestomach (Thomas *et al.*, 1967). Stroobandt & Brucher (1968) have observed mainly neurogenic malignant tumours. A single intragastric dose of 90 mg/kg bw produced benign and malignant tumours of the kidney, the forestomach, the small and large intestine, the skin (keratoacanthomas) and the jaw (odontomas) (Leaver *et al.*, 1969). Odontogenic neoplasms were found in 2/10 rats after a single i.g. administration of 90 mg/kg bw (Ebling *et al.*, 1973).

Hamster: I.g. administration of 1 mg NMU/animal twice weekly for 4 months to Syrian golden hamsters produced odontogenic tumours and epidermoid carcinomas of the oral cavity in 6/9 animals and 5 adenocarcinomas of the small and 1 of the large intestine, many of which metastasized to lymph nodes (Herrold, 1968, 1969).

Guinea-pig: Doses of 2.5 mg/kg bw NMU in the drinking-water produced malignant tumours in 12/26 animals: 3 carcinomas and 2 sarcomas of the stomach, 2 adenocarcinomas of the pancreas, 2 malignant tumours of the ear duct, 1 neurinoma of the lumbar nerve and 2 leukaemias were seen (Druckrey *et al.*, 1968). Similar results were obtained by Bücheler & Thomas (1971).

When inbred guinea-pigs (NIH 13 strain) were treated with weekly i.g. administrations of 10 mg/kg bw NMU, 13/24 died within 6 months; 4/11 survivors developed adenocarcinomas of the pancreas, the first of which appeared 28 weeks after commencement of treatment (Reddy *et al.*, 1974). Of 74 guinea-pigs of the same strain treated similarly with NMU, 10/34 survivors at 27 weeks had adenocarcinomas of the pancreas, 2 adenocarcinomas of the stomach, 1 of the colon, 3 lymphomas of the mesenteric lymph nodes and 1 hepatocellular carcinoma (Reddy & Rao, 1975).

Pig: Ten Hanford minipigs received 10 mg/kg bw NMU at fortnightly intervals for 4½ years. All of the 9 animals that lived 50 months developed benign and some malignant tumours of the stomach (Stavrou *et al.*, 1976).

Monkey: Three species of monkeys, *Macaca mulatta, M. fascicularis* and *Cercopithecus aethiops* were administered NMU orally, beginning within one week of birth, on 5 days/week at doses of 10, 20 or 40 mg/kg bw for lifetime. In this study, which is still in progress, 41 monkeys had received NMU since its initiation, and 11 animals were necropsied during the following 7-year period; 5 of these were found to have squamous-cell carcinomas of the oropharynx and/or oesophagus. Parallels were noted between these tumours and human oesophageal carcinoma, including the clinical manifestations of the tumour and its complicated radiographic appearance and morphology (Adamson *et al.*, 1977).

(b) Skin application

Mouse: Topical application of a 0.5% solution of NMU in acetone 3 times/week for 18 weeks produced malignant skin tumours in 30/43 animals (Graffi *et al.*, 1967).

Single doses of 100 µg-6 mg NMU applied to the shaved dorsal skin of BALB/c mice induced papillomas in only a few animals. A higher tumorigenic response was seen after repeated administrations of 400 µg NMU for 6-18 weeks at total doses of 2 mg/animal or more. NMU had a tumour-initiating effect when given as a single dose or as three doses of 400 µg but was a complete carcinogen when 5 or more applications were made (Waynforth & Magee, 1975).

Newborn mouse: One application of 50-100 mg/kg bw to 125 newborn mice induced mainly lymphatic leukaemias in about 50% of treated animals (Graffi & Hoffmann, 1966a).

Rat: Application to Wistar rats of a 0.5% solution of NMU in acetone 3 times/week for 30 weeks (1.75 mg/dose) produced multiple squamous- and basal-cell carcinomas of the skin in 9/9 animals, the first tumour appearing at 20 weeks (Graffi & Hoffmann, 1966b; Graffi *et al.*, 1967).

Hamster: Treatment of 20 Syrian golden hamsters with a 0.5% solution of NMU in acetone 3 times/week for 13 weeks (0.35 mg/dose) produced squamous-cell carcinomas of the skin in 18/18 animals, the first tumour appearing at 8 weeks (Graffi & Hoffmann, 1966b; Graffi *et al.*, 1967).

(c) Inhalation and/or intratracheal administration

Hamster: Weekly intratracheal instillations to Syrian golden hamsters of 0.5 mg/animal NMU for 2.5 months produced epidermoid carcinomas in the nasopharyngeal tube, pharynx, larynx, trachea, bronchi, oesophagus and forestomach (Herrold, 1970).

Tracheal tumours (15 epidermoid carcinomas, 3 large-cell anaplastic carcinomas) were found in 18/18 male Syrian golden hamsters alive at 15 weeks following bi-weekly exposure of a circumscribed region of the trachea to 1 ml of a 1% solution of NMU in 10% ethanol-water by means of a special catheter for 15 weeks. Tumours were observed within 15-40 weeks (Schreiber *et al.*, 1975).

(d) Subcutaneous and/or intramuscular administration

Mouse: Treatment of 24 12-week-old male Swiss mice with single doses of 50 or 100 mg/kg bw NMU produced 10 malignant lymphomas and 1 local s.c. sarcoma in 13 mice that died after the 24th week of life; 11 were still alive at 50 weeks of age (Terracini & Stramignoni, 1967).

Newborn mouse: Newborn Swiss mice received single injections of 0.05 mg/animal NMU (33 mg/kg bw); of those alive at 5 weeks of age, 15/19 had developed poorly differentiated lymphosarcomas involving the thymus, myocardium, lung, spleen, lymph nodes, liver, kidney and bone marrow (Terracini & Stramignoni, 1967). Leukaemias (25-80%) and pulmonary tumours (81-100%) were induced after s.c. injection of 0.05-0.2 mg NMU in newborn (BALB/CxDBA/2)F_1 and random-bred albino mice (Kelly *et al.*, 1968).

Newborn rat: Single s.c. injections of NMU (dose unspecified) within 24 hours *post partum* to newborn hooded rats resulted in a total of 233 nervous system tumours in 96/145 animals (Güthert & Warzok, 1974).

Hamster: In 10 Syrian golden hamsters, weekly s.c. injections of 0.5-1 mg NMU/animal for 3-4 months induced sarcomas at the site of injection in all animals; 6 tumours metastasized to the lung or lymph nodes. Benign tumours of the forestomach (2), ovary (3) and vagina (2) were also seen (Herrold, 1966).

Treatment of 30 male and 30 female European hamsters with weekly s.c. injections of 1/5, 1/10 or 1/20 of the LD_{50} (LD_{50}: 113 mg/kg bw) for 18 weeks resulted in fibrosarcomas, carcinosarcomas and epidermal carcinomas at the injection site. A few papillomas of the forestomach were also seen (Mohr *et al.*, 1974). Fibrosarcomas at the injection site were seen in similarly treated Chinese hamsters (LD_{50}: 49 mg/kg bw) (Reznik *et al.*, 1976). In similarly treated Syrian golden hamsters (LD_{50}: 71 mg/kg bw),

Haas *et al.* (1973) found sarcomas at the injection site and a few papillomas of the forestomach (7%).

(e) Intraperitoneal administration

Adult and newborn mouse: I.p. injection of various single doses (25-100 mg/kg bw) into newborn or 6-8-week-old CFW/D mice produced high yields of thymic lymphomas (7-72%) and pulmonary adenomas (Frei, 1970; Joshi & Frei, 1970a,b). Fractionated dose schedules, with total doses ranging from 50-250 mg/kg bw, resulted in malignant lymphomas in up to 93% of the animals (Joshi & Frei, 1970b). Newborn and 5-week-old mice were treated with a single dose of 50 mg/kg bw; newborn animals were more susceptible to the induction of lymphosarcomas, lung adenomas and hepatomas; and tumours of the forestomach were more frequent in 5-week-old mice (Terracini & Testa, 1970).

Once-weekly i.p. injections of 5-15 mg/kg bw NMU over 10 months to A mice and 7.5 mg/kg bw over the same period to C3H mice resulted in tumours in 18/60 A mice and 3/20 C3H mice; most of these were bronchial adenomas, although 2 mice had malignant lung tumours which metastasized into the liver and the kidney (Eckert & Seidler, 1971).

C3HF/Dp mice were given single i.p. injections of 5, 25 or 50 mg/kg bw NMU at 1 or 70 days of age and 50 mg/kg bw on day 21; the 2 higher dose levels produced tumours in the thymus, forestomach, lung, liver (males only), kidneys, ovaries and orbital glands (Terracini *et al.*, 1976).

Adult or newborn rat: Repeated weekly i.p. injections of 10 mg/kg bw NMU to Wistar rats produced malignant tumours in the peritoneal cavity; some of these were neurogenic tumours arising from peripheral nerves (Thomas *et al.*, 1968). After a single i.p. injection of 50 mg/kg bw NMU, newborn Wistar rats developed renal anaplastic tumours and forestomach tumours more readily than did 5-week-old animals. No significant difference between adult and newborn rats was seen in the induction of lymphosarcomas, intestinal adenocarcinomas or mammary tumours (Terracini & Testa, 1970).

Following i.p. injections of 10 or 20 mg/kg bw NMU (total doses, 180-200 mg/kg bw) to hooded and Wistar rats, the incidences of nervous system tumours were 76% and 41% in the two strains, respectively (Schreiber *et al.*, 1972a).

Hamster: Weekly i.p. injections of 1 mg/animal to Syrian golden hamsters for 4-5 months produced adenocarcinomas of the large and small intestine, some of which metastazised to the lymph nodes (Herrold, 1969).

Guinea-pig: Once-weekly i.p. administrations of 10 mg/kg bw NMU to 42 guinea-pigs of the NIH 13 strain for 18 weeks resulted in tumours in 11/22 animals that survived beyond 22 weeks. Tumours included 2 adenocarcinomas of the pancreas, 2 fibrosarcomas of the mesentery, 2 angiosarcomas of the mesentery, a mesothelioma of the peritoneum, 2 tumours of the small intestine, and a haemangiosarcoma of the liver (Rao & Reddy, 1977).

Monkey: In a study still in progress, no tumours had been observed after 5 years in 2 *Macaca mulatta* monkeys whose mothers had received *N*-nitroso-*N*-ethylurea as a single dose during pregnancy and who received 19-20 i.p. injections of 10 mg/kg bw NMU at fortnightly intervals starting at 2 weeks of age (Jänisch *et al.*, 1977).

(f) Intravenous administration

Mouse: In 2/19 C3HeB/FeJ mice treated with i.v. injections of 25 mg/kg bw NMU every 4 weeks up to a total dose of 175 mg/kg bw, tumours developed in the stomach (7), lung (9), liver (2), lymphoid organs (3) and brain (2). One brain tumour was an oligodendroglioma of the diencephalon, the other was described as a mixed neuroblastoma-glioma of the cerebellum (Denlinger *et al.*, 1974).

Fifty female BDF1 mice given single i.v. injections of 50 mg/kg bw NMU developed a high incidence (45/50, 90%) of leukaemia, 50% of them within 200 days. No cases of leukaemia occurred among 40 untreated controls (Dexter *et al.*, 1974).

Rat: Repeated i.v. injections of NMU produced malignant tumours of the brain, spinal cord and peripheral nervous system in B rats. Histologically, the brain tumours were diagnosed as various types of gliomas, ependymomas, medulloblastomas and intracranial sarcomas; the tumours of the spinal cord were spongioblastomas, medulloblastomas and gliomas; and those of the peripheral nervous system were neurinomas. Dosage was usually 5-10 mg/kg bw/week, with total doses between 180 and 230 mg/kg bw, and the median induction time was 300 days (Druckrey *et al.*, 1964a, 1965; Fried & Fried, 1966; Jänisch *et al.*, 1967; Schiffer *et al.*, 1970; Wechsler *et al.*, 1969; Weiss *et al.*, 1970). Single doses of 70-100 mg/kg bw produced malignant and benign tumours in various organs, including the forestomach, large and small intestine, kidney and brain (Druckrey *et al.*, 1963, 1964b).

A single i.v. injection of 70 mg/kg bw NMU to Wistar rats induced tumours at multiple sites in 22/28 treated males and in 21/23 females (Murthy *et al.*, 1973).

Mammary carcinomas were seen in 206/240 (89%) BUF/N females, in 19/26 (73%) Sprague-Dawley females and in 25/28 (89%) F344 females given 3 i.v. injections of 50 mg/kg bw NMU at 4-week intervals to 50-day-old animals. Metastases to bone and spleen were found consistently. Mean latent periods were 77, 86 and 94 days, respectively (Gullino *et al.*, 1975). In Lewis rats, repeated i.v. injections of 25 mg/kg bw NMU at 4-week intervals resulted exclusively in mammary gland tumours in 23/35 animals (Bots & Willighagen, 1975).

In 17/18 Sprague-Dawley and 17/17 Fischer rats, 33 and 38 neurogenic tumours, respectively, were produced after weekly i.v. injections of 5 mg/kg bw NMU over a period of 36 weeks. The tumours were classified as astrocytomas, oligodendrogliomas, mixed gliomas, anaplastic gliomas, gliosarcomas and differentiated and anaplastic neurinomas (Swenberg *et al.*, 1972).

Hamster: In Syrian golden hamsters, three to four injections of 2.5-5 mg NMU/animal produced adenocarcinomas of the small and large intestine, odontogenic tumours and epidermoid carcinomas of the oral cavity (Herrold, 1968, 1969).

Weekly sublingual i.v. injections of NMU to a group of 15 male and 15 female European hamsters at doses of 1/5, 1/10 or 1/20 LD_{50} (LD_{50}: 50 mg/kg bw), up to total doses of 45, 90 or 180 mg/kg bw, resulted in tumour incidences of 20-93%. The main tumour types were sarcomas of the heart and squamous-cell carcinomas of the stomach (Ketkar *et al.*, 1977).

Gerbil: Two groups of 12 male and 12 female gerbils (*Meriones unguiculatus*) were given sublingual i.v. injections of 1/5 or 1/10 LD_{50} (5 or 2.5 mg/kg bw) once weekly for 15 weeks. Carcinomas and papillomas of the oral cavity and carcinomas and adenomas of the midventral sebaceous gland were induced (Haas *et al.*, 1975).

Rabbit: I.v. doses of 10 or 20 mg/kg bw NMU given every 2 weeks to 64 rabbits produced polymorphous gliomas and sarcomas in 33/48 animals; no tumours of peripheral nerves were seen. Adenocarcinomas of the small intestine and vascular tumours of different organs were also found (Jänisch & Schreiber, 1967; Schreiber *et al.*, 1969). The morphology of the malignant gliomas has been described by Kleihues *et al.* (1970).

Carcinomas of the small intestine were produced in 61/127 crossbred rabbits injected with 10 or 20 mg/kg bw NMU every 2 or 4 weeks. Injections of 20 mg/kg bw every 4 weeks to 67 rabbits led to a significantly higher frequency of small-intestine tumours (68.7%) than did 10 mg/kg bw every 2 weeks to 60 rabbits (25%). In 50% of the animals with tumours of the intestine, tumours of the central nervous system were also found. Malignant haemangioendotheliomas were found in 19 animals, and vascular tumours, localized particularly in the uterus, were found in 15 others (Schreiber & Jänisch, 1973; Schreiber *et al.*, 1972b).

Dog: Monthly injections of 20 mg/kg bw NMU for 12-18 months produced brain tumours (sarcomas or multiform glioblastomas) in 4/10 dogs. Four dogs developed sarcomas and haemangioendotheliomas of the lung, spleen and heart; 2 dogs also had brain tumours (Warzok *et al.*, 1970).

In a study described as a preliminary report, a group of 10 dogs received 20 mg/kg bw NMU every 4 weeks for life, while 13 others were treated with 15 mg/kg bw every 4 weeks for 48 weeks. Seven brain tumours were observed in 16 dead animals (5 from the first group, 2 from the second group) (Schneider & Warzok, 1972).

Four tumours of the peripheral nervous system and 2 brain tumours were found in 6/10 mongrel dogs that received monthly i.v. injections of 20 mg/kg bw NMU. The mean latency for these neoplasms was 25 months (Stavrou *et al.*, 1975).

It was reported in an abstract that 14/20 boxer dogs developed anaplastic neurinomas in various organs and that the other 6 developed non-neural tumours after receiving i.v. injections of 5 mg/kg bw NMU over a period of 36 weeks. The average survival time was 29±5 months (Koestner *et al.*, 1976).

Monkey: Two male and 4 female *Macaca mulatta* monkeys were given 8-16 monthly i.v. injections of 20 mg/kg bw NMU starting at 4-6 years of age (total dose, 688-1435 mg/animal). Two animals died 1 and 2.5 years after the start of treatment with no tumours; at the time of reporting, the remaining animals were still alive, with a maximum survival time of 10 years (Jänisch *et al.*, 1977) [The Working Group noted the low dose used].

(g) Other experimental systems

Various routes

The different organotropic effects of NMU depend upon dose levels and administration times; these have been summarized by Thomas & Bollmann (1969), who showed that tumours could be produced in nearly all organs of rats by selective NMU treatment. The different oncogenic effects of NMU, which depend upon route of administration and dose level, have been studied by Swenberg *et al.* (1974, 1975).

Malignant extraneural tumours were induced in hooded and Wistar rats by i.v., i.p. and i.g. administration of different dose levels, up to total doses of 70-250 mg/kg bw NMU. The main localizations were: stomach (36.9%), tongue (10.6%), colon (4.3%), mesenterium, pelvis and abdominal wall (17.2%), heart (8.9%), ear duct (5.8%), mediastinum (4.1%), neck (3%) and kidney (2.7%) (Schreiber *et al.*, 1972c).

Prenatal exposure

Two-month-old C3HA mice were injected with 25-100 mg/kg bw NMU during the last days of pregnancy. During the following 12-14 months, 53% of the offspring developed pulmonary adenomas and 20%, hepatomas (Likhachev, 1972; Smetanin, 1971).

Tumours of the nervous system and kidney were observed in the offspring of rats treated with NMU during the last third of pregnancy. Mammary tumours also occurred in the treated mothers (Alexandrov, 1969, 1974).

A single i.v. dose of 50 mg/kg bw NMU to 11 pregnant Donryu rats on the 20th day of gestation caused tumours in 60/110 offspring surviving for longer than 163 days. Of a total of 93 tumours induced, 61 (65.6%) arose from the nervous sytem (Ishida *et al.*, 1975).

A single i.v. dose of NMU to hooded rats during the last days of pregnancy resulted in tumours of the nervous system, mainly of the central nervous system, in 249/306 offspring (Güthert & Warzok, 1974).

Tumours of the mammary gland were observed in 5 and a lymphoma in 1 of 8 BD-IV female rats which received a single i.p. injection of 20 mg/kg bw NMU during pregnancy. A variety of tumours were seen in their 54 F_1 descendants, including 5 tumours of the nervous tissue in 5 animals, and 5 mesenchymal tumours and 1 carcinoma of the kidney in 6 animals. Kidney tumours (1 mesenchymal and 1 tubular adenoma) were seen in 2 and a nervous tissue tumour in 1 of 120 F_2 descendants; and 2 nervous tissue tumours were seen in 2/88 F_3 descendants. F_2 and F_3 generations received no other treatment. No kidney or nervous tissue tumours were seen in 64 controls (Tomatis *et al.*, 1975).

Bladder instillation

Papillomas and transitional-cell carcinomas of the bladder occurred in all of 100 female Wistar rats 30 weeks after administration of 4 doses of 1.5 mg/animal NMU on alternate weeks by urethral catheterization (Hicks & Wakefield, 1972). Total doses of 6 mg/animal NMU induced bladder papillomas in 16/23 rats within 9-56 weeks (Vlasov *et al.*, 1976).

Intrarectal administration

Two groups of 30 female ICR/Ha Swiss mice received a total dose of 9 mg/animal NMU either as 6 doses of 1.5 mg (group I) or as 30 doses of

0.3 mg (group II0, all given intrarectally 3 times/week. Tumours of the large intestine (adenomas and adenocarcinomas of the distal colon and rectum, squamous-cell carcinomas of the anal canal) developed in 14/30 mice in group I and 18/28 mice in group II; lung adenomas and lymphomas were also seen. Animals in group II had a lower yield of lymphomas and a higher yield of intestinal neoplasms when compared to those in group I (Narisawa & Weisburger, 1975; Narisawa *et al.*, 1976).

Groups of male Charles River CD-Fischer rats, 9 or 18 weeks of age, received intrarectal administrations of 1 or 2.5 mg/animal NMU 3 times/ week for 10 weeks. Tumours of the large bowel, including adenomas, adenocarcinomas and carcinomas, occurred in 25/29 and 27/27 rats at each dose level, respectively, within 20-35 weeks (Narisawa *et al.*, 1976).

Large-bowel adenocarcinomas were induced in 9/10 female inbred strain-2 guinea-pigs 38-56 weeks after intrarectal administration of 1.25 mg NMU twice weekly for 42 weeks (Narisawa *et al.*, 1975).

Intracerebral injection

A single intracerebral injection of 0.2-0.4 mg/animal to newborn rats or 0.05-0.8 mg/animal to newborn mice did not induce brain tumours in either species but produced some kidney fibrosarcomas and 1 mammary gland carcinoma in the rats and leukaemias (8-100%) and pulmonary tumours (67-100%) in the mice (Kelly *et al.*, 1968).

(h) Carcinogenicity of precursors

Of 26 Swiss mice given 5.4 g/kg of diet methylurea and 1 g/l sodium nitrite in the drinking-water, 16 (61%) developed lung adenomas, compared with 14% in untreated controls (Mirvish *et al.*, 1972).

A level of 0.3% sodium nitrite given simultaneously in the diet with 0.01 or 0.03% methylurea in drinking-water for 2 years to a group of 20 Sprague-Dawley rats caused nervous system tumours in 15 and 45% of animals, respectively. With the dose of 0.03%, there was also a 25% increase in lymphomas (Koestner & Wechsler, 1974; Koestner *et al.*, 1975).

(i) Factors that modify carcinogenicity in animals

Swiss mice given single s.c. injections of 50 μg NMU/animal at birth and thymectomized at 12 days of age developed no tumours of the lymphatic system; these occurred in NMU-treated, intact animals (Palestro & Stramignoni, 1975).

A single i.p. injection of 45-90 mg/kg bw NMU to female albino rats during the period of increased DNA synthesis after partial hepatectomy caused liver-cell adenomas in up to 50% of the animals (Craddock, & Frei, 1974).

Tumours of the salivary (5/39) and mammary gland tissues (29/39) were observed after stimulating DNA synthesis by i.p. injection of 310 mg/kg bw isoprenaline sulphate to 50 female Wistar rats and giving subsequent i.v. injections of 77 mg/kg bw NMU; no salivary and 6/9 mammary gland tumours were seen in NMU-treated controls (Parkin & Neale, 1976).

When female Wistar rats were pretreated with single intravesicular instillations of 2 mg/animal NMU followed by 2 or 4 g/kg bw sodium saccharin/day or 1 or 2 g/kg bw sodium cyclamate/day in the diet, more than half of the animals developed bladder tumours from 10 weeks onwards (46/79 with saccharin and 31/54 with cyclamate). In this experiment, instillations of 2 mg/animal NMU alone to 124 rats did not cause bladder cancers. Sodium saccharin and sodium cyclamate, alone, produced 4/253 and 3/228 bladder tumours, respectively (Hicks *et al.*, 1973, 1975).

3.2 Other relevant biological data

(a) Experimental systems

Toxic effects

The acute LD_{50} of NMU in rats was 110 mg/kg bw whether given orally or by i.v. injection (Druckrey *et al.*, 1967). The LD_{50} by s.c. injection in European hamsters was 110 mg/kg bw (Mohr *et al.*, 1974), in Chinese hamsters, 50 mg/kg bw (Reznik *et al.*, 1976) and in Syrian golden hamsters, 70 mg/kg bw (Haas *et al.*, 1973). The i.v. LD_{50} in European hamsters was 50 mg/kg bw (Ketkar *et al.*, 1977).

The major toxic effects result from severe damage to haematopoietic, lymphoid and other tissues that have rapid rates of cell turnover (Magee & Barnes, 1967; Magee & Swann, 1969). Acute treatment with NMU has been shown to inhibit protein and nucleic acid synthesis in various tissues (Magee *et al.*, 1975; Pegg, 1977). A dose of 50 mg/kg bw NMU produced pancreatic damage and diabetes in Chinese hamsters. Higher doses were required to produce hyperglycaemia in golden hamsters, rats and mice; no diabetic effects were apparent in guinea-pigs or sand rats (Wilander & Gunnarsson, 1975; Wilander & Tjälve, 1975).

Embryotoxicity and teratogenicity

A single i.p. dose of 5-10 mg/kg bw NMU to rats on days 3, 4 or 5 of gestation resulted in a high rate of foetal resorptions (Alexandrov, 1973); 10-40 mg/kg bw NMU given on day 9 of gestation led to a dose-dependent embryolethal effect. When treated before or after day 9, embryo mortality fell sharply (Koyama *et al.*, 1970).

Administration of a single i.p. dose of 10 mg/kg bw to rats on day 9 of gestation produced abnormalities of the brain in most of the surviving foetuses. Treatment with the same dose on days 11-16 caused malformations of the limbs (days 11-13) in 100% of the foetuses, micrognathia (days 13-14), hydrocephaly (day 12) and microcephaly, which increased with treatment on day 12-16. The surviving foetuses from dams treated with NMU during organogenesis showed significantly retarded growth (Koyama *et al.*, 1970; Napalkov & Alexandrov, 1968).

Daily injections of 3 mg/kg bw NMU to rats during the first week of pregnancy induced no teratogenic lesions; 20 mg/kg bw administered on day 21 of gestation induced malformation of the brain in all of the offspring (Napalkov, 1971).

Absorption, distribution and excretion

NMU was not detected in the blood of rats 15 minutes after an i.v. injection of 100 mg/kg bw (Swann, 1968). The compound was widely distributed in rats shortly after i.v. administration (Kleihues & Patzschke, 1971).

Metabolism

The high chemical reactivity of NMU renders it unlikely that enzymic catalysis is involved in its decomposition. NMU is a direct alkylating agent and alkylates nucleic acids both *in vitro* and *in vivo*. Such alkylation has been detected in a number of tissues, including brain, lung, kidney, liver, intestine, thymus and spleen, in a number of species, including mice, rats, hamsters and mini-pigs (Frei & Lawley, 1975; Lawley, 1974; Magee *et al.*, 1976; Margison & Kleihues, 1975; Pegg, 1977; Swann & Magee, 1968). All three hydrogen atoms in the methyl group of NMU are retained in the methylated nucleosides formed in nucleic acids after alkylation by NMU *in vivo* (Lijinsky *et al.*, 1972).

The major methylated product is 7-methylguanine, but other, minor products are also formed. These products are similar to those produced in liver after administration of *N*-nitroso-*N*-dimethylamine and include 1-methyl-, 3-methyl- and 7-methyladenines, 3-methyl- and O^6-methylguanines, 3-methylcytosine, 3-methyl- and O^4-methylthymine and methylphosphate triesters (Frei & Lawley, 1975; Lawley, 1974; Margison & Kleihues, 1975; Pegg, 1977; Swenson *et al.*, 1976). Removal of O^6-methylguanine from the DNA of the brain and, to a lesser extent, from that of the kidney, organs which are relatively susceptible to the carcinogenic action of NMU, is slower than from the liver, which is relatively insensitive to carcinogenesis by NMU (Bücheler & Kleihues 1977; Kleihues & Margison, 1974; Margison & Kleihues, 1975; Pegg, 1977; Pegg & Nicoll, 1976).

In vivo formation of NMU was shown by methylation of guanine at N^7 after feeding of the precursors methylurea and sodium nitrite (Montesano & Magee, 1971).

The importance of cellular proliferation in carcinogenesis by NMU is suggested by studies in which liver tumours were produced by NMU only if its administration was preceded by partial hepatectomy (Craddock & Frei, 1974) and by the finding that the DNA of neuronal cells of the brains of young rats treated with NMU was alkylated to the same extent as the DNA from glial cells. In these rats, the brain tumours are produced by NMU from the glial cells, which divide, and not from the neuronal cells which do not (Kleihues *et al.*, 1973).

The cyanate ion produced by decomposition of NMU at physiological pH can react with proteins by carbamoylation. Such a reaction with serum proteins was responsible for some of the toxic effects of NMU on the growth of cells in culture (Knox, 1976).

Mutagenicity and other short-term tests

The genetic activity of NMU has been demonstrated in bacterial phage, *Escherichia coli*, *Salmonella typhimurium*, *Saccharomyces cerevisiae*, *Serratia marcescens*, Chinese hamster cells and *Drosophila melanogaster*, inducing forward and reverse mutations and gene conversions (for reviews, see Montesano & Bartsch, 1976; Neale, 1976).

Sister chromatid exchanges were found in Chinese hamster cells exposed to NMU (Abe & Sasaki, 1977).

NMU at an i.p. dose of 50 mg/kg bw caused dominant lethal mutations in mice during the first 3-4 weeks after administration (Parkin *et al.*, 1973). NMU induced chromosome and chromatid aberrations (single breaks and exchanges) in bone marrow of mice injected intraperitoneally with 0.8 or 0.08 mM (Frei & Venitt, 1975). I.p. injection of 100 mg/kg bw or 50 mg/kg bw NMU, administered as two injections at an interval of 4 hours, produced chromosome fragmentation and translocations in spermatocytes and spermatogonia from Wistar rats (Goetz, 1973).

Human fibroblasts, mouse C3H 10T½ fibroblasts and rat hepatocytes in culture treated with NMU showed unscheduled DNA synthesis. There was no significant difference in DNA repair in the three cell lines (Zardi *et al.*, 1977).

Transformation of cultured fibroblasts from hamster (Sanders & Burford, 1967), mouse (Frei & Oliver, 1972) and rat embryos (Kirkland *et al.*, 1975) by NMU *in vitro* gives rise to cells which produce tumours on transplantation into experimental animals.

(b) Humans

Nausea and vomiting were seen after i.v. injection of 4 mg/kg bw NMU to patients (Kolarić, 1977).

3.3 Case reports and epidemiological studies

No data were available to the Working Group.

4. Summary of Data Reported and Evaluation

4.1 Experimental data

N-Nitroso-*N*-methylurea is carcinogenic in all animal species tested: mice, rats, Syrian golden, Chinese and European hamsters, guinea-pigs, rabbits, gerbils, pigs, dogs and monkeys. It induces benign and malignant tumours following its administration by different routes, including ingestion. It produces tumours at different sites, including the nervous tissue, stomach, oesophagus, pancreas, respiratory tract, intestine, lymphoreticular tissues, skin and kidney. It is carcinogenic following its administration prenatally and in single doses.

4.2 Human data

No case reports or epidemiological studies were available to the Working Group. Except for reported investigation of its use as a chemotherapeutic agent, no information on the occurrence or use of *N*-nitroso-*N*-methylurea was available.

4.3 Evaluation

There is *sufficient evidence* of a carcinogenic effect of *N*-nitroso-*N*-methylurea in several experimental animal species. Although no epidemiological data were available, *N*-nitroso-*N*-methylurea should be regarded for practical purposes as if it were carcinogenic to humans.

5. References

Abe, S. & Sasaki, M. (1977) Chromosome aberrations and sister chromatid exchanges in Chinese hamster cells exposed to various chemicals. J. nat. Cancer Inst., 58, 1635-1641

Adamson, R.H., Krolikowski, F.J., Correa, P., Sieber, S.M. & Dalgard, D.W. (1977) Carcinogenicity of 1-methyl-1-nitrosourea in nonhuman primates. J. nat. Cancer Inst., 59, 415-422

Alexandrov, V.A. (1969) Transplacental blastomogenic action of *N*-nitrosomethylurea on rat offspring. Vop. Onkol., 15, 55-61

Alexandrov, V.A. (1973) Embryotoxic and teratogenic effects of chemical carcinogens. In: Tomatis, L. & Mohr, U., eds, Transplacental Carcinogenesis, Lyon (IARC Scientific Publications No. 4), pp. 112-126

Alexandrov, V.A. (1974) Embryotoxic, teratogenic and carcinogenic effects of *N*-nitrosomethyl urea in rats. Vop. Onkol., 20, 76-82

Bots, G.T.A.M. & Willighagen, R.G.J. (1975) Tumours in the mammary gland induced in Lewis rats by intravenous methylnitrosourea. Brit. J. Cancer, 31, 372-374

Bücheler, J. & Kleihues, P. (1977) Excision of O^6-methylguanine from DNA of various mouse tissues following a single injection of *N*-methyl-*N*-nitrosourea. Chem.-biol. Interact., 16, 325-333

Bücheler, J. & Thomas, C. (1971) Experimentell erzeugte Drüsenmagentumoren bei Meerschweinchen und Ratte. Beitr. path. Anat., 142, 194-209

Craddock, V.M. & Frei, J.V. (1974) Induction of liver cell adenomata in the rat by a single treatment with *N*-methyl-*N*-nitrosourea given at various times after partial hepatectomy. Brit. J. Cancer, 30, 503-511

Denlinger, R.H., Koestner, A. & Wechsler, W. (1974) Induction of neurogenic tumors in C3HeB/FeJ mice by nitrosourea derivatives: observations by light microscopy, tissue culture, and electron microscopy. Int. J. Cancer, 13, 559-571

Dexter, T.M., Schofield, R., Lajtha, L.G. & Moore, M. (1974) Studies on the mechanisms of chemical leukaemogenesis. Brit. J. Cancer, 30, 325-331

Druckrey, H., Preussmann, R., Schmähl, D. & Müller, M. (1961) Erzeugung von Magenkrebs durch Nitrosamide an Ratten. Naturwissenschaften, 48, 165

Druckrey, H., Steinhoff, D., Preussmann, R. & Ivankovic, S. (1963) Krebserzeugung durch einmalige Dosis von Methylnitrosoharnstoff und verschiedenen Dialkylnitrosaminen. Naturwissenschaften, 50, 735

Druckrey, H., Ivankovic, S. & Preussmann, R. (1964a) Selektive Erzeugung von Hirntumoren bei Ratten durch Methylnitrosoharnstoff. Naturwissenschaften, 51, 144

Druckrey, H., Steinhoff, D., Preussmann, R. & Ivankovic, S. (1964b) Erzeugung von Krebs durch eine einmalige Dosis von Methylnitroso-Harnstoff und verschiedenen Dialkylnitrosaminen an Ratten. Z. Krebsforsch., 66, 1-10

Druckrey, H., Ivankovic, S. & Preussmann, R. (1965) Selektive Erzeugung maligner Tumoren im Gehirn und Rückenmark von Ratten durch *N*-Methyl-*N*-nitrosoharnstoff. Z. Krebsforsch., 66, 389-408

Druckrey, H., Preussmann, R., Ivankovic, S. & Schmähl, D. (1967) Organotrope carcinogene Wirkungen bei 65 verschiedenen *N*-Nitroso-Verbindungen an BD-Ratten. Z. Krebsforsch., 69, 103-201

Druckrey, H., Ivankovic, S., Bücheler, J., Preussmann, R. & Thomas, C. (1968) Erzeugung von Magen- und Pankreas-Krebs beim Meerschweinchen durch Methylnitroso-harnstoff und -urethan. Z. Krebsforsch., 72, 167-182

Ebling, H., Barbachan, J.J.D., Castro do Valle, J.G. & de Oliveira, L.Y. (1973) *N*-Methyl-*N*-nitrosourea-induced odontogenic neoplasms in rats. J. dent. Res., 52, 177

Eckert, H. & Seidler, E. (1971) Zur tumorerzeugenden Wirkung von Methylnitrosoharnstoff an der Maus. Arch. Geschwulstforsch., 38, 7-14

Fine, D.H., Rounbehler, D.P., Silvergleid, A. & Ross, R. (1977) Trace analysis of polar and apolar *N*-nitroso compounds by combined high-performance liquid chromatography and thermal energy analysis. In: Tinbergen, B.J. & Krol, B., eds, Proceedings of the Second International Symposium on Nitrite in Meat Products, Zeist, 1976, Wageningen, Centre for Agricultural Publishing and Documentation, pp. 191-199

Frei, J.V. (1970) Toxicity, tissue changes, and tumor induction in inbred Swiss mice by methylnitrosamine and -amide compounds. Cancer Res., 30, 11-17

Frei, J.V. & Lawley, P.D. (1975) Methylation of DNA in various organs of C57Bl mice by a carcinogenic dose of *N*-methyl-*N*-nitrosourea and stability of some methylation products up to 18 hours. Chem.-biol. Interact., 10, 413-427

Frei, J.V. & Oliver, J. (1972) Early enhancement of plating efficiency of primary mouse embryo cells by the carcinogen methylnitrosourea. Cancer Res., 32, 2747-2752

Frei, J.V. & Venitt, S. (1975) Chromosome damage in the bone marrow of mice treated with the methylating agents methyl methanesulphonate and *N*-methyl-*N*-nitrosourea in the presence or absence of caffeine, and its relationship with thymoma induction. Mutation Res., 29, 89-96

Fried, R. & Fried, L.W. (1966) The induction of brain tumors in rats by administration of methyl-nitroso-urea (Abstract No. 3070). Fed. Proc., 25, 734

Garrett, E.R., Goto, S. & Stubbins, J.F. (1965) Kinetics of solvolyses of various *N*-alkyl-*N*-nitrosoureas in neutral and alkaline solutions. J. pharm. Sci., 54, 119-123

Goetz, P. (1973) Chromosomal aberrations induced by methylnitrosourea on the germ cells of male rats (Abstract No. 21). Mutation Res., 21, 34

Graffi, A. & Hoffmann, F. (1966a) Starke leukämogene Wirkung von *N*-Methyl-*N*-nitroso-Harnstoff bei der Maus nach einmaliger Applikation an neugeborene Tiere. Acta biol. med. germ., 17, K33-K35

Graffi, A. & Hoffmann, F. (1966b) Starke kanzerogene Wirkung von *N*-Methyl-*N*-nitroso-Harnstoff auf die Hamster- und Rattenhaut im Tropfungsversuch. Arch. Geschwulstforsch., 28, 234-248

Graffi, A., Hoffmann, F. & Schütt, M. (1967) *N*-Methyl-*N*-nitrosourea as a strong topical carcinogen when painted on skin of rodents. Nature (Lond.), 214, 611

Gullino, P.M., Pettigrew, H.M. & Grantham, F.H. (1975) *N*-Nitrosomethylurea as mammary gland carcinogen in rats. J. nat. Cancer Inst., 54, 401-414

Güthert, H. & Warzok, R. (1974) Zur karzinogenen Wirkung von Methyl- und Äthylnitrosoharnstoff bei Ratten nach transplazentarer und postnataler Applikation. Zbl. allg. Path., 118, 115-123

Haas, H., Mohr, U. & Krüger, F.W. (1973) Comparative studies with different doses of *N*-nitrosomorpholine, *N*-nitrosopiperidine, *N*-nitrosomethylurea, and dimethylnitrosamine in Syrian golden hamsters. J. nat. Cancer Inst., 51, 1295-1301

Haas, H., Hilfrich, J., Kmoch, N. & Mohr, U. (1975) Specific carcinogenic effect of *N*-methyl-*N*-nitrosourea on the midventral sebaceous gland of the gerbil (*Meriones unguiculatus*). J. nat. Cancer Inst., 55, 637-640

Herrold, K.M. (1966) Carcinogenic effect of *N*-methyl-*N*-nitrosourea administered subcutaneously to Syrian hamsters. J. Path. Bact., 92, 35-41

Herrold, K.M. (1968) Odontogenic tumors and epidermoid carcinomas of the oral cavity. An experimental study in Syrian hamsters. Oral Surg., 25, 262-272

Herrold, K.M. (1969) Adenocarcinomas of the intestine induced in Syrian hamsters by *N*-methyl-*N*-nitrosourea. Path. Vet., 6, 403-412

Herrold, K.M. (1970) Upper respiratory tract tumors induced in Syrian hamsters by *N*-methyl-*N*-nitrosourea. Int. J. Cancer, 6, 217-222

Hicks, R.M. & Wakefield, J.St J. (1972) Rapid induction of bladder cancer in rats with *N*-methyl-*N*-nitrosourea. I. Histology. Chem.-biol. Interact., 5, 139-152

Hicks, R.M., Wakefield, J.St J. & Chowaniec, J. (1973) Co-carcinogenic action of saccharin in the chemical induction of bladder cancer. Nature (Lond.), 243, 347-349

Hicks, R.M., Wakefield, J.St J. & Chowaniec, J. (1975) Evaluation of a new model to detect bladder carcinogens or co-carcinogens: results obtained with saccharin, cyclamate and cyclophosphamide. Chem.-biol. Interact., 11, 225-233

IARC (1972) IARC Monographs on the Evaluation of Carcinogenic Risk of Chemicals to Man, 1, Lyon, pp. 125-134

Ishida, Y., Tamura, M., Kanda, H. & Okamoto, K. (1975) Histopathological studies of the nervous system tumors in rats induced by *N*-nitrosomethyl-urea. Acta path. jap., 25, 385-401

Jänisch, W. & Schreiber, D. (1967) Experimentelle Hirngeschwülste bei Kaninchen nach Injektion von Methylnitrosoharnstoff. Naturwissenschaften, 54, 171-172

Jänisch, W., Schreiber, D., Stengel, R. & Steffen, V. (1967) Die Induktion von experimentellen Hirngeschwülsten bei Ratten mit Methylnitrosoharnstoff. Exp. Path., 1, 243-255

Jänisch, W., Schreiber, D., Warzok, R. & Scholtze, P. (1977) Versuche mit den Kanzerogenen Methyl- und Äthylnitrosoharnstoff bei *Macaca mulatta*. Arch. Geschwulstforsch., 47, 123-126

Joshi, V.V. & Frei, J.V. (1970a) Gross and microscopic changes in the lymphoreticular system during genesis of malignant lymphoma induced by a single injection of methylnitrosourea in adult mice. J. nat. Cancer Inst., 44, 379-394

Joshi, V.V. & Frei, J.V. (1970b) Effects of dose and schedule of methylnitrosourea on incidence of malignant lymphoma in adult female mice. J. nat. Cancer Inst., 45, 335-339

Kelly, M.G., O'Gara, R.W., Yancey, S.T. & Botkin, C. (1968) Carcinogenicity of 1-methyl-1-nitrosourea in newborn mice and rats. J. nat. Cancer Inst., 41, 619-626

Kerkadze, I.G., Zoz, N.N., Kontridze, A.N. & Pirtskhalaishvili, B.I. (1974) Penetration of chemical mutagens into plant seeds. In: Rapoport, I.A., ed., Proceedings on Chemical Mutagenesis, Moscow, Nauka, pp. 137-140 [Chem. Abstr., 83, 54437c]

Ketkar, M., Reznik, G., Haas, H., Hilfrich, J. & Mohr, U. (1977) Tumors of the heart and stomach induced in European hamsters by intravenous administration of *N*-methyl-*N*-nitrosourea. J. nat. Cancer Inst., 58, 1695-1699

Kirkland, D.J., Armstrong, C. & Harris, R.J.C. (1975) Spontaneous and chemically induced transformation of rat embryo cell cultures. Brit. J. Cancer, 31, 329-337

Kleihues, P. & Margison, G.P. (1974) Carcinogenicity of *N*-methyl-*N*-nitrosourea: possible role of excision repair of O^6-methylguanine from DNA. J. nat. Cancer Inst., 53, 1839-1841

Kleihues, P. & Patzschke, K. (1971) Verteilung von *N*-[^{14}C]-Methyl-*N*-nitrosoharnstoff in der Ratte nach systemischer Applikation. Z. Krebsforsch., 75, 193-200

Kleihues, P., Zülch, K.J., Matsumoto, S. & Radke, U. (1970) Morphology of malignant gliomas induced in rabbits by systemic application of *N*-methyl-*N*-nitrosourea. Z. Neurol., 198, 65-78

Kleihues, P., Magee, P.N., Austoker, J., Cox, D. & Mathias, A.P. (1973) Reaction of *N*-methyl-*N*-nitrosourea with DNA of neuronal and glial cells *in vivo*. FEBS Lett., 32, 105-108

Knox, P. (1976) Carcinogenic nitrosamides and cell cultures. Nature (Lond.), 259, 671-673

Koestner, A. & Wechsler, W. (1974) Induction of neurogenic- and non-neurogenic neoplasms by feeding precursors of methyl- and ethylnitrosourea to adult rats (Abstract No. 39). J. Neuropath. exp. Neurol., 33, 178

Koestner, A., Denlinger, R.H. & Wechsler, W. (1975) Induction of neurogenic and lymphoid neoplasms by the feeding of threshold levels of methyl- and ethylnitrosourea precursors to adult rats. Fd Cosmet. Toxicol., 13, 605-609

Koestner, A., Denlinger, R. & Swenberg, J.A. (1976) Carcinogenicity of methylnitrosourea (MNU) in boxer dogs (Abstract No. 325). Proc. Amer. Ass. Cancer Res., 17, 82

Kolarić, K. (1977) Combination chemotherapy with 1-methyl-1-nitrosourea (MNU) and cyclophosphamide in solid tumors. Z. Krebsforsch., 89, 311-319

Koyama, T., Handa, J., Handa, H. & Matsumoto, S. (1970) Methylnitrosourea-induced malformations of brain in SD-JCL rat. Arch. Neurol., 22, 342-347

Lawley, P.D. (1974) Some chemical aspects of dose-response relationships in alkylation mutagenesis. Mutation Res., 23, 283-295

Leaver, D.D., Swann, P.F. & Magee, P.N. (1969) The induction of tumours in the rat by a single oral dose of *N*-nitrosomethylurea. Brit. J. Cancer, 23, 177-187

Lijinsky, W., Garcia, H., Keefer, L., Loo, J. & Ross, A.E. (1972) Carcinogenesis and alkylation of rat liver nucleic acids by nitrosomethylurea and nitrosoethylurea administered by intraportal injection. Cancer Res., 32, 893-897

Likhachev, A.Y. (1972) Blastomogenesis in mice in combined transplacental and postnatal action of *N*-nitrosomethylurea and *N*-nitrosodiethylamine. Vop. Onkol., 18, 71-76

Magee, P.N. & Barnes, J.M. (1967) Carcinogenic nitroso compounds. Adv. Cancer Res., 10, 163-246

Magee, P.N. & Swann, P.F. (1969) Nitroso compounds. Brit. med. Bull., 25, 240-244

Magee, P.N., Pegg, A.E. & Swann, P.F. (1975) Molecular mechanisms of chemical carcinogenesis. In: Altmann, H.-W., *et al.*, eds, Handbuch der Allgemeinen Pathologie, Vol. 6, Berlin, Springer, pp. 329-419

Magee, P.N., Montesano, R. & Preussmann, R. (1976) *N*-Nitroso compounds and related carcinogens. In: Searle, C.E., ed., Chemical Carcinogens (ACS Monographs 173), Washington DC, American Chemical Society, pp. 491-625

Margison, G.P. & Kleihues, P. (1975) Chemical carcinogenesis in the nervous system. Preferential accumulation of O^6-methylguanine in rat brain deoxyribonucleic acid during repetitive administration of *N*-methyl-*N*-nitrosourea. Biochem. J., 148, 521-525

McCalla, D.R., Reuvers, A. & Kitai, R. (1968) Inactivation of biologically active *N*-methyl-*N*-nitroso compounds in aqueous solution: effect of various conditions of pH and illumination. Canad. J. Biochem., 46, 807-811

Mirvish, S.S., Greenblatt, M. & Choudari Kommineni, V.R. (1972) Nitrosamide formation *in vivo*: induction of lung adenomas in Swiss mice by concurrent feeding of nitrite and methylurea or ethylurea. J. nat. Cancer Inst., 48, 1311-1315

Mirvish, S.S., Karlowski, K., Sams, J.P. & Arnold, S.D. (1978) Studies related to nitrosamide formation: nitrosation in solvent:water and solvent systems, nitrosomethylurea formation in the rat stomach, and analysis of a fish product for ureas. In: Walker, E.A., Castegnaro, M., Griciute, L. & Lyle, R.E., eds, Environmental Aspects of *N*-Nitroso Compounds, Lyon (IARC Scientific Publications No. 19) (in press)

Mohr, U., Haas, H. & Hilfrich, J. (1974) The carcinogenic effects of dimethylnitrosamine and nitrosomethylurea in European hamsters (*Cricetus cricetus* L.). Brit. J. Cancer, 29, 359-364

Montesano, R. & Bartsch, H. (1976) Mutagenic and carcinogenic *N*-nitroso compounds: possible environmental hazards. Mutation Res., 32, 179-228

Montesano, R. & Magee, P.N. (1971) Evidence of formation of *N*-methyl-*N*-nitrosourea in rats given *N*-methylurea and sodium nitrite. Int. J. Cancer, 7, 249-255

Montgomery, J.A., Johnston, T.P., Thomas, H.J., Piper, J.R. & Temple, C., Jr (1977) The use of microparticulate reverse-phase packing in high pressure liquid chromatography of compounds of biological interest. Adv. Chromatogr., 15, 169-195

Murthy, A.S.K., Vawter, G.F. & Bhaktaviziam, A. (1973) Neoplasms in Wistar rats after an *N*-methyl-*N*-nitrosourea injection. Arch. Path., 96, 53-57

Napalkov, N.P. (1971) Experimentation on transplacental blastomogenesis as a tool for study of etiopathogenesis of tumours in children. Vop. Onkol., 17, 3-15

Napalkov, N.P. & Alexandrov, V.A. (1968) On the effects of blastomogenic substances on the organism during embryogenesis. Z. Krebsforsch., 71, 32-50

Narisawa, T. & Weisburger, J.H. (1975) Colon cancer induction in mice by intrarectal instillation of *N*-methylnitrosourea. Proc. Soc. exp. Biol. (N.Y.), 148, 166-169

Narisawa, T., Wong, C.-Q. & Weisburger, J.H. (1975) Induction of carcinoma of the large intestine in guinea pigs by intrarectal instillation of *N*-methyl-*N*-nitrosourea. J. nat. Cancer Inst., 54, 785-787

Narisawa, T., Wong, C.-Q., Maronpot, R.R. & Weisburger, J.H. (1976) Large bowel carcinogenesis in mice and rats by several intrarectal doses of methylnitrosourea and negative effect of nitrite plus methylurea. Cancer Res., 36, 505-510

Neale, S. (1976) Mutagenicity of nitrosamides and nitrosamidines in micro-organisms and plants. Mutation Res., 32, 229-266

Nikiforova, I.L. (1972) Characteristics of M_5 mutants of barley produced under the action of chemical mutagens. In: Rapoport, I.A., ed., Proceedings on Selection of Chemical Mutagens, Moscow, Nauka, pp. 250-253 [Chem. Abstr., 80, 34121g]

Palestro, G. & Stramignoni, A. (1975) Nitrosomethylurea-induced lymphomas in thymectomized mice, in relation to thymus-dependent and independent systems. Oncology, 31, 115-122

Parkin, R. & Neale, S. (1976) The effect of isoprenaline on induction of tumours by methyl nitrosourea in the salivary and mammary glands of female Wistar rats. Brit. J. Cancer, 34, 437-443

Parkin, R., Waynforth, H.B. & Magee, P.N. (1973) The activity of some nitroso compounds in the mouse dominant-lethal mutation assay. I. Activity of *N*-nitroso-*N*-methylurea, *N*-methyl-*N*-nitroso-*N*'-nitrosoguanidine and *N*-nitrosomorpholine. Mutation Res., 21, 155-161

Pegg, A.E. (1977) Formation and metabolism of alkylated nucleosides: possible role in carcinogenesis by nitroso compounds and alkylating agents. Adv. Cancer Res., 25, 195-269

Pegg, A.E. & Nicoll, J.W. (1976) Nitrosamine carcinogenesis: the importance of the persistence in DNA of alkylated bases in the organotropism of tumour induction. In: Montesano, R., Bartsch, H. & Tomatis, L., eds, Screening Tests in Chemical Carcinogenesis, Lyon (IARC Scientific Publications No. 12), pp. 571-592

Prager, B., Jacobson, P., Schmidt, P. & Stern, D., eds (1922) Beilsteins Handbuch der Organischen Chemie, 4th ed., Vol. 4, Syst. No. 335, Berlin, Springer, p. 85

Rao, M.S. & Reddy, J.K. (1977) Pathology of tumors developed in guinea pigs given intraperitoneal injections of *N*-methyl-*N*-nitrosourea. Neoplasma, 24, 57-62

Reddy, J.K. & Rao, M.S. (1975) Pancreatic adenocarcinoma in inbred guinea pigs induced by *N*-methyl-*N*-nitrosourea. Cancer Res., 35, 2269-2277

Reddy, J.K., Svoboda, D.J. & Rao, M.S. (1974) Susceptibility of an inbred strain of guinea pigs to the induction of pancreatic adenocarcinoma by *N*-methyl-*N*-nitrosourea. J. nat. Cancer Inst., 52, 991-993

Reznik, G., Mohr, U. & Kmoch, N. (1976) Carcinogenic effects of different nitroso-compounds in Chinese hamsters: *N*-dibutylnitrosamine and *N*-nitrosomethylurea. Cancer Lett., 1, 183-188

Sanders, F.K. & Burford, B.O. (1967) Morphological conversion of cells *in vitro* by *N*-nitrosomethylurea. Nature (Lond.), 213, 1171-1173

Schiffer, D., Fabiani, A., Grossi-Paoletti, E. & Paoletti, P. (1970) Experimental brain tumours induced in rats by nitrosourea derivatives. I. Morphological aspects of methylnitrosourea tumours. J. neurol. Sci., 11, 559-572

Schneider, J. & Warzok, R. (1972) Induktion von Hirntumoren durch Methylnitrosoharnstoff beim Hund. Z. inn. Med., 27, 580-582

Schreiber, D. & Jänisch, W. (1967) Geschwülste bei Ratten nach wiederholter Applikation von *N*-Methyl-*N*-nitrosoharnstoff durch die Magensonde. Exp. Path., 1, 331-338

Schreiber, D. & Jänisch, W. (1973) Tumoren des Gefässsystems bei Kaninchen nach Applikation von Methylnitrosoharnstoff (MNH). Zbl. allg. Path., 117, 99-105

Schreiber, D., Jänisch, W., Warzok, R. & Tausch, H. (1969) Die Induktion von Hirn- und Rückenmarktumoren bei Kaninchen mit *N*-Methyl-*N*-nitrosoharnstoff. Z. ges. exp. Med., 150, 76-86

Schreiber, D., Scholtze, P., Jänisch, W. & Batka, H. (1972a) Tumoren des Nervensystems bei Ratten nach intraperitonealer Injektion von Methylnitrosoharnstoff. Zbl. allg. Path., 115, 3-7

Schreiber, D., Lageman, A. & Geyer, M. (1972b) Erzeugung von Dünndarmkarzinomen bei Kaninchen mit Methylnitrosoharnstoff. Zbl. allg. Path., 115, 40-47

Schreiber, D., Warzok, R., Scholtze, P., Schneider, J., Lageman, A. & Batka, H. (1972c) Das Spektrum extraneuraler Tumoren bei Ratten nach Applikation von *N*-Methyl-*N*-nitrosoharnstoff. Zbl. allg. Path., 115, 48-61

Schreiber, H., Schreiber, K. & Martin, D.H. (1975) Experimental tumor induction in a circumscribed region of the hamster trachea: correlation of histology and exfoliative cytology. J. nat. Cancer Inst., 54, 187-197

Singer, G.M., Singer, S.S. & Schmidt, D.G. (1977) A nitrosamide-specific detector for use with high-pressure liquid chromatography. J. Chromat., 133, 59-66

Smetanin, E.E. (1971) On transplacental blastomogenic effect of dimethyl nitrosamine and nitrosomethyl urea. Vop. Onkol., 17, 75-81

Stavrou, D., Haglid, K.G. & Weidenbach, W. (1975) Experimentelle Induktion neurogener Tumoren beim Hund durch chronische parenterale Applikation von Methylnitrosoharnstoff. In: Proceedings of the VIIth International Congress of Neuropathology, Budapest, 1974, Amsterdam, Excerpta Medica, pp. 425-431

Stavrou, D., Dahme, E. & Kalich, J. (1976) Gastroonkogene Wirkung von Methylnitrosoharnstoff beim Miniaturschwein. Res. exp. Med., 169, 33-43

Stroobandt, G. & Brucher, J.M. (1968) Etude de tumeurs nerveuses obtenues par l'administration de méthylnitrosourée au rat. Neuro-chirurgie, 14, 515-535

Swann, P.F. (1968) The rate of breakdown of methyl methanesulphonate, dimethyl sulphate and *N*-methyl-*N*-nitrosourea in the rat. Biochem. J., 110, 49-52

Swann, P.F. & Magee, P.N. (1968) Nitrosamine-induced carcinogenesis. The alkylation of nucleic acids of the rat by *N*-methyl-*N*-nitrosourea, dimethylnitrosamine, dimethyl sulphate and methyl methanesulphonate. Biochem. J., 110, 39-47

Swenberg, J.A., Koestner, A. & Wechsler, W. (1972) The induction of tumors of the nervous system with intravenous methylnitrosourea. Lab. Invest., 26, 74-85

Swenberg, J.A., Koestner, A. & Wechsler, W. (1974) Differential neuro-oncogenic effects of methylnitrosourea: the influence of route, dose, sex and strain (Abstract no. 116). J. Neuropath. exp. Neurol., 33, 194

Swenberg, J.A., Koestner, A., Wechsler, W., Brunden, M.N. & Abe, H. (1975) Differential oncogenic effects of methylnitrosourea. J. nat. Cancer Inst., 54, 89-96

Swenson, D.H., Farmer, P.B. & Lawley, P.D. (1976) Identification of the methyl phosphotriester of thymidylyl(3'-5')thymidine as a product from reaction of DNA with the carcinogen *N*-methyl-*N*-nitrosourea. Chem.-biol. Interact., 15, 91-100

Terracini, B. & Stramignoni, A. (1967) Malignant lymphomas and renal changes in Swiss mice given nitrosomethylurea. Europ. J. Cancer, 3, 435-436

Terracini, B. & Testa, M.C. (1970) Carcinogenicity of a single administration of *N*-nitrosomethylurea: a comparison between newborn and 5-week-old mice and rats. Brit. J. Cancer, 24, 588-598

Terracini, B., Testa, M.C., Cabral, J.R. & Rossi, L. (1976) The roles of age at treatment and dose in carcinogenesis in C3Hf/Dp mice with a single administration of *N*-nitroso-*N*-methylurea. Brit. J. Cancer, 33, 427-439

Thomas, C. & Bollmann, R. (1969) Untersuchungen zur Organotropie der krebserzeugenden Wirkung des *N*-Nitroso-*N*-methyl-Harnstoffes (NMH) an Ratten. Experientia, 25, 50-51

Thomas, C., Sierra, J.L. & Kersting, G. (1967) Hirntumoren bei Ratten nach oraler Gabe von *N*-Nitroso-*N*-methyl-harnstoff. Naturwissenschaften, 54, 228

Thomas, C., Sierra, J.L. & Kersting, G. (1968) Neurogene Tumoren bei Ratten nach intraperitonealer Applikation von *N*-Nitroso-*N*-methyl-harnstoff. Naturwissenschaften, 55, 183

Tomatis, L., Hilfrich, J. & Turusov, V. (1975) The occurrence of tumours in F_1, F_2 and F_3 descendants of BD rats exposed to *N*-nitrosomethylurea during pregnancy. Int. J. Cancer, 15, 385-390

Veleminský, J., Osterman-Golkar, S. & Ehrenberg, L. (1970) Reaction rates and biological action of *N*-methyl- and *N*-ethyl-*N*-nitrosourea. Mutation Res., 10, 169-174

Vlasov, N.N., Balanski, R.M. & Khudoley, V.V. (1976) Papillomas of the urinary bladder induced by *N*-nitroso-*N*-methylurea in rats. Vop. Onkol., 22, 58-61

Warzok, R., Schneider, J., Schreiber, D. & Jänisch, W. (1970) Experimental brain tumours in dogs. Experientia, 26, 303-304

Waynforth, H.B. & Magee, P.N. (1975) The effect of various doses and schedules of administration of *N*-methyl-*N*-nitrosourea, with and without croton oil promotion, on skin papilloma production in BALB/c mice. Gann Mongr. Cancer Res., 17, 439-448

Wechsler, W., Kleihues, P., Matsumoto, S., Zülch, K.J., Ivankovic, S., Preussmann, R. & Druckrey, H. (1969) Pathology of experimental neurogenic tumors chemically induced during prenatal and postnatal life. Ann. N.Y. Acad. Sci., 159, 360-408

Weiss, J.F., Grossi Paoletti, E., Paoletti, P., Schiffer, D. & Fabiani, A. (1970) Occurrence of desmosterol in tumors of the nervous system induced in the rat by nitrosourea derivatives. Cancer Res., 30, 2107-2109

Wilander, E. & Gunnarsson, R. (1975) Diabetogenic effects of *N*-nitrosomethylurea in the Chinese hamster. Acta path. microbiol. scand., Sect. A, 83, 206-212

Wilander, E. & Tjälve, H. (1975) Diabetogenic effects of *N*-nitrosomethylurea with special regard to species variations. Exp. Path., 11, 133-141

Zardi, L., St Vincent, L., Barbin, A., Montesano, R. & Margison, G.P. (1977) Effect of split doses of *N*-methyl-*N*-nitrosourea on DNA repair synthesis in cultured mammalian cells. Cancer Lett., 3, 183-188

Zhuravel, B.N. & Shlyapunov, V.N. (1972) Use of chemical mutagens and γ-rays in the breeding of corn for cold hardiness. In: Rapoport, I.A., ed., Proceedings on Selection of Chemical Mutagens, Moscow, Nauka, pp. 253-256 [Chem. Abstr., 80, 34122h]

N-NITROSOMETHYLVINYLAMINE

1. Chemical and Physical Data

1.1 Synonyms and trade names

Chem. Abstr. Services Reg. No.: 4549-40-0

Chem. Abstr. Name: *N*-Methyl-*N*-nitroso-ethenylamine

N-Methyl-*N*-nitrosovinylamine; methylvinylnitrosamine; NMVA

1.2 Structural and molecular formulae and weight

$O{=}N{-}N(CH_3){-}CH{=}CH_2$

$C_3H_6N_2O$ Mol. wt: 86.1

1.3 Chemical and physical properties of the pure substance

(a) Description: Yellow liquid

(b) Boiling-point: 47-48° C (30 mm)

(c) Refractive index: n_D^{25} 1.4920

(d) Spectroscopy data: λ_{max} 200, 270, 376 nm (E_1^1 = 519, 786, 20) in water (Druckrey *et al.*, 1967); mass spectroscopy data are given by Pensabene *et al.* (1972) and Rainey *et al.* (1978).

(e) Solubility: Soluble in water (3%) and in organic solvents and lipids

(f) Volatility: Very volatile; can be steam-distilled (Eisenbrand *et al.*, 1970)

(g) Stability: Relatively unstable; a concentration decrease of more than 10% has been observed in aqueous solution over 24 hours (Druckrey *et al.*, 1967); light-sensitive, especially to ultra-violet light

1.4 Technical products and impurities

No data were available to the Working Group.

2. Production, Use, Occurrence and Analysis

2.1 Production and use

(a) Production

N-Nitrosomethylvinylamine (NMVA) has been prepared by the reaction of β-chloroethylmethylnitrosamine with either sodium ethoxide (Workman, 1955) or a solution of potassium hydroxide in methanol (Ogimachi & Kruse, 1961). It can be prepared by reaction of methylvinylamine with sodium nitrite at 60°C (Druckrey *et al.*, 1967). No evidence was found that NMVA has been produced commercially.

(b) Use

No data were available to the Working Group.

2.2 Occurrence

A preliminary report indicates that NMVA may be present in apple brandy (IARC, 1977).

2.3 Analysis

Gas chromatography/thermal energy analysis (TEA), high-pressure liquid chromatography/TEA and gas chromatography/mass spectrometry have been used for the analysis of NMVA (Preussmann *et al.*, 1978).

3. Biological Data Relevant to the Evaluation of Carcinogenic Risk to Man

3.1 Carcinogenicity and related studies in animals

(a) Oral administration

Rat: Of a group of 19 BD rats given *N*-nitrosomethylvinylamine (NMVA) in drinking-water at doses of 0.3 or 0.6 mg/kg bw/day, 2 developed papillomas and 17, nodular and widely distributed squamous-cell carcinomas of the oesophagus. In addition, 4 animals had carcinomas of the tongue and

5 animals, carcinomas of the pharynx; 8 rats showed bile-duct proliferation and cysts in the liver. The average induction time for the tumours of the upper digestive tract was 390 or 270 days, respectively; the average total dose that caused tumours in 50% of the animals was 0.11 or 0.16 g/kg bw (Druckrey *et al.*, 1967; Thomas & So, 1969).

(b) Inhalation and/or intratracheal administration

Rat: Two BD rats that survived a single exposure to 18 mg/kg bw NMVA died 277 and 374 days later with carcinomas of the nasal cavities. Ten of 18 BD rats exposed chronically to 25 or 50 ppm in air twice weekly for 30 minutes (~1 or 2 mg/kg bw) died early as a result of severe inflammation of the respiratory tract. Of the remaining 8 rats, 3 developed squamous-cell carcinomas and 2, tumours described as cholesteatomas in the nasal cavity. One animal had an aesthesioneuroepithelioma of the ethmoturbinals, 1, a carcinoma of the pharynx, and 2, an oesophageal papilloma (Druckrey *et al.*, 1967; Thomas, 1965; Thomas & So, 1969).

3.2 Other relevant biological data

(a) Experimental systems

Toxic effects

The oral LD_{50} of NMVA in BD rats was 24 mg/kg bw and that by inhalation, 22 mg/kg bw (Druckrey *et al.*, 1967).

No data on the metabolism, embryotoxicity or teratogenicity of this compound were available to the Working Group.

Mutagenicity and other short-term tests

NMVA causes X-linked recessive lethal mutations in *Drosophila melanogaster* (Pasternak, 1964).

(b) Humans

No data were available to the Working Group.

3.3 Case reports and epidemiological studies

No data were available to the Working Group.

4. Summary of Data Reported and Evaluation

4.1 Experimental data

N-Nitrosomethylvinylamine is carcinogenic in rats, the only species tested. It produces carcinomas of the oesophagus, tongue and pharynx after its continuous oral administration and carcinomas of the nasal cavities after inhalation exposure.

4.2 Human data

No case reports or epidemiological studies were available to the Working Group. Insufficient information on the occurrence or use of this compound was available to permit identification of exposed groups.

4.3 Evaluation

There is *sufficient evidence* of a carcinogenic effect of *N*-nitrosomethylvinylamine in one experimental animal species. Although no epidemiological data were available, *N*-nitrosomethylvinylamine should be regarded for practical purposes as if it were carcinogenic to humans.

5. References

Druckrey, H., Preussmann, R., Ivankovic, S. & Schmähl, D. (1967) Organotrope carcinogene Wirkungen bei 65 verschiedenen *N*-Nitroso-Verbindungen an BD-Ratten. Z. Krebsforsch., 69, 103-201

Eisenbrand, G., Hodenberg, A. von & Preussmann, R. (1970) Trace analysis of *N*-nitroso compounds. II. Steam distillation at neutral, alkaline and acid pH under reduced and atmospheric pressure. Z. analyt. Chem., 251, 22-24

IARC (1977) Annual Report 1977, Lyon, International Agency for Research on Cancer, p. 56

Ogimachi, N.N. & Kruse, H.W. (1961) Preparation and reduction of methylvinylnitrosamine. J. org. Chem., 26, 1642-1644

Pasternak, L. (1964) Untersuchungen über die mutagene Wirkung verschiedener Nitrosamin- und Nitrosamid-Verbindungen. Arzneimittel-Forsch., 14, 802-804

Pensabene, J.W., Fiddler, W., Dooley, C.J., Doerr, R.C. & Wasserman, A.E. (1972) Spectral and gas chromatographic characteristics of some *N*-nitrosamines. J. agric. Fd Chem., 20, 274-277

Preussmann, R., Walker, E.A., Wasserman, A.E. & Castegnaro, M., eds (1978) Environmental Carcinogens - Selected Methods of Analysis, Vol. 1, Nitrosamines, Lyon (IARC Scientific Publications No. 18) (in press)

Rainey, W.T., Christie, W.H. & Lijinsky, W. (1978) Mass spectrometry of *N*-nitrosamines. Biomed. Mass Spectrom. (in press)

Thomas, C. (1965) Zur Morphologie der Nasenhöhlentumoren bei der Ratte. Z. Krebsforsch., 67, 1-10

Thomas, C. & So, B.T. (1969) Zur Morphologie der durch *N*-Nitroso-Verbindungen erzeugten Tumoren im oberen Verdauungstrakt der Ratte. Arzneimittel-Forsch., 19, 1077-1081

Workman, W.R. (1955) Unusual reactions of methylvinylnitrosamine and β-chloroethylmethylnitrosamine. Diss. Abstr., 15, 1733

N-NITROSOMORPHOLINE

1. Chemical and Physical Data

1.1 Synonyms and trade names

Chem. Abstr. Services Reg. No.: 59-89-2

Chem. Abstr. Name: 4-Nitrosomorpholine

NMOR

1.2 Structural and molecular formulae and weight

O=N—N(morpholine ring)O

$C_4H_8N_2O_2$ Mol. wt: 116.1

1.3 Chemical and physical properties of the pure substance

(a) Description: Yellow crystals

(b) Boiling-point: 224-225°C (747 mm); 96°C (6 mm)

(c) Melting-point: 29°C

(d) Spectroscopy data: λ_{max} 237 and 346 nm (E^1_1 = 685 and 7.3) in water (Druckrey *et al.*, 1967); mass spectroscopy data are given by Pensabene *et al.* (1972) and Rainey *et al.* (1978).

(e) Solubility: Miscible in water in all proportions; soluble in organic solvents

(f) Stability: Stable at room temperature for more than 14 days in neutral and alkaline aqueous solutions in the dark (Druckrey *et al.*, 1967); slightly less stable in acidic solutions; light-sensitive, especially to ultra-violet light

(g) Reactivity: Strong oxidants (peracids) oxidize it to the corresponding nitramine; can be reduced to the corresponding hydrazine and/or amine; relatively resistant to hydrolysis but can be split by hydrogen bromide in acetic acid (Eisenbrand & Preussmann, 1970). Photochemically reactive (Fridman *et al.*, 1971)

1.4 Technical products and impurities

No data were available to the Working Group.

2. Production, Use, Occurrence and Analysis

2.1 Production and use

For background information on this section, see preamble, p. 22.

(a) Production

N-Nitrosomorpholine (NMOR) was prepared by Knorr in 1907 and by Bellamy *et al.* in 1961 by the reaction of sodium nitrite with a solution of morpholine in sulphuric acid (Prager & Jacobson, 1937); it has also been prepared by the reaction of nitrogen trioxide with morpholine (Levering & Maury, 1962).

No evidence was found that NMOR has been manufactured commercially.

(b) Use

Patents have been issued for the use of NMOR as a solvent for polyacrylonitrile (Kowalik *et al.*, 1954) and as a chemical intermediate in the synthesis of *N*-aminomorpholine (Zimmer *et al.*, 1955). It has also been found to be effective against microbial infections (Bellamy *et al.*, 1961). No evidence was found that it has been used commercially for these purposes.

2.2 Occurrence

Eisenbrand *et al.* (1978) demonstrated the presence of NMOR in 3/11 batches of analytical grade dichloromethane at the 10-32 μg/l level and in 4/10 batches of analytical grade chloroform at the 2-376 μg/l level. It was not present in less pure grades of these solvents.

2.3 Analysis

An IARC manual gives selected methods for the analysis of volatile *N*-nitrosamines, including *N*-nitrosomorpholine (Preussmann *et al.*, 1978).

3. Biological Data Relevant to the Evaluation of Carcinogenic Risk to Man

3.1 Carcinogenicity and related studies in animals

(a) Oral administration

Mouse: A group of 58 male NMRI mice received *N*-nitrosomorpholine (NMOR) in the drinking-water at concentrations of 100 mg/l (corresponding to approximately 16 mg/kg bw/day at the beginning of the experiment) for life. Sixteen mice developed benign hepatocellular tumours after total doses of 58-150 mg/animal; 1 animal had a haemangioendothelioma, and 2 had benign haemangiomas of the liver. In addition to liver tumours, numerous lung adenomas and 1 squamous-cell carcinoma of the lung were observed. Of 17 controls, only 1 had a small adenoma of the lung (Bannasch & Müller, 1964; Müller, 1964).

Rat: A group of 16 BD rats were given NMOR in the drinking-water at doses of 8 mg/kg bw/day for life. Fourteen animals developed hepatocellular carcinomas after an average induction time of 165 days (average total dose that induced tumours in 50% of the animals, 1.3 g/kg bw); another animal had a haemangioendothelioma of the liver (Druckrey *et al.*, 1967). After a short-term treatment consisting of 6 oral applications of 30 mg/kg bw NMOR, 1/9 surviving BD rats developed a renal carcinoma, 1, a hepatoma, and 2, carcinomas of the ovary at the 540th, 590th and 600th day, respectively (Druckrey *et al.*, 1964a). The induction of liver tumours by NMOR has been confirmed in BD rats (Bannasch & Müller, 1964), Sprague-Dawley rats (Bannasch & Reiss, 1971; Lijinsky & Taylor, 1975; Newberne & Shank, 1973) and MRC Wistar rats (Mirvish *et al.*, 1976).

Detailed light and electron microscope investigations of the morphogenesis of hepatocellular tumours were performed in 102 BD rats which received NMOR in the drinking-water at concentrations of 60, 120 or 200 mg/l for 7-12 weeks or for life. Foci of hepatocellular alterations (clear, acidophilic, basophilic or vacuolated cells) consistently preceded the development of hepatocellular carcinomas (Bannasch, 1968, 1975).

A total of 272 Sprague-Dawley rats were given NMOR in the drinking-water at a concentration of 500 mg/l for 3 weeks. A high incidence of cholangiocellular tumours (cystadenomas, cholangiofibromas, cholangio-carcinomas) was induced after a latent period of several weeks or months. In addition to cholangiocellular tumours, benign and malignant hepatocellular tumours and haemangiosarcomas were seen. The morphogenesis of the cholangiocellular tumours was followed in detail (Bannasch & Reiss, 1971; Bannasch & Massner, 1976). Electron microscope investigations of 11 cholangiofibromas induced by NMOR support the view that this type of tumour originates from the intrahepatic bile ductules (Bannasch & Massner, 1978).

Sequential investigations of the morphogenesis of epithelial kidney tumours were performed in 165 Sprague-Dawley rats which received NMOR in the drinking-water at concentrations of 120 mg/l or 500 mg/l for 3-14 weeks. No kidney tumours were observed in 66 animals that were killed up to 5 weeks after withdrawal of the carcinogen. Only 1/21 animals that were killed between 7 and 18 weeks after removal of the carcinogen had a microscopic adenoma. However, 22-97 weeks after stopping the carcinogenic treatment, 47/69 animals (68%) had epithelial kidney tumours. Histologically, all of the types of epithelial kidney tumours seen in humans were observed, namely, clear-cell tumours, acidophilic tumours, basophilic tumours and oncocytomas (Bannasch *et al.*, 1974). In addition to epithelial kidney tumours, putative preneoplastic tubular changes (clear, chromophobic, oncocytic and basophilic cells instead of normal epithelia) were observed in most animals (Bannasch & Schacht, 1968, 1970; Bannasch *et al.*, 1971).

Groups of 30 male Sprague-Dawley rats were given NMOR-[3,3,5,5-d_4] or unlabelled NMOR in the drinking-water at concentrations of 41.5 or 8.3 mg/l labelled NMOR or 40 or 8 mg/l unlabelled NMOR (corresponding to 0.35 and 0.07×10^{-3}M) for 30 weeks. Of animals given the higher dose of unlabelled NMOR, 16/30 had hepatocellular tumours, and 2 had haemangioendotheliomas of the liver; in the lower dose group, 11/30 rats developed hepatocellular tumours, and 1 had a haemangioendothelioma of the liver. The higher dose of the labelled NMOR induced hepatocellular tumours in 5/30 animals, whereas the lower dose induced these tumours in 3/30 rats. No haemangioendotheliomas of the liver occurred in either group administered the labelled compound (Lijinsky *et al.*, 1976).

(b) Subcutaneous and/or intramuscular administration

Hamster: Of 18 Syrian golden hamsters treated subcutaneously with 0.5 ml of 1:125 solution of NMOR in water twice weekly for more than 2 months, 14 developed multiple papillary tumours of the trachea (Dontenwill & Mohr, 1962).

Groups of 20 male and 20 female 8-week-old Syrian golden hamsters were given weekly s.c. injections of 1/5, 1/10 or 1/20th of the LD_{50} (LD_{50}: males, 492 mg/kg bw; females, 562 mg/kg bw) for life. The incidence of tumours in the respiratory system (mainly nasal cavities and trachea) ranged from 69-100%. The total incidence of neoplasms was dose-dependent. Multiple adenomas were located in the lung parenchyma of 4 hamsters. The neoplasms of the nasal cavities were usually multicentric in origin and of different histological types (squamous-cell papillomas, squamous-cell carcinomas, anaplastic carcinomas, adenocarcinomas, mixed tumours and olfactory neuroepitheliomas) (Haas *et al.*, 1973). Similar results were obtained in European (Mohr *et al.*, 1974) and Chinese hamsters (Reznik *et al.*, 1976), in which, in addition, benign and/or malignant tumours of the oesophagus and forestomach were seen.

Groups of 5 male and 5 female Syrian golden hamsters were injected subcutaneously with single doses of 50, 100, 200 or 400 mg/kg bw NMOR. The majority of neoplasms were found in the trachea, but some tumours were also observed in the nasal cavities, larynx and bronchi. Epidermoid carcinomas and adenocarcinomas were found in the nasal cavities (Althoff *et al.*, 1974).

(c) Intravenous administration

Rat: Of 7 BD rats injected intravenously once weekly with 5 or 10 mg/kg bw NMOR, 2 developed hepatocellular carcinomas and 5, carcinomas of the ethmoturbinals after an induction time of 400-450 days (Druckrey *et al.*, 1964b).

(d) Other experimental systems

Immersion

NMOR was added to the water of tanks containing 20 zebra fish (*Danio rerio*) and 30 guppies (*Lebistes reticulatus*) at concentrations of 100-320 mg/l or 75-250 mg/l for 28 weeks. Surviving fish were killed at 31 weeks. Eight out of 9 guppies had hepatic lesions (4 hepatocellular carcinomas, 3 hepatic adenomas, 1 cystic cholangioma) after an average latent period of 30 weeks. Four out of 13 zebra fish had hepatocellular carcinomas, and 1 intestinal adenocarcinoma, 1 adenocarcinoma of the liver and 1 mesenchymal tumour in the abdominal cavity were also observed; the average latent period was 16 weeks (Pliss & Khudoley, 1975).

(e) Carcinogenicity of precursors

Groups of 20 male and 20 female Swiss mice were given 0.08 g/l NMOR in the drinking-water for life. Corresponding groups received 6.33 g/kg of diet morpholine concurrently with 1.0 g/l sodium nitrite in the drinking-water. Controls were treated with the same concentrations of morpholine or sodium nitrite alone or left untreated. At 40 weeks, all survivors were killed. Of those treated with NMOR, 16/22 animals (73%) developed lung adenomas (total number, 106); in addition, 4 liver carcinomas and 1 papillary adenoma of the bile duct were observed. Of those that received concurrent administration of morpholine and sodium nitrite, 20/35 (57%) had a total of 41 lung adenomas. Treatment with morpholine alone or with sodium nitrite alone produced no effects in the mice when compared with untreated controls (Greenblatt *et al.*, 1971).

The addition of 5.75, 11.5 or 23.0 g/kg of diet sodium ascorbate to A mice resulted in 72-89% inhibition of adenoma induction by 6.33 g/kg of diet morpholine plus 2.0 g/l of drinking-water sodium nitrite. Moreover, adenoma induction by the combination was strongly inhibited (86%) by gallic acid (5.45 or 21.8 g/kg of diet), moderately inhibited (65%) by caffeine (1.0 g/kg of diet) and unaffected by sodium thiocyanate (1.0 g/kg of diet) (Mirvish *et al.*, 1975).

Groups of 7 female Sprague-Dawley rats (120 g) were given morpholine and sodium nitrite concurrently in the diet at concentrations of 0.5% each for 8 weeks and were observed until they died. Equal numbers of animals received 0.5% morpholine or 0.5% sodium nitrite alone for 8 weeks. All animals that received morpholine plus nitrite developed hepatocellular adenomas and, with one exception, hepatocellular carcinomas. Two animals had haemangioendotheliomas of the liver, and 1 animal had a liver tumour diagnosed as a cyst-adenocarcinoma. Renal adenomas were found in 1 animal. Morpholine or nitrite given alone did not induce tumours (Sander & Bürkle, 1969).

Comprehensive investigations in Sprague-Dawley rats with different doses of sodium nitrite and morpholine have been performed by Newberne & Shank (1973) and Shank & Newberne (1976). Details are given in Table 1. Histologically, the liver tumours induced by NMOR and by nitrite plus morpholine were identical. A great variety of tumours other than hepato-cellular carcinomas and haemangiosarcomas developed in experimental and control animals; tumour sites were the glandular and non-glandular epithe-lium, lymphoreticular system, nervous system, muscles, connective tissue and embryonal or mixed tissues. Of 104 controls that received 1000 mg/kg of diet morpholine, 3 developed hepatocellular carcinomas and 2, lung angiosarcomas. The diet of these animals contained no detectable nitrite, and they were given only distilled water; thus, either morpholine itself is weakly carcinogenic or nitrite reached the stomach from an unknown source. Animals in this group also developed two malignant brain gliomas, a rare finding in this species. Control animals fed the high nitrite diet (1000 mg/kg of diet) showed a high incidence of tumours in the lymphoreti-cular system (27%, compared with 6% in untreated controls) and a high total number of tumours other than hepatomas and haemangiosarcomas (60%, compared with 18% in untreated controls) (Newberne & Shank, 1973; Shank & Newberne, 1976).

Table 1

Incidence of hepatocellular carcinomas and angiosarcomas among rats fed experimental diets[1]

Mg/kg of diet			Number of rats	Incidence (%)					Age at death with liver carcinoma (weeks)	
Sodium nitrite	Morpholine	NMOR		Liver-cell carcinomas	Liver haemangio-sarcomas	Lung angio-sarcomas	Other angio-sarcomas	Metastases from liver to lung	First death	Median
0	0	0	156	0	0	0	0	-	-	-
1000	0	0	96	1	0	0	1	0	123	-
0	1000	0	104	3	0	2	1	0	68	-
1000	1000	0	159	97	14	23	1	49	19	38
1000	50	0	117	59	5	6	0	17	47	111
1000	5	0	154	28	12	8	1	7	24	-
50	1000	0	109	3	2	1	0	0	89	-
5	1000	0	172	1	2	1	1	0	64	-
50	50	0	152	2	1	1	1	0	65	-
5	5	0	125	1	2	2	1	0	88	-
0	0	5	128	58	15	9	1	22	53	106
0	0	50	94	93	21	20	1	58	30	56

[1]From Shank & Newberne, 1976

Groups of 40 male MRC Wistar rats were treated for 2 years with either 10 g/kg of diet morpholine plus 3 g/l of drinking-water sodium nitrite or with 0.15 g/l of drinking-water NMOR. In both cases, one group of rats were also given sodium ascorbate (22.7 g/kg of diet). The results of treatment with morpholine plus nitrite or with NMOR were similar to those reported above. When ascorbate was present, the liver tumours induced by morpholine plus nitrite had a longer induction period (93 *versus* 54 weeks), a slightly lower incidence (49% *versus* 65%) and no metastases to the lungs; however, ascorbate did not affect liver tumour induction by preformed NMOR. Of those treated with morpholine, nitrite and ascorbate, 21/39 animals developed forestomach tumours (14 squamous-cell papillomas, 7 squamous-cell carcinomas) (Mirvish *et al.*, 1976).

Syrian golden hamsters were fed sodium nitrite plus morpholine at concentrations of 5-1000 mg/kg of diet. Hepatocellular carcinomas and haemangiosarcomas of the liver developed in animals given the higher dose levels; while in those given the lower dose levels, liver lesions diagnosed as nodular hyperplasia developed in some animals (Shank & Newberne, 1976).

(f) Carcinogenicity of derivatives

2,6-Dimethylnitrosomorpholine

Oral administration: A group of 30 male Sprague-Dawley rats were given 40 mg/l NMOR, and a group of 15 male and 15 female Sprague-Dawley rats were given 50 mg/l 2,6-dimethylnitrosomorpholine, in the drinking-water at equimolar concentrations on 5 days/week for 30 weeks. Animals treated with 2,6-dimethylnitrosomorpholine died within 35 weeks after initiation of treatment, while those treated with NMOR lived considerably longer and were killed at 104 weeks. After treatment with NMOR, 16/30 rats developed hepatocellular tumours, and 2 developed Kupffer-cell sarcomas. 2,6-Dimethylnitrosomorpholine induced tumours in the nasal cavities (28 adenocarcinomas), trachea (5 papillomas), oesophagus (28 papillomas and carcinomas) and stomach (5 papillomas and carcinomas), but only 1 hepatocellular carcinoma (Lijinsky & Taylor, 1975).

Four groups of 15 male and 15 female Syrian golden hamsters were given 1/5, 1/10, or 1/20 the LD_{50} intragastrically once weekly for life (LD_{50}:

367 mg/kg bw). Pancreatic-duct carcinomas and adenomas occurred in 71% of animals; some tumours metastasized to the lungs. Tumours were also induced in the nasal cavities, respiratory tract and kidneys (Mohr *et al.*, 1977).

(g) Factors that modify carcinogenicity in animals

A group of 96 BR 46 rats of both sexes received NMOR, *N*-nitrosodiethylamine (NDEA) and *N*-nitrosodimethylamine (NDMA) in the drinking-water at doses of 0.2, 0.05 and 0.01 mg/kg bw, respectively, concurrently with 3 mg/kg bw 4-dimethylaminoazobenzene (DAB) in their food for 580 days (total doses: NMOR, 114 mg/kg bw; NDEA, 29 mg/kg bw; NDMA, 5.8 mg/kg bw; DAB, 1630 mg/kg bw). These doses were derived from the literature and were assumed to be not high enough to induce tumours under the experimental conditions used. After an average induction time of 700±110 days, 29/86 animals (34%) developed malignant liver tumours (20 hepatocellular carcinomas, 9 haemangioendotheliomas and/or haemangiosarcomas); 8 animals also had benign hepatocellular tumours. Only 1 animal showed liver cirrhosis, and 12 animals had a variety of malignant extrahepatic tumours. Of 100 untreated control animals, 2 had tumours of the mammary gland described as sarcomas, 1, a lung carcinoma, 6, mammary fibrosarcomas and 5, benign thymomas (Schmähl, 1970) [No concurrent controls of animals treated with the individual carcinogens were carried out].

An unexpected increase (15-30%) in the induction of lung adenomas in mice by administration of 20 mg/l NMOR in the drinking-water was observed after the addition of sodium ascorbate (5.75-23 g/kg of diet). The authors suggested that the mice treated with sodium ascorbate consumed more NMOR solution (Mirvish *et al.*, 1975).

3.2 Other relevant biological data

(a) Experimental systems

Toxic effects

In rats, the LD_{50} of NMOR was 320 mg/kg bw by oral and i.p. administration and 100 mg/kg bw by i.v. injection (Druckrey *et al.*, 1967; Lee & Lijinsky, 1966). The s.c. LD_{50} in Syrian golden hamsters was about

500 mg/kg bw (Haas *et al.*, 1973), that in Chinese hamsters about 170 mg/kg bw (Reznik *et al.*, 1976) and that in European hamsters 450 mg/kg bw (Mohr *et al.*, 1974). The oral LD_{50} in Syrian golden hamsters was 360 mg/kg bw (Mohr *et al.*, 1977).

In rats, NMOR causes centrolobular hepatic necrosis and a variety of cytoplasmic and nuclear changes (Bannasch, 1968, 1975; Stewart *et al.*, 1975).

No data on the embryotoxicity or teratogenicity of this compound were available to the Working Group.

Absorption, distribution and excretion

After i.p. injection of 400 mg/kg bw [3-^{14}C]-NMOR to rats, 3.3% of the label was excreted as $^{14}CO_2$ and 81% in the urine over 24 hours; 24% of the radioactivity was recovered as unchanged NMOR and 15% as *N*-nitrosodiethanolamine (Stewart *et al.*, 1974).

Metabolism

Acid hydrolysis of the liver RNA and DNA isolated from the rats in the above experiment gave 6 distinct radioactive products, one of which was probably 7-(2-hydroxyethyl)guanine (Stewart *et al.*, 1974). Oral administration of ^{3}H-NMOR and NMOR-[3,5-d_4] to rats also led to reaction with liver DNA and RNA, yielding products which were not identified (Lijinsky *et al.*, 1973).

After i.p. administration of 100 mg/kg bw NMOR to rats, the repair of liver DNA was determined by velocity sedimentation in both alkaline and neutral sucrose gradients. The repair of double-strand breaks was rapid, but repair of single-strand breaks was not complete after 14 days (Stewart & Farber, 1973).

Mutagenicity and other short-term tests

N-Nitrosomorpholine was mutagenic in *Salmonella typhimurium* TA 1530, TA 1535, TA 1537 and TA 1538 in the presence of liver microsomal fractions from phenobarbital-treated rats and human biopsies (Bartsch *et al.*, 1976; Gomez *et al.*, 1974). NMOR induced reverse mutations in *Escherichia coli* when liver microsomes from phenobarbital-treated or untreated rats were used (Elespuru & Lijinsky, 1976; Nakajima *et al.*, 1974).

In the presence of a liver microsomal system from phenobarbital-pretreated rats, NMOR induced 8-azaguanine resistant mutants in Chinese hamster V79 cells (Kuroki *et al.*, 1977). In BHK-21 cells, NMOR induced 8-azaguanine resistant mutants as well as chromatid breaks and rearrangements (Kimble *et al.*, 1973).

In the host-mediated assay, 100 mg/kg bw NMOR given intramuscularly or orally to mice was mutagenic to *S. typhimurium* G-46 injected intraperitoneally into the mice (Zeiger & Legator, 1971).

Induction of X-linked recessive lethal mutations and translocations was noted in *Drosophila melanogaster* (Henke *et al.*, 1964, 1965). Doses of 50 and 100 mg/kg bw NMOR injected intraperitoneally to male mice did not increase the incidence of dominant lethal mutations (Parkin *et al.*, 1973).

(b) Humans

No data were available to the Working Group.

3.3 Case reports and epidemiological studies

No data were available to the Working Group.

4. Summary of Data Reported and Evaluation

4.1 Experimental data

N-Nitrosomorpholine is carcinogenic in mice, rats, Syrian golden, Chinese and European hamsters and various fish. Following its oral administration, it produces benign and malignant tumours of the liver and lung in mice, of the liver, kidney and blood vessels in rats and of the liver in hamsters. After its subcutaneous injection it produces tumours of the upper digestive and respiratory tracts in hamsters; it is carcinogenic after its administration in single doses. It produces liver tumours in rats following its intravenous injection. It produces liver tumours in various fish following its administration in tank-water. A study in hamsters has been reported in which a dose-response relationship was established.

4.2 Human data

No case reports or epidemiological studies were available to the Working Group. Insufficient information on the occurrence of *N*-nitrosomorpholine was available to permit identification of exposed groups.

4.3 Evaluation

There is *sufficient evidence* for a carcinogenic effect of *N*-nitrosomorpholine in several experimental animal species. Although no epidemiological data were available, *N*-nitrosomorpholine should be regarded for practical purposes as if it were carcinogenic to humans.

5. References

Althoff, J., Wilson, R., Cardesa, A. & Pour, P. (1974) Comparative studies of neoplastic response to a single dose of nitroso compounds. III. The effect of *N*-nitrosopiperidine and *N*-nitrosomorpholine in Syrian golden hamsters. Z. Krebsforsch., 81, 251-259

Archer, M.C. & Wishnok, J.S. (1976) Nitrosamine formation in corrosion-inhibiting compositions containing nitrite salts of secondary amines. J. environm. Sci. Hlth, A11, 583-590

Bannasch, P. (1968) The cytoplasm of hepatocytes during carcinogenesis. Electron- and lightmicroscopical investigations of the nitrosomorpholine-intoxicated rat liver. Recent Results Cancer Res., 19, 1-100

Bannasch, P. (1975) Die Cytologie der Hepatocarcinogenese. In: Altmann, H.-W. *et al.*, eds, Handbuch der Allgemeinen Pathologie, Vol. 6, Berlin, Springer, pp. 123-276

Bannasch, P. & Massner, B. (1976) Histogenese und Cytogenese von Cholangiofibromen und Cholangiocarcinomen bei Nitrosomorpholin-vergifteten Ratten. Z. Krebsforsch., 87, 239-255

Bannasch, P. & Massner, B. (1978) Die Feinstruktur des Nitrosomorpholin-induzierten Cholangiofibroms der Ratte. Virchows Arch., Abt. B Zellpath. (in press)

Bannasch, P. & Müller, H.-A. (1964) Lichtmikroskopische Untersuchungen über die Wirkung von *N*-Nitrosomorpholin auf die Leber von Ratte und Maus. Arzneimittel-Forsch., 14, 805-814

Bannasch, P. & Reiss, W. (1971) Histogenese und Cytogenese cholangiocellulärer Tumoren bei Nitrosomorpholin-vergifteten Ratten. Zugleich ein Beitrag zur Morphogenese der Cystenleber. Z. Krebsforsch., 76, 193-215

Bannasch, P. & Schacht, U. (1968) Nitrosamin-induzierte tubuläre Glykogenspeicherung und Geschwulstbildung in der Rattenniere. Virchows Arch., Abt. B Zellpath., 1, 95-97

Bannasch, P. & Schacht, U. (1970) Morphogenese und Mikromorphologie experimenteller Nierentumoren vom Typ des sogenannten Hypernephroms. Verh. dtsch. Ges. Path., 54, 464-470

Bannasch, P., Schacht, U., Weidner, R. & Storch, E. (1971) Morphogenese und Mikromorphologie basophiler und onkozytärer Nierentumoren bei Nitrosamin-vergifteten Ratten. Verh. dtsch. Ges. Path., 55, 665-670

Bannasch, P., Schacht, U. & Storch, E. (1974) Morphogenese und Mikromorphologie epithelialer Nierentumoren bei Nitrosomorpholin-vergifteten Ratten. I. Induktion und Histologie der Tumoren. Z. Krebsforsch., 81, 311-331

Bartsch, H., Camus, A. & Malaveille, C. (1976) Comparative mutagenicity of *N*-nitrosamines in a semi-solid and in a liquid incubation system in the presence of rat or human tissue fractions. Mutation Res., 37, 149-162

Bellamy, E.A., Hayes, K.J. & Michels, J.G. (1961) *N*-(5-Nitro-2-furfurylidene)aminoheterocycles. US Patent 3,001,992, 26 September (to Norwich Pharmacal Co.) [Chem. Abstr., 57, 11201]

Dontenwill, W. & Mohr, U. (1962) Die organotrope Wirkung der Nitrosamine. Z. Krebsforsch., 65, 166-167

Druckrey, H., Steinhoff, D., Preussmann, R. & Ivankovic, S. (1964a) Erzeugung von Krebs durch eine einmalige Dosis von Methylnitroso-Harnstoff und verschiedenen Dialkylnitrosaminen an Ratten. Z. Krebforsch., 66, 1-10

Druckrey, H., Ivankovic, S., Mennel, H.D. & Preussmann, R. (1964b) Selektive Erzeugung von Carcinomen der Nasenhöhle bei Ratten durch *N*,*N*'-Di-Nitrosopiperazin, Nitrosopiperidin, Nitrosomorpholin, Methyl-ally-, Dimethyl- und Methyl-vinyl-nitrosamin. Z. Krebsforsch., 66, 138-150

Druckrey, H., Preussmann, R., Ivankovic, S. & Schmähl, D. (1967) Organotrope carcinogene Wirkungen bei 65 verschiedenen *N*-Nitroso-Verbindungen an BD-Ratten. Z. Krebsforsch., 69, 103-201

Eisenbrand, G. & Preussmann, R. (1970) Eine neue Methode zur kolorimetrischen Bestimmung von Nitrosaminen nach Spaltung der *N*-Nitrosogruppe mit Bromwasserstoff in Eisessig. Arzneimittel-Forsch., 20, 1513-1517

Eisenbrand, G., Spiegelhalder, B., Janzowski, C., Kann, J. & Preussmann, R. (1978) Volatile and non-volatile *N*-nitroso compounds in foods and other environmental media. In: Walker, E.A., Castegnaro, M., Griciute, L. & Lyle, R.E., eds, Environmental Aspects of *N*-Nitroso Compounds, Lyon (IARC Scientific Publications No. 19) (in press)

Elespuru, R.K. & Lijinsky, W. (1976) Mutagenicity of cyclic nitrosamines in *Escherichia coli* following activation with rat liver microsomes. Cancer Res., 36, 4099-4101

Fridman, A.L., Mukhametshin, F.M. & Novikov, S.S. (1971) Advances in the chemistry of aliphatic *N*-nitrosamines. Russ. chem. Rev., 40, 34-50

Gomez, R.F., Johnston, M. & Sinskey, A.J. (1974) Activation of nitrosomorpholine and nitrosopyrrolidine to bacterial mutagens. Mutation Res., 24, 5-7

Greenblatt, M., Mirvish, S. & So, B.T. (1971) Nitrosamine studies: induction of lung adenomas by concurrent administration of sodium nitrite and secondary amines in Swiss mice. J. nat. Cancer Inst., 46, 1029-1034

Haas, H., Mohr, U. & Krüger, F.W. (1973) Comparative studies with different doses of *N*-nitrosomorpholine, *N*-nitrosopiperidine, *N*-nitrosomethylurea, and dimethylnitrosamine in Syrian golden hamsters. J. nat. Cancer Inst., 51, 1295-1301

Henke, H., Höhne, G. & Künkel, H.A. (1964) Über die mutagene Wirkung von Röntgenstrahlen, *N*-nitroso-*N*-methyl-urethan und *N*-nitroso-morpholin bei *Drosophila melanogaster*. Biophysik, 1, 418-421

Henke, H., Höhne, G., Künkel, H.A. & Trams, A. (1965) Zur Frage der differentiellen Mutationswirkung einiger neuer organotroper Cancerogene. Arch. Gynäkol., 202, 475-479

Kimble, C.E., Sinsky, A.J. & Gorczyca, P. (1973) Mutagenesis of BHK-21 cells by *N*-nitroso compounds and ultraviolet light (Abstract No. 149). In Vitro, 8, 442-443

Kowalik, E.J., Downing, J. & Drewitt, J.G.N. (1954) Solvents for acrylonitrile polymers. US Patent 2,697,698, 21 December (to British Celanese Ltd) [Chem. Abstr., 49, 5854]

Kuroki, T., Drevon, C. & Montesano, R. (1977) Microsome-mediated mutagenesis in V79 Chinese hamster cells by various nitrosamines. Cancer Res., 37, 1044-1050

Lee, K.Y. & Lijinsky, W. (1966) Alkylation of rat liver RNA by cyclic *N*-nitrosamines *in vivo*. J. nat. Cancer Inst., 37, 401-407

Levering, D.R. & Maury, L.G. (1962) Nitrosamines. US Patent 3,062,887, 6 November (to Hercules Powder Co.) [Chem. Abstr., 59, 1486]

Lijinsky, W. & Taylor, H.W. (1975) Increased carcinogenicity of 2,6-dimethylnitrosomorpholine compared with nitrosomorpholine in rats. Cancer Res., 35, 2123-2125

Lijinsky, W., Keefer, L., Loo, J. & Ross, A.E. (1973) Studies of alkylation of nucleic acids in rats by cyclic nitrosamines. Cancer Res., 33, 1634-1641

Lijinsky, W., Taylor, H.W. & Keefer, L.K. (1976) Reduction of rat liver carcinogenicity of 4-nitrosomorpholine by α-deuterium substitution. J. nat. Cancer Inst., 57, 1311-1313

Mirvish, S.S., Cardesa, A., Wallcave, L. & Shubik, P. (1975) Induction of mouse lung adenomas by amines or ureas plus nitrite and by *N*-nitroso compounds: effect of ascorbate, gallic acid, thiocyanate, and caffeine. J. nat. Cancer Inst., 55, 633-636

Mirvish, S.S., Pelfrene, A.F., Garcia, H. & Shubik, P. (1976) Effect of sodium ascorbate on tumor induction in rats treated with morpholine and sodium nitrite, and with nitrosomorpholine. Cancer Lett., 2, 101-108

Mohr, U., Reznik, G. & Reznik-Schüller, H. (1974) Carcinogenic effects of *N*-nitrosomorpholine and *N*-nitrosopiperidine on European hamster (*Cricetus cricetus*). J. nat. Cancer Inst., 53, 231-237

Mohr, U., Reznik, G., Emminger, E. & Lijinsky, W. (1977) Induction of pancreatic duct carcinomas in the Syrian hamster with 2,6-dimethyl-nitrosomorpholine. J. nat. Cancer Inst., 58, 429-432

Müller, H.-A. (1964) Morphologische Untersuchungen zur Wirkung von *N*-Nitrosomorpholin auf die Lunge der Maus. Z. Krebsforsch., 66, 303-309

Nakajima, T., Tanaka, A. & Tojyo, K.-I. (1974) The effect of metabolic activation with rat liver preparations on the mutagenicity of several *N*-nitrosamines on a streptomycin-dependent strain of *Escherichia coli*. Mutation Res., 26, 361-366

Newberne, P.M. & Shank, R.C. (1973) Induction of liver and lung tumours in rats by the simultaneous administration of sodium nitrite and morpholine. Fd Cosmet. Toxicol., 11, 819-825

Parkin, R., Waynforth, H.B. & Magee, P.N. (1973) The activity of some nitroso compounds in the mouse dominant-lethal mutation assay. I. Activity of *N*-nitroso-*N*-methylurea, *N*-methyl-*N*-nitroso-*N*'-nitroso-guanidine and *N*-nitrosomorpholine. Mutation Res., 21, 155-161

Pensabene, J.W., Fiddler, W., Dooley, C.J., Doerr, R.C. & Wasserman, A.E. (1972) Spectral and gas chromatographic characteristics of some *N*-nitrosamines. J. agric. Fd Chem., 20, 274-277

Pliss, G.B. & Khudoley, V.V. (1975) Tumor induction by carcinogenic agents in aquarium fish. J. nat. Cancer Inst., 55, 129-136

Prager, B. & Jacobson, P., eds (1937) Beilsteins Handbuch der Organischen Chemie, 4th ed., Vol. 27, Syst. No. 4190, Berlin, Springer, p. 8

Preussmann, R., Walker, E.A., Wasserman, A.E. & Castegnaro, M., eds (1978) Environmental Carcinogens - Selected Methods of Analysis, Vol. 1, Nitrosamines, Lyon (IARC Scientific Publications No. 18) (in press)

Rainey, W.T., Christie, W.H. & Lijinsky, W. (1978) Mass spectrometry of *N*-nitrosamines. Biochem. Mass Spectrom. (in press)

Reznik, G., Mohr, U. & Kmoch, N. (1976) Carcinogenic effects of different nitroso-compounds in Chinese hamsters. II. *N*-Nitrosomorpholine and *N*-nitrosopiperidine. Z. Krebsforsch., 86, 95-102

Sander, J. & Bürkle, G. (1969) Induktion maligner Tumoren bei Ratten durch gleichzeitige Verfütterung von Nitrit und sekundären Aminen. Z. Krebsforsch., 73, 54-66

Schmähl, D. (1970) Experimentelle Untersuchungen zur Syncarcinogenese. VI. Addition minimaler Dosen von vier verschiedenen hepatotropen Carcinogenen bei der Leberkrebserzeugung bei Ratten. Z. Krebsforsch., 74, 457-466

Shank, R.C. & Newberne, P.M. (1976) Dose-response study of the carcinogenicity of dietary sodium nitrite and morpholine in rats and hamsters. Fd Cosmet. Toxicol., 14, 1-8

Stewart, B.W. & Farber, E. (1973) Strand breakage in rat liver DNA and its repair following administration of cyclic nitrosamines. Cancer Res., 33, 3209-3215

Stewart, B.W., Swann, P.F., Holsman, J.W. & Magee, P.N. (1974) Cellular injury and carcinogenesis. Evidence for the alkylation of rat liver nucleic acids *in vivo* by *N*-nitrosomorpholine. Z. Krebsforsch., 82, 1-12

Stewart, B.W., Hicks, R.M. & Magee, P.N. (1975) Acute biochemical and morphological effects of *N*-nitrosomorpholine in comparison to dimethyl- and diethylnitrosamine. Chem.-biol. Interact., 11, 413-429

Zeiger, E. & Legator, M.S. (1971) Mutagenicity of *N*-nitrosomorpholine in the host-mediated assay. Mutation Res., 12, 469-471

Zimmer, H., Audrieth, L.F., Zimmer, M. & Rowe, R.A. (1955) The synthesis of unsymmetrically disubstituted hydrazines. J. Amer. chem. Soc., 77, 790-793

1 pharyngeal papilloma and 3 carcinomas of the nasal cavity with invasion of the brain were observed; 19 untreated controls were free of tumours (Hoffmann *et al.*, 1975).

A group of 15 18-week-old female Sprague-Dawley rats were given 7 mg/rat/day NNN in the drinking-water (354 mg/l) on 5 days/week for 44 weeks. All rats died within 46 weeks, and all had olfactory adenocarcinomas. In addition, 1 squamous papilloma of the oesophagus, 1 squamous papilloma of the forestomach and 1 hepatocellular tumour occurred in 3 rats surviving 43 or more weeks (Singer & Taylor, 1976).

(b) Skin application

Mouse: A group of 20 female Swiss (Ha/ICR/mil) mice received 0.1 ml of a 0.03% solution of NNN in acetone thrice weekly for 50 weeks. No skin tumours developed (Hoffmann *et al.*, 1976) [No data are available on tumours in other organs].

(c) Subcutaneous and/or intramuscular administration

Hamster: Groups of 10 male and 10 female Syrian golden hamsters were injected thrice weekly with 5 mg/animal NNN in aqueous solution for 25 weeks (total dose administered, 375 mg/animal). Of 19 effective animals, 12 developed single papillary tumours of the trachea within 83 weeks (first tumour after 38 weeks). One animal had an adenocarcinoma of the nasal cavity after 45 weeks (Hilfrich *et al.*, 1977).

(d) Intraperitoneal administration

Mouse: Groups of 20 male and 20 female mice (Chester Beatty stock strain), approximately 6-weeks-old, were injected intraperitoneally once weekly with 0.1 ml NNN dissolved in arachis oil (2%) for 41 weeks; 14 males and 11 females died during the first 7 months of treatment without showing tumours. Of 8 animals that died after the 8th month, 7 (5 females and 2 males) had multiple pulmonary adenomas (Boyland *et al.*, 1964). These results were confirmed by Hoffmann *et al.* (1976).

3.2 Other relevant biological data

(a) Experimental systems

Toxic effects

The s.c. LD_{50} of NNN in male rats (8 days' observation) was more than 1000 mg/kg bw. Haemorrhages in the lungs and abdominal organs and epithelial-cell necrosis in the posterior nasal cavities and liver were observed (Hoffmann *et al.*, 1975).

No data on the embryotoxicity, teratogenicity, metabolism or mutagenicity of this compound were available to the Working Group.

(b) Humans

No data were available to the Working Group.

3.3 Case reports and epidemiological studies

No data were available to the Working Group.

4. Summary of Data Reported and Evaluation

4.1 Experimental data

N'-Nitrosonornicotine is carcinogenic in rats, mice and Syrian golden hamsters. Following its oral administration to rats, it produces carcinomas of the upper digestive tract, mainly the oesophagus, and of the nasal cavities. In hamsters, its subcutaneous injection produces mainly tracheal tumours. In mice, its intraperitoneal injection produces lung tumours.

4.2 Human data

No case reports or epidemiological studies were available to the Working Group. Available information on occurrence suggests that tobacco users are exposed to *N*'-nitrosonornicotine together with other *N*-nitroso compounds.

4.3 Evaluation

There is *sufficient evidence* of a carcinogenic effect of *N*'-nitrosonornicotine in several experimental animal species. Although no epidemiological data were available, *N*'-nitrosonornicotine should be regarded for practical purposes as if it were carcinogenic to humans.

5. References

Bharadwaj, V.P., Takayama, S., Yamada, T. & Tanimura, A. (1975) *N*'-Nitrosonornicotine in Japanese tobacco products. Gann, 66, 585-586

Boyland, E., Roe, F.J.C. & Gorrod, J.W. (1964) Induction of pulmonary tumours in mice by nitrosonornicotine, a possible constituent of tobacco smoke. Nature (Lond.), 202, 1126

Hecht, S.S., Ornaf, R.M. & Hoffmann, D. (1975) Determination of *N*'-nitrosonornicotine in tobacco by high speed liquid chromatography. Analyt. Chem., 47, 2046-2048

Hecht, S.S., Chen, C.B. & Hoffmann, D. (1978) Chemical studies on tobacco smoke. LVI. Tobacco specific nitrosamines: origins, carcinogenicity and metabolism. In: Walker, E.A., Castegnaro, M., Griciute, L. & Lyle, R.E., eds, Environmental Aspects of *N*-Nitroso Compounds, Lyon (IARC Scientific Publications No. 19) (in press)

Hilfrich, J., Hecht, S.S. & Hoffmann, D. (1977) A study of tobacco carcinogenesis. XV. Effects of *N*'-nitrosonornicotine and *N*'-nitrosoanabasine in Syrian golden hamsters. Cancer Lett., 2, 169-176

Hoffmann, D., Rathkamp, G. & Liu, Y.Y. (1974) Chemical studies on tobacco smoke. XXVI. On the isolation and identification of volatile and non-volatile *N*-nitrosamines and hydrazines in cigarette smoke. In: Bogovski, P. & Walker, E.A., eds, *N*-Nitroso Compounds in the Environment, Lyon (IARC Scientific Publications No. 9), pp. 159-165

Hoffmann, D., Raineri, R., Hecht, S.S., Maronpot, R. & Wynder, E.L. (1975) A study of tobacco carcinogenesis. XIV. Effects of *N*'-nitrosonornicotine and *N*'-nitrosoanabasine in rats. J. nat. Cancer Inst., 55, 977-981

Hoffmann, D., Hecht, S.S., Ornaf, R.M., Wynder, E.L. & Tso, T.C. (1976) Chemical studies on tobacco smoke. XLII. Nitrosonornicotine: presence in tobacco, formation and carcinogenicity. In: Walker, E.A., Bogovski, P. & Griciute, L., eds, Environmental *N*-Nitroso Compounds Analysis and Formation, Lyon (IARC Scientific Publications No. 14), pp. 307-320

Hoffmann, D., Dong, M. & Hecht, S.S. (1977) Origin in tobacco smoke of *N*'-nitrosonornicotine, a tobacco-specific carcinogen: brief communication. J. nat. Cancer Inst., 58, 1841-1844

Hu, M.W., Bondinell, W.E. & Hoffmann, D. (1974) Chemical studies on tobacco smoke. XXIII. Synthesis of carbon-14 labelled myosmine, nornicotine and *N*'-nitrosonornicotine. J. labelled Compds, 10, 79-88

Klus, H. & Kuhn, H. (1975) Untersuchungen über die nichtflüchtigen *N*-Nitrosamine der Tabakalkaloide. Fachl. Mitt. Oesterreich. Tabakwerke, 16, 307-317

Rainey, W.T., Christie, W.H. & Lijinsky, W. (1978) Mass spectrometry of *N*-nitrosamines. Biochem. Mass Spectrom. (in press)

Singer, G.M. & Taylor, H.W. (1976) Carcinogenicity of *N*'-nitrosonornicotine in Sprague-Dawley rats. J. nat. Cancer Inst., 57, 1275-1276

N-NITROSOPIPERIDINE

1. Chemical and Physical Data

1.1 Synonyms and trade names

Chem. Abstr. Services Reg. No.: 100-75-4

Chem. Abstr. Name: 1-Nitroso-piperidine

NO-Pip; *N*-Pip; NPip; NPIP

1.2 Structural and molecular formulae and weight

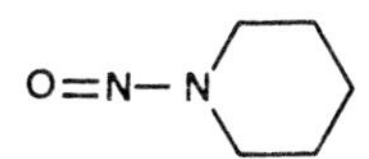

$C_5H_{10}N_2O$ Mol. wt: 114.2

1.3 Chemical and physical properties of the pure substance

(a) Description: Yellow oil

(b) Boiling-point: 215°C (721 mm); 100°C (14 mm)

(c) Density: $d_4^{18.5}$ 1.0631

(d) Refractive index: $n_D^{18.5}$ 1.4933

(e) Spectroscopy data: λ_{max} 235 and 337 (E_1^1 = 837 and 6.4) in water (Druckrey *et al.*, 1967); mass spectrometry data are given by Pensabene *et al.* (1972) and Rainey *et al.* (1978).

(f) Solubility: Soluble in water (7.7%) and in organic solvents and lipids

(g) Volatility: Slightly volatile; can be steam-distilled quantitatively (Eisenbrand *et al.*, 1970)

(h) Stability: Stable at room temperature for more than 14 days in neutral or alkaline solutions in the dark (Druckrey *et al.*, 1967); slightly less stable in acidic solutions; light-sensitive, especially to ultra-violet light

(i) Reactivity: Strong oxidants (peracids) oxidize it to the corresponding nitramine; can be reduced to the corresponding hydrazine and/or amine; relatively resistant to hydrolysis but can be split by hydrogen bromide in acetic acid (Eisenbrand & Preussmann, 1970)

1.4 Technical products and impurities

No data were available to the Working Group.

2. Production, Use, Occurrence and Analysis

2.1 Production and use

For background information on this section, see preamble, p. 22.

(a) Production

N-Nitrosopiperidine (NPIP) was first prepared by Wertheim in 1863 by the action of nitrogen dioxide on piperidine (Prager & Jacobson, 1935). Numerous patents have been issued for the production of NPIP, most of which involve the reaction of piperidine with nitrogen dioxide (Levering & Maury, 1963; Reilly, 1964) or nitric oxide (Hercules Powder Co., 1958; Reilly, 1960, 1961) under pressure and in the presence of suitable catalysts.

NPIP is produced by one US manufacturer of laboratory chemicals (Pfaltz & Bauer, Inc., 1976), but no evidence was found that it has been manufactured on a commercial scale.

(b) Use

No data were available to the Working Group.

2.2 Occurrence

(a) Tobacco smoke

McCormick *et al.* (1973) reported 1-9 ng/cigarette NPIP in 5/11 samples of tobacco smoke condensate. Klimsch *et al.* (1976) reported levels of 0.5-8 ng/cigarette. The vapour phase of the smoke of hand-rolled cigarettes contained 2-63 ng NPIP/cigarette (Groenen & ten Noever de Brauw, 1975).

Brunnemann & Hoffmann (1978), Hoffmann *et al.* (1974) and IARC (1977) found no NPIP in tobacco smoke.

(b) Water

Cohen & Bachman (1978) reported levels of 0.03 µg/l[1] NPIP in waste-water from 1/19 chemical factories.

(c) Food and feed

Cheese: Sen *et al.* (1978) found NPIP in 3/62 samples of various cheeses at levels of 2-11 µg/kg.

Fish: NPIP has been found at levels of less than 1.0 µg/kg[1] in smoked cod (Alliston *et al.*, 1972).

Meat: NPIP has been found in cooking-fat from fried bacon at levels less than 1.0 µg/kg[1] (Alliston *et al.*, 1972). It has also been found at various concentrations in meat products such as fried smoked back rashers (less than 1 µg/kg) (Crosby *et al.*, 1972) and Mettwurst sausages (20-60 µg/kg) (Sen *et al.*, 1973). Sen *et al.* (1976) reported 14-50 µg/kg in 6/8 bolognas, 15-50 µg/kg in 2/3 wieners and 50 µg/kg in meatloaf.

Stephany *et al.* (1976) reported levels of 0-8.2 µg/kg NPIP in various processed and preserved meats. Fine & Rounbehler (1976) reported 0.2 µg/kg[1] in raw bacon and 1 µg/kg[1] in cooked bacon. Eisenbrand *et al.* (1977) reported 2-64 µg/kg in 14/52 meat samples; the concentration was observed to increase substantially after cooking. Groenen *et al.* (1977) reported 0.4-7 µg/kg in 13/48 assorted raw or cooked meats. Gough (1978) reported levels of 0.08-0.25 µg/kg[1] in all of 8 samples of cooked bacon and 0.1 µg/kg[1] in all cured meats which were examined.

Spices: Dry, premixed cures containing spices and sodium nitrite were found to contain up to 3000 µg/kg NPIP (Gough & Goodhead, 1975; Havery *et al.*, 1976). Similar results were obtained by Sen *et al.* (1973).

---

[1]These results were not confirmed by mass spectroscopy (see also 'General Remarks on the Substances Considered', p. 40).

d: Kann *et al.* (1978) found NPIP at a level of 4 μg/kg in 1/10 f rabbit diet. A maximum of 210 μg/kg NPIP has been found in erimental animal feed (IARC, 1977). Mirna *et al.* (1976) reported 1 μg/kg in 2/5 fishmeal samples.

2.3 Analysis

An IARC Manual gives selected methods for the analysis of volatile *N*-nitrosamines, including *N*-nitrosopiperidine (Preussmann *et al.*, 1978).

3. Biological Data Relevant to the Evaluation of Carcinogenic Risk to Man

3.1 Carcinogenicity and related studies in animals

(a) Oral administration

Mouse: A group of 33 male ICR mice were fed a diet containing *N*-nitrosopiperidine (NPIP) at a concentration of 50 mg/kg of diet for 12 months. Of 24 surviving mice, 18 had squamous-cell carcinomas of the forestomach, 2, papillomas of the oesophagus, 11, liver tumours (2 hepatocellular carcinomas, 3 haemangioendotheliomas, 6 liver adenomas) and 10, lung adenomas. Of the 30 control animals, 2 had lung adenomas and 1, a lymphocytic leukaemia (Takayama, 1969).

A group of 20 male and 20 female Swiss mice were given 0.01% NPIP in the drinking-water (total dose, 65 mg/animal) for 26 weeks; 42.5% of the animals developed lung adenomas (Greenblatt & Lijinsky, 1972).

Rat: Groups of 10 and 20 BD rats received in NPIP at concentrations equivalent to doses of 5 and 20 mg/kg bw/day in the drinking-water. Of those given the high dose, 17/20 animals died early during treatment without tumours; the remaining 3 rats developed hepatocellular carcinomas metastasizing to the lungs, and 1 animal also had a squamous-cell carcinoma of the oesophagus. Of those given the lower dose level, 9/10 animals developed oesophageal tumours (8 carcinomas, 1 papilloma), and 3 had liver tumours. The average induction time for these tumours was 280 days (average total dose that induced tumours in 50% of the animals, 1.4 g/kg bw) (Druckrey *et al.*, 1967; Thomas & So, 1969). Similar results were obtained in albino rats (Chester Beatty strain) (Boyland *et al.*, 1964) and in MRC rats (Garcia

& Lijinsky, 1972); in the latter, additional tumours were observed in the trachea, pharynx, larynx, nasal cavity, tongue and stomach.

A detailed study has been made of the histogenesis of the oesophageal tumours induced in Wistar rats by NPIP (Ito *et al.*, 1971).

Monkey: It was reported in an abstract that hepatocellular carcinomas were observed in 3 animals which received NPIP orally (O'Gara *et al.*, 1970).

(b) Subcutaneous and/or intramuscular administration

Rat: A group of 25 BD rats were injected subcutaneously with twice-weekly injections of 10 mg/kg bw NPIP. Twenty-two animals developed tumours of the nasal cavities, described as aesthesioneuroepitheliomas (10), squamous-cell carcinomas (10), cholesteatomas (3) and neuroblastomas (1). In addition, 15 animals had oesophageal squamous-cell tumours (5 papillomas, 10 carcinomas). The average induction time for the tumours was 365 days (average total dose that induced tumours in 50% of animals, 0.85 g/kg bw) (Druckrey *et al.*, 1967; Thomas, 1965; Thomas & So, 1969).

Hamster: Of 21 Syrian golden hamsters that received s.c. injections of 0.5 ml of a 1:250 solution of NPIP in water 3 times/week for life, 16 developed tumours of the trachea. Two animals had squamous-cell carcinomas of the lung (Dontenwill & Mohr, 1962).

Groups of 20 male and 20 female 8-week-old Syrian golden hamsters were treated subcutaneously once a week for life with 1/5, 1/10 or 1/20th of the LD_{50} (LD_{50}: males, 324 mg/kg bw; females, 283 mg/kg bw). The incidences of papillomas and carcinomas of the respiratory system, mostly in the trachea, were 65-100% (Haas *et al.*, 1973). Tumours, mainly of the nasal cavities, lung, tongue, palate, oesophagus, forestomach and liver, were observed in Chinese hamsters (Reznik *et al.*, 1976). Tumours, mainly of the nasal cavity, lung and forestomach, were seen in European hamsters (Mohr *et al.*, 1974).

Groups of 5 male and 5 female Syrian golden hamsters were given single s.c. injections of 25, 50, 100 or 200 mg/kg bw NPIP. The majority of neoplasms were found in the trachea (23), but some tumours were also observed in the nasal cavities (1), larynx (3) and bronchi (3). The tracheal tumours were diagnosed as polyps and papillary polyps. A variety of other tumours were also found (Althoff *et al.*, 1974).

(c) Intraperitoneal administration

Mouse: A group of 30 9-13-week-old SWR mice of both sexes were injected intraperitoneally with single doses of 107 mg/kg bw NPIP. Sixteen mice developed adenomas of the lung, as compared with 10 lung adenomas in 36 untreated controls; the multiplicity of lung tumours was higher in the treated group (Mirvish & Kaufman, 1970).

(d) Intravenous administration

Rat: A group of 15 BD rats were injected intravenously with 10 mg/kg bw NPIP twice weekly. Twelve animals developed carcinomas of the oesophagus and pharynx after an average induction time of 366 days (average total dose that induced tumours in 50% of animals, 0.75 g/kg bw). One animal had an adenocarcinoma of the glandular stomach (Druckrey *et al.*, 1967; Thomas & So. 1969).

(e) Other experimental systems

Prenatal exposure: Offspring of Syrian golden hamsters that had been treated on days 8, 10, 12 or 14 of pregnancy with a single dose of 100 mg/kg bw NPIP were observed for life. A low incidence (2-7%) of tumours of the upper respiratory tract was observed in the offspring (highest incidence in those treated on day 14). A high incidence (54%) of respiratory tract tumours was observed in the treated mothers (Althoff *et al.*, 1977).

(f) Carcinogenicity of derivatives

The available studies are summarized in Table 1.

3.2 Other relevant biological data

(a) Experimental systems

Toxic effects

The oral LD_{50} of NPIP in BD rats was 200 mg/kg bw, the s.c. LD_{50}, 100 mg/kg bw and the i.v. LD_{50}, is 60 mg/kg bw (Druckrey *et al.*, 1967); the i.p. LD_{50} in Wistar rats was 85 mg/kg bw (Lee & Lijinsky, 1966).

Table 1

Carcinogenicity of derivatives of *N*-nitrosopiperidine in Sprague-Dawley rats

Compound	Main tumour sites	References
N-Nitroso-4-hydroxypiperidine	Nasal cavity, liver	Lijinsky & Taylor, 1975a
N-Nitroso-4-piperidone	Nasal cavity, liver	" " "
N-Nitroso-3-hydroxypiperidine	Nasal cavity, tongue, pharynx, oesophagus, liver	" " "
N-Nitroso-2-methylpiperidine	Nasal cavity, oesophagus, forestomach, pharynx, tongue, liver	Lijinsky & Taylor, 1975b
N-Nitroso-3-methylpiperidine	Nasal cavity, oesophagus, forestomach, pharynx, tongue	" " "
N-Nitroso-4-methylpiperidine	Nasal cavity, oesophagus, forestomach, pharynx, tongue	" " "
N-Nitroso-2,6-dimethylpiperidine	Negative	" " "
N-Nitroso-2,2,6,6,-tetramethylpiperidine	Negative	" " "

The s.c. LD_{50} was 110 mg/kg in Chinese hamsters (Reznik *et al.*, 1976), about 300 mg/kg bw in Syrian golden hamsters (Haas *et al.*, 1973) and 230 mg/kg bw in European hamsters (Mohr *et al.*, 1974).

No data on the embryotoxicity or teratogenicity of this compound were available to the Working Group.

Absorption, distribution and excretion

^{3}H-NPIP injected into the bladder of rats or Syrian golden hamsters was absorbed, and radioactivity was found in the liver and kidneys of both species and in the stomach, small intestine and lungs of hamsters (Hawksworth & Hill, 1974).

Metabolism

NPIP was oxidized by rat liver microsomes to 4-hydroxynitrosopiperidine (Rayman *et al.*, 1975).

Administration of ^{3}H-NPIP or deuterated NPIP to rats led to reaction with DNA and RNA in the liver, but the products were not characterized (Lee & Lijinsky, 1966; Lijinsky *et al.*, 1973). After administration of 50 mg/kg bw NPIP, repair of single-strand breaks in rat liver DNA, as determined by velocity sedimentation in an alkaline sucrose gradient, was not complete after 6 days (Stewart & Farber, 1973).

Mutagenicity and other short-term tests

NPIP caused reverse mutations in *Escherichia coli* and in *Salmonella typhimurium* TA 100, TA 1530 and TA 1535 in the presence of liver microsomal fractions from phenobarbital- or Aroclor 1254-treated rats or from human biopsies (Bartsch *et al.*, 1976; Elespuru & Lijinsky, 1976; McCann *et al.*, 1975; Nakajima *et al.*, 1974; Rao *et al.*, 1977; Stoltz & Sen, 1977). In Chinese hamster V79 cells, NPIP induced 8-azaguanine-resistant mutants in the presence of a liver microsomal fraction from phenobarbital-treated rats (Kuroki *et al.*, 1977).

(b) Humans

No data were available to the Working Group.

3.3 Case reports and epidemiological studies

No data were available to the Working Group.

4. Summary of Data Reported and Evaluation

4.1 Experimental data

N-Nitrosopiperidine is carcinogenic in mice, rats, Syrian golden, European and Chinese hamsters and monkeys after its administration by oral and other routes. It produces benign and malignant tumours of the liver, lung, forestomach and oesophagus in mice, of the liver, oesophagus and respiratory system in rats, and of the upper digestive tract, respiratory system and liver in hamsters; it produces hepatocellular carcinomas in monkeys. It is carcinogenic in mice and hamsters after its administration in single doses.

4.2 Human data

No case reports or epidemiological studies were available to the Working Group. Available information on occurrence suggests that the general population may be exposed sporadically to low levels of *N*-nitrosopiperidine; however, no exposed group suitable for an epidemiological investigation has yet been identified.

4.3 Evaluation

There is *sufficient evidence* of a carcinogenic effect of *N*-nitrosopiperidine in several experimental animal species. Although no epidemiological data were available, *N*-nitrosopiperidine should be regarded for practical purposes as if it were carcinogenic to humans.

5. References

Alliston, T.G., Cox, G.B. & Kirk, R.S. (1972) The determination of steam-volatile *N*-nitrosamines in foodstuffs by formation of electron-capturing derivatives from electrochemically derived amines. Analyst, 97, 915-920

Althoff, J., Wilson, R., Cardesa, A. & Pour, P. (1974) Comparative studies of neoplastic response to a single dose of nitroso compounds. III. The effect of *N*-nitrosopiperidine and *N*-nitrosomorpholine in Syrian golden hamsters. Z. Krebsforsch., 81, 251-259

Althoff, J., Grandjean, C., Marsh, S., Pour, P. & Takahashi, M. (1977) Transplacental effects of nitrosamines in Syrian hamsters. II. Nitrosopiperidine. Z. Krebsforsch., 90, 71-77

Bartsch, H., Camus, A. & Malaveille, C. (1976) Comparative mutagenicity of *N*-nitrosamines in a semi-solid and in a liquid incubation system in the presence of rat or human tissue fractions. Mutation Res., 37, 149-162

Boyland, E., Roe, F.J.C., Gorrod, J.W. & Mitchley, B.C.V. (1964) The carcinogenicity of nitrosoanabasine, a possible constituent of tobacco smoke. Brit. J. Cancer, 18, 265-270

Brunnemann, K.D. & Hoffmann, D. (1978) Chemical studies on tobacco smoke. LIX. Analysis of volatile nitrosamines in tobacco smoke and polluted indoor environments. In: Walker, E.A., Castegnaro, M., Griciute, L. & Lyle, R.E., eds, Environmental Aspects of *N*-Nitroso Compounds, Lyon (IARC Scientific Publications No. 19) (in press)

Cohen, J.B. & Bachman, J.D. (1978) Measurement of environmental nitrosamines. In: Walker, E.A., Castegnaro, M., Griciute, L. & Lyle, R.E., eds, Environmental Aspects of *N*-Nitroso Compounds, Lyon (IARC Scientific Publications No. 19) (in press)

Crosby, N.T., Foreman, J.K., Palframan, J.F. & Sawyer, R. (1972) Estimation of steam-volatile *N*-nitrosamines in foods at the 1 μg/kg level. Nature (Lond.), 238, 342-343

Dontenwill, W. & Mohr, U. (1962) Die organotrope Wirkung der Nitrosamine. Z. Krebsforsch., 65, 166-167

Druckrey, H., Preussmann, R., Ivankovic, S. & Schmähl, D. (1967) Organotrope carcinogene Wirkungen bei 65 verschiedenen *N*-Nitroso-Verbindungen an BD-Ratten. Z. Krebsforsch., 69, 103-201

Eisenbrand, G. & Preussmann, R. (1970) Eine neue Methode zur kolorimetrischen Bestimmung von Nitrosaminen nach Spaltung der *N*-Nitrosogruppe mit Bromwasserstoff in Eisessig. Arzneimittel-Forsch., 20, 1513-1517

Eisenbrand, G., Hodenberg, A. von & Preussmann, R. (1970) Trace analysis of *N*-nitroso compounds. II. Steam distillation at neutral, alkaline and acid pH under reduced and atmospheric pressure. Z. analyt. Chem., 251, 22-24

Eisenbrand, G., Janzowski, C. & Preussmann, R. (1977) Analysis, formation and occurrence of volatile and non-volatile *N*-nitroso compounds: recent results. In: Tinbergen, B.J. & Krol, B., eds, Proceedings of the Second International Symposium on Nitrite in Meat Products, Zeist, 1976, Wageningen, Centre for Agricultural Publishing and Documentation, pp. 155-169

Elespuru, R.K. & Lijinsky, W. (1976) Mutagenicity of cyclic nitrosamines in *Escherichia coli* following activation with rat liver microsomes. Cancer Res., 36, 4099-4101

Fine, D.H. & Rounbehler, D.P. (1976) Analysis of volatile *N*-nitroso compounds by combined gas chromatography and thermal energy analysis. In: Walker, E.A., Bogovski, P. & Griciute, L., eds, Environmental *N*-Nitroso Compounds Analysis and Formation, Lyon (IARC Scientific Publications No. 14), pp. 117-127

Garcia, H. & Lijinsky, W. (1972) Tumorigenicity of five cyclic nitrosamines in MRC rats. Z. Krebsforsch., 77, 257-261

Gough, T.A. (1978) An examination of some foodstuff for trace amounts of volatile nitrosamines using the thermal energy analyser. In: Walker, E.A., Castegnaro, M., Griciute, L. & Lyle, R.E., eds, Environmental Aspects of *N*-Nitroso Compounds, Lyon (IARC Scientific Publications No. 19) (in press)

Gough, T.A. & Goodhead, K. (1975) Occurrence of volatile nitrosamines in spice premixes. J. Sci. Fd Agric., 26, 1473-1478

Greenblatt, M. & Lijinsky, W. (1972) Failure to induce tumors in Swiss mice after concurrent administration of amino acids and sodium nitrite. J. nat. Cancer Inst., 48, 1389-1392

Groenen, P.J. & ten Noever de Brauw, M.C. (1975) Determination of volatile *N*-nitrosamines in the vapour phase of the smoke from various tobacco products. Beitr. Tabakforsch., 8, 113-123

Groenen, P.J., de Cock-Bethbeder, M.W., Jonk, R.J.G. & van Ingen, C. (1977) Further studies on the occurrence of volatile *N*-nitrosamines in meat products by combined gas chromatography and mass spectrometry. In: Tinbergen, B.J. & Krol, B., eds, Proceedings of the Second International Symposium on Nitrite in Meat Products, Zeist, 1976, Wageningen, Centre for Agricultural Publishing and Documentation, pp. 227-237

Haas, H., Mohr, U. & Krüger, F.W. (1973) Comparative studies with different doses of *N*-nitrosomorpholine, *N*-nitrosopiperidine, *N*-nitrosomethylurea, and dimethylnitrosamine in Syrian golden hamsters. J. nat. Cancer Inst., 51, 1295-1301

Havery, D.C., Kline, D.A., Miletta, E.M., Joe, F.L., Jr & Fazio, T. (1976) Survey of food products for volatile *N*-nitrosamines. J. Ass. off. analyt. Chem., 59, 540-546

Hawksworth, G. & Hill, M.J. (1974) The *in vivo* formation of *N*-nitrosamines in the rat bladder and their subsequent absorption. Brit. J. Cancer, 29, 353-358

Hercules Powder Co. (1958) Nitrosamines. British Patent 789,702, 29 January [Chem. Abstr., 52, 13805]

Hoffmann, D., Rathkamp, G. & Liu, Y.Y. (1974) Chemical studies on tobacco smoke. XXVI. On the isolation and identification of volatile and non-volatile *N*-nitrosamines and hydrazines in cigarette smoke. In: Bogovski, P. & Walker, E.A., eds, *N*-Nitroso Compounds in the Environment, Lyon (IARC Scientific Publications No. 9), pp. 159-165

IARC (1977) Annual Report 1977, Lyon, International Agency for Research on Cancer, p. 63

Ito, N., Kamamoto, Y., Hiasa, Y., Makiura, S., Marugami, M., Yokota, Y., Sugihara, S. & Hirao, K. (1971) Histopathological and ultrastructural studies on esophageal tumors in rats treated with *N*-nitrosopiperidine. Gann, 62, 445-451

Kann, J., Spiegelhalder, B., Eisenbrand, G. & Preussmann, R. (1978) Occurrence of volatile *N*-nitrosamines in animal diets. Z. Krebsforsch. (in press)

Klimsch, H.-J., Stadler, L. & Brahm, S. (1976) Quantitative Bestimmung flüchtiger Nitrosamine in Zigarettenrauchkondensat. Z. Lebensmittel-Untersuch., 162, 131-138

Kuroki, T., Drevon, C. & Montesano, R. (1977) Microsome-mediated mutagenesis in V79 Chinese hamster cells by various nitrosamines. Cancer Res., 37, 1044-1050

Lee, K.Y. & Lijinsky, W. (1966) Alkylation of rat liver RNA by cyclic *N*-nitrosamines *in vivo*. J. nat. Cancer Inst., 37, 401-407

Levering, D.R. & Maury, L.G. (1963) Nitrosamines. US Patent 3,090,786, 21 May (to Hercules Powder Co.) [Chem. Abstr., 59, 12770]

Lijinsky, W. & Taylor, H.W. (1975a) Tumorigenesis by oxygenated nitrosopiperidines in rats. J. nat. Cancer Inst., 55, 705-708

Lijinsky, W. & Taylor, H.W. (1975b) Carcinogenicity of methylated nitrosopiperidines. Int. J. Cancer, 16, 318-322

Lijinsky, W., Keefer, L., Loo, J. & Ross, A.E. (1973) Studies of alkylation of nucleic acids in rats by cyclic nitrosamines. Cancer Res., 33, 1634-1641

McCann, J., Choi, E., Yamasaki, E. & Ames, B.N. (1975) Detection of carcinogens as mutagens in the *Salmonella*/microsome test: assay of 300 chemicals. Proc. nat. Acad. Sci. (Wash.), 72, 5135-5139

McCormick, A., Nicholson, M.J., Baylis, M.A. & Underwood, J.G. (1973) Nitrosamines in cigarette smoke condensate. Nature (Lond.), 244, 237-238

Mirna, A., Harada, K., Rapp, U. & Kaufmann, H. (1976) *N*-Nitrosamine in Futtermitteln. Fleischwirtschaft, 56, 1014

Mirvish, S.S. & Kaufman, L. (1970) A study of nitrosamines and *S*-carboxyl derivatives of cysteine as lung carcinogens in adult SWR mice. Int. J. Cancer, 6, 69-73

Mohr, U., Reznik, G. & Reznik-Schüller, H. (1974) Carcinogenic effects of *N*-nitrosomorpholine and *N*-nitrosopiperidine on European hamster (*Cricetus cricetus*). J. nat. Cancer Inst., 53, 231-237

Nakajima, T., Tanaka, A. & Tojyo, K.-I. (1974) The effect of metabolic activation with rat liver preparations on the mutagenicity of several *N*-nitrosamines on a streptomycin-dependent strain of *Escherichia coli*. Mutation Res., 26, 361-366

O'Gara, R.W., Adamson, R.H. & Dalgard, D.W. (1970) Induction of tumors in subhuman primates by two nitrosamine compounds (Abstract No. 236). Proc. Amer. Ass. Cancer Res., 11, 60

Pensabene, J.W., Fiddler, W., Dooley, C.J., Doerr, R.C. & Wasserman, A.E. (1972) Spectral and gas chromatographic characteristics of some *N*-nitrosamines. J. agric. Fd Chem., 20, 274-277

Pfaltz & Bauer, Inc. (1976) Research Chemicals Catalog, Stamford, Connecticut, p. 310

Prager, B. & Jacobson, P., eds (1935) Beilsteins Handbuch der Organischen Chemie, 4th ed., Vol. 20, Syst. No. 3038, Berlin, Springer, p. 83

Preussmann, R., Walker, E.A., Wasserman, A.E. & Castegnaro, M., eds (1978) Environmental Carcinogens - Selected Methods of Analysis, Vol. 1, Nitrosamines, Lyon (IARC Scientific Publications No. 18) (in press)

Rainey, W.T., Christie, W.H. & Lijinsky, W. (1978) Mass spectrometry of *N*-nitrosamines. Biomed. Mass Spectrom. (in press)

Rao, T.K., Hardigree, A.A., Young, J.A., Lijinsky, W. & Epler, J.L. (1977) Mutagenicity of *N*-nitrosopiperidines with *Salmonella typhimurium*/ microsomal activation system. Mutation Res., 56, 131-145

Rayman, M.P., Challis, B.C., Cox, P.J. & Jarman, M. (1975) Oxidation of *N*-nitrosopiperidine in the Udenfriend model system and its metabolism by rat-liver microsomes. Biochem. Pharmacol., 24, 621-626

Reilly, E.L. (1960) Nitrosamines. German Patent 1,085,166, 14 July (to E.I. du Pont de Nemours & Co.) [Chem. Abstr., 56, 4594]

Reilly, E.L. (1961) Disubstituted nitrosamines and ammonium nitrites and amine-nitric oxide addition compounds. British Patent 867,992, 10 May (to E.I. du Pont de Nemours & Co.) [Chem. Abstr., 55, 25755]

Reilly, E.L. (1964) Nitrosamine manufacture. US Patent 3,153,094, 13 October (to E.I. du Pont de Nemours & Co.) [Chem. Abstr., 62, 5192]

Reznik, G., Mohr, U. & Kmoch, N. (1976) Carcinogenic effects of different nitroso-compounds in Chinese hamsters. II. *N*-Nitrosomorpholine and *N*-nitrosopiperidine. Z. Krebsforsch., 86, 95-102

Sen, N.P., Miles, W.F., Donaldson, B., Panalaks, T. & Iyengar, J.R. (1973) Formation of nitrosamines in a meat curing mixture. Nature (Lond.), 245, 104-105

Sen, N.P., Iyengar, J.R., Miles, W.F. & Panalaks, T. (1976) Nitrosamines in cured meat products. In: Walker, E.A., Bogovski, P. & Griciute, L., eds, Environmental *N*-Nitroso Compounds Analysis and Formation, Lyon (IARC Scientific Publications No. 14), pp. 333-342

Sen, N.P., Donaldson, B.A., Seaman, S., Iyengar, J.R. & Miles, W.F. (1978) Recent studies in Canada on the analysis and occurrence of volatile and non-volatile *N*-nitroso compounds in foods. In: Walker, E.A., Castegnaro, M., Griciute, L. & Lyle, R.E., eds, Environmental Aspects of *N*-Nitroso Compounds, Lyon (IARC Scientific Publications No. 19) (in press)

Stephany, R.W., Freudenthal, J. & Schuller, P.L. (1976) Quantitative and qualitative determination of some volatile nitrosamines in various meat products. In: Walker, E.A., Bogovski, P. & Griciute, L., eds, Environmental *N*-Nitroso Compounds Analysis and Formation, Lyon (IARC Scientific Publications No. 14), pp. 343-354

Stewart, B.W. & Farber, E. (1973) Strand breakage in rat liver DNA and its repair following administration of cyclic nitrosamines. Cancer Res., 33, 3209-3215

Stoltz, D.R. & Sen, N.P. (1977) Mutagenicity of five cyclic *N*-nitrosamines: assay with *Salmonella typhimurium*. J. nat. Cancer Inst., 58, 393-394

Takayama, S. (1969) Induction of tumors in ICR mice with *N*-nitrosopiperidine, especially in forestomach. Naturwissenschaften, 56, 142

Thomas, C. (1965) Zur Morphologie der Nasenhöhlentumoren bei der Ratte. Z. Krebsforsch., 67, 1-10

Thomas, C. & So, B.T. (1969) Zur Morphologie der durch *N*-Nitroso-Verbindungen erzeugten Tumoren im oberen Verdauungstrakt der Ratte. Arzneimittel-Forsch., 19, 1077-1081

N-NITROSOPROLINE and *N*-NITROSOHYDROXYPROLINE

1. Chemical and Physical Data

N-Nitrosoproline

1.1 Synonyms and trade names

Chem. Abstr. Services Reg. No.: 7519-36-0

Chem. Abstr. Name: 1-Nitroso-L-proline

NO-Pro; *N*-Pro; NPRO

1.2 Structural and molecular formulae and weight

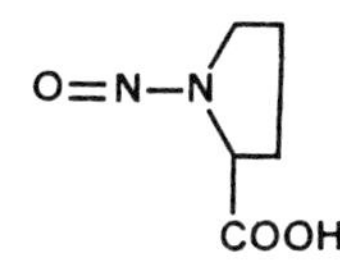

$C_5H_8N_2O_3$ Mol. wt: 144

1.3 Chemical and physical properties of the pure substance

From Lijinksy *et al.* (1970), unless otherwise specified

(a) Description: Pale-yellow crystals

(b) Melting-point: 100-101°C (decomposition)

(c) Optical rotation: $[\alpha]_D^{25}$ -185°C

(d) Spectroscopy data: λ_{max} 238 and 343 nm (E_1^1 = 451 and 6.3) in water; mass spectroscopy data are given by Rainey *et al.* (1978); the nuclear magnetic resonance spectrum has been given.

(e) Solubility: Very soluble in water; soluble in polar organic solvents; insoluble in non-polar organic solvents

(f) Reactivity: Partially decarboxylates on heating above 170°C to form *N*-nitrosopyrrolidine (Eisenbrand *et al.*, 1978)

1.4 Technical products and impurities

No data were available to the Working Group.

N-Nitrosohydroxyproline

1.1 Synonyms and trade names

Chem. Abstr. Services Reg. No.: 30310-80-6

Chem. Abstr. Name: *trans*-4-Hydroxy-1-nitroso-L-proline

1.2 Structural and molecular formulae and weight

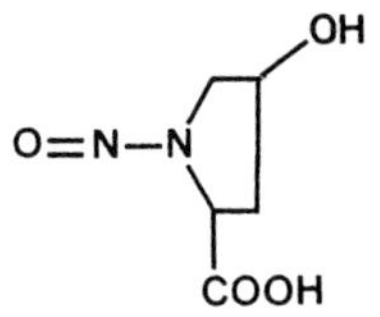

O=N—N (pyrrolidine ring) with OH and COOH

$C_5H_8N_2O_4$ Mol. wt: 160

1.3 Chemical and physical properties of the pure substance

From Lijinsky *et al.* (1970), unless otherwise specified

(a) Description: Colourless crystals

(b) Melting-point: 114-115°C

(c) Optical rotation: $[\alpha]_D^{25}$ -192°C

(d) Spectroscopy data: Mass and nuclear magnetic resonance spectra have been given

(e) Reactivity: Decarboxylates on heating at 170°C to form *N*-nitroso-3-hydroxypyrrolidine (Eisenbrand *et al.*, 1977; Lee *et al.*, 1977)

1.4 Technical products and impurities

No data were available to the Working Group.

2. Production, Use, Occurrence and Analysis

2.1 Production and use

(a) Production

N-Nitrosoproline (NPRO) and *N*-nitrosohydroxyproline (NHPRO) have been prepared for laboratory use by the reaction of sodium nitrite with a solution of proline or hydroxyproline in hydrochloric acid (Hamilton & Ortiz, 1950; Lijinsky *et al.*, 1970; Sander, 1967).

No evidence was found that NPRO or NHPRO has been manufactured commercially.

(b) Use

No data were available to the Working Group.

2.2 Occurrence

Dhont & van Ingen (1976) found NPRO in uncooked cured meat products, such as bacon and smoked meat, at levels of 340-440 μg/kg. Kushnir *et al.* (1975) found levels of 380-1180 μg/kg[1] in uncooked bacon; Sen *et al.* (1978) reported 24-44 μg/kg in 4/8 uncooked bacon samples; and Green *et al.* (1977) reported 70 or 80 μg/kg (depending upon the method of analysis) in only one sample of raw bacon. Eisenbrand *et al.* (1978) found 8/9 meat products to be positive: ham, 2 and 172 μg/kg; boiled ham, 49 and 124 μg/kg; bologna, 42 and 401 μg/kg; meatloaf, 5 and 16 μg/kg.

One sample of meatloaf contained 8 μg/kg NHPRO (Eisenbrand *et al.*, 1978).

2.3 Analysis

Eisenbrand *et al.* (1976) formed the trimethylsilyl derivative and used gas chromatography-mass spectrometry to look at single ions. Dhont & van Ingen (1976) extracted meat samples with methanol:water, separated the amino acids on an ion-exchange column and then converted them into the methyl ester for final analysis by gas chromatography-low-resolution mass spectrometry. Dhont (1977) and Kushnir *et al.* (1975) also prepared methyl esters and used gas chromatography-flame ionization detector and gas chromatography-

[1]This result was not confirmed by mass spectroscopy (see also 'General Remarks on the Substances Considered', p. 40).

high-resolution mass spectrometry for analysis; recovery was 20-25%. The methyl-ester technique has been further improved by Sen *et al.* (1978). Wolfram *et al.* (1977) denitrosated and then derivatized with 7-chloro-4-nitrobenzo-2-oxa-1,3-diazole; the highly fluorescent derivative was analysed by either thin-layer or high-pressure liquid chromatography (HPLC).

Chromatographic conditions suitable for use with HPLC-thermal energy analysis are described by Fan *et al.* (1978). Separation of *syn-anti* conformers by HPLC-ultra-violet spectroscopy is described by Iwaoka & Tannenbaum (1976). Green *et al.* (1977) used HPLC with detection by photo-hydrolysis.

A collaborative study on several analytical methods for 3 *N*-nitroso amino acids, including NPRO and NHPRO showed good agreement between the methods (Castegnaro & Walker, 1978).

3. Biological Data Relevant to the Evaluation of Carcinogenic Risk to Man

3.1 Carcinogenicity studies in animals

(a) Oral administration

Mouse: Two groups of 30 male and 30 female 5-7-week-old Swiss mice received *N*-nitrosoproline (NPRO) in the drinking-water at concentrations of 0.05% or 0.1% for 26 weeks (total doses, 325 or 650 mg/mouse). All survivors were killed at 38 weeks. No more lung adenomas were found in treated animals as compared with 30 male and 30 female controls; administration of *N*-nitrosopiperidine as a positive control gave a significantly increased incidence dence of lung adenomas (Greenblatt & Lijinsky, 1972) [The Working Group noted the short duration of the experiment and the low dose used].

Rat: Two groups of 15 male and 15 female MRC rats, 8-10-weeks old, were given NPRO or NHPRO in the drinking-water at a concentration of 0.015% for 75 weeks. Survival of the treated animals was similar to that of 30 untreated controls. No significant difference was observed between untreated and treated animals in proportion of tumour-bearing animals or in proportion of tumours commonly found in control rats (Garcia & Lijinsky, 1973) [The Working Group noted the low dose used].

No carcinogenic effects were seen in groups of 26 male weanling Wistar rats given NPRO or NHPRO intragastrically once weekly for 4 weeks (total dose, 290 mg/animal) and observed for lifespan (Nixon *et al.*, 1976) [The Working Group noted the limited duration of dosing].

(b) Carcinogenicity of derivatives

A group of 18 BD rats were given *N*-nitrosoproline-ethylester in the drinking-water at concentrations of 50 or 100 mg/kg bw/day up to a total dose of 19 or 38 g/kg bw, respectively. One animal which died after 790 days had papillomas of the oesophagus; no other tumours were observed (Druckrey *et al.*, 1967).

3.2 Other relevant biological data

(a) Experimental systems

No data on the toxic effects, embryotoxicity or teratogenicity of NPRO or NHPRO were available to the Working Group.

Absorption, distribution, excretion and metabolism

All of an oral dose of 10 mg ^{14}C-NPRO was absorbed from the gastro-intestinal tract of rats within 24-48 hours. When the rats were fasted, 98% of the radioactivity appeared in the urine and 1-2% in the faeces. In rats fed normally, 71% had appeared in the urine and 20% in the faeces after 4 days; some was excreted in the urine up to 7 days. Only 2% of the radioactivity was excreted as CO_2; trace amounts were found in the tissues (Dailey *et al.*, 1975).

Mutagenicity and other short-term tests

NPRO was not mutagenic in *Salmonella typhimurium* TA 1535 either in the presence or absence of a liver microsomal fraction from Aroclor 1254-treated rats (Stolz & Sen, 1977).

(b) Humans

No data were available to the Working Group.

3.3 Case reports and epidemiological studies

No data were available to the Working Group.

4. Summary of Data Reported and Evaluation

4.1 Experimental data

N-Nitrosoproline has been tested in mice and rats and *N*-nitrosohydroxyproline in rats by oral administration. Although these studies did not indicate a carcinogenic effect, they were inadequate with regard to dose and/or duration.

4.2 Human data

No case reports or epidemiological studies were available to the Working Group. Available information on occurrence suggests that the general population may be exposed to low levels of *N*-nitrosoproline and *N*-nitrosohydroxyproline; however, no exposed group suitable for an epidemiological investigation has yet been identified.

4.3 Evaluation

No evaluation of the carcinogenicity of *N*-nitrosoproline or *N*-nitrosohydroxyproline could be made on the basis of the available data.

5. References

Castegnaro, M. & Walker, E.A. (1978) New data on collaborative studies on analysis of nitrosamines. In: Walker, E.A., Castegnaro, M., Griciute, L. & Lyle, R.E., eds, Environmental Aspects of *N*-Nitroso Compounds, Lyon (IARC Scientific Publications No. 19) (in press)

Dailey, R.E., Braunberg, R.C. & Blaschka, A.M. (1975) The absorption, distribution, and excretion of [^{14}C]nitrosoproline by rats. Toxicology, 3, 23-28

Dhont, J.H. (1977) Development of a method of estimating *N*-nitrosamino acids and its use on some meat products, In: Tinbergen, B.J. & Krol, B., eds, Proceedings of the Second International Symposium on Nitrite in Meat Products, Zeist, 1976, Wageningen, Centre for Agricultural Publishing and Documentation, pp. 221-225

Dhont, J.H. & van Ingen, C. (1976) Identification and quantitative determination of nitrosoproline and nitrososarcosine and preliminary investigations on nitrosohydroxyproline in cured meat products. In: Walker, E.A., Bogovski, P. & Griciute, L., eds, Environmental *N*-Nitroso Compounds Analysis and Formation, Lyon (IARC Scientific Publications No. 14), pp. 355-360

Druckrey, H., Preussmann, R., Ivankovic, S. & Schmähl, D. (1967) Organotrope carcinogene Wirkungen bei 65 verschiedenen *N*-Nitroso-Verbindungen an BD-Ratten. Z. Krebsforsch., 69, 103-201

Eisenbrand, G., Janzowski, C. & Preussmann, R. (1976) Gas chromatographic determination of nitrosoamino acids by trimethylsilylation and single-ion monitoring in a gas chromatography-mass spectrometry system. In: Walker, E.A., Bogovski, P. & Griciute, L., eds, Environmental *N*-Nitroso Compounds Analysis and Formation, Lyon (IARC Scientific Publications No. 14), pp. 21-26

Eisenbrand, G., Janzowski, C. & Preussmann, R. (1977) Analysis, formation and occurrence of volatile and non-volatile *N*-nitroso compounds: recent results. In: Tinbergen, B.J. & Krol, B., eds, Proceedings of the Second International Symposium on Nitrite in Meat Products, Zeist, 1976, Wageningen, Centre for Agricultural Publishing and Documentation, pp. 155-166

Eisenbrand, G., Spiegelhalder, B., Janzowski, C., Kann, J. & Preussmann, R. (1978) Volatile and non-volatile *N*-nitroso compounds in foods and other environmental media. In: Walker, E.A., Castegnaro, M., Griciute, L. & Lyle, R.E., eds, Environmental Aspects of *N*-Nitroso Compounds, Lyon (IARC Scientific Publications No. 19) (in press)

Fan, S.T., Krull, I.S., Ross, R.D., Wolff, M.H. & Fine, D.H. (1978) Comprehensive analytical procedures for the determination of volatile and nonvolatile, polar and nonpolar *N*-nitroso compounds. In: Walker, E.A., Castegnaro, M., Griciute, L. & Lyle, R.E., eds, Environmental Aspects of *N*-Nitroso Compounds, Lyon (IARC Scientific Publications No. 19) (in press)

Garcia, H. & Lijinsky, W. (1973) Studies of the tumorigenic effect in feeding of nitrosamine acids and of low doses of amines and nitrite to rats. Z. Krebsforsch., 79, 141-144

Green, C., Hansen, T.J., Iwaoka, W.T. & Tannenbaum, S.R. (1977) Specific detection systems for the chromatographic analysis of nitrosamines. In: Tinbergen, B.J. & Krol, B., eds, Proceedings of the Second International Symposium on Nitrite in Meat Products, Zeist, 1976, Wageningen, Centre for Agricultural Publishing and Documentation, pp. 145-153

Greenblatt, M. & Lijinsky, W. (1972) Failure to induce tumors in Swiss mice after concurrent administration of amino acids and sodium nitrite. J. nat. Cancer Inst., 48, 1389-1392

Hamilton, P.B. & Ortiz, P.J. (1950) Proline and hydroxyproline, purification, reaction with ninhydrin, and some properties of their *N*-nitroso derivatives. J. biol. Chem., 184, 607-615

Iwaoka, W. & Tannenbaum, S.R. (1976) Liquid chromatography of *N*-nitrosoamino acids and their *syn* and *anti* conformers. J. Chromat., 124, 105-110

Kushnir, I., Feinberg, J.I., Pensabene, J.W., Piotrowski, E.G., Fiddler, W. & Wasserman, A.E. (1975) Isolation and identification of nitrosoproline in uncooked bacon. J. Fd Sci., 40, 427-428

Lee, J.S., Bills, D.D., Scanlan, R.A. & Libbey, L.M. (1977) 3-Hydroxy-*N*-nitrosopyrrolidine. Isolation from heated 4-hydroxy-*N*-nitrosoproline. J. agric. Fd Chem., 25, 422-423

Lijinsky, W., Keefer, L. & Loo, J. (1970) The preparation and properties of some nitrosamino acids. Tetrahedron, 26, 5137-5153

Nixon, J.E., Wales, J.H., Scanlan, R.A., Bills, D.D. & Sinnhuber, R.O. (1976) Null carcinogenic effect of large doses of nitrosoproline and nitrosohydroxyproline in Wistar rats. Fd Cosmet. Toxicol., 14, 133-135

Rainey, W.T., Christie, W.H. & Lijinsky, W. (1978) Mass spectrometry of *N*-nitrosamines. Biomed. Mass Spectrom. (in press)

Sander, J. (1967) Eine Methode zum Nachweis von Nitrosaminen. Hoppe-Seyler's Z. physiol. Chem., 348, 852-854

Sen, N.P., Donaldson, B.A., Seaman, S., Iyengar, J.R. & Miles, W.F. (1978) Recent studies in Canada on the analysis and occurrence of volatile and non-volatile *N*-nitroso compounds in foods. In: Walker, E.A., Castegnaro, M., Griciute, L. & Lyle, R.E., eds, Environmental Aspects of *N*-Nitroso Compounds, Lyon (IARC Scientific Publications No. 19) (in press)

Stoltz, D.R. & Sen, N.P. (1977) Mutagenicity of five cyclic *N*-nitrosamines: assay with *Salmonella typhimurium*. J. nat. Cancer Inst., 58, 393-394

Wolfram, J.H., Feinberg, J.I., Doerr, R.C. & Fiddler, W. (1977) Determination of *N*-nitrosoproline at the nanogram level. J. Chromat., 132, 37-43

N-NITROSOPYRROLIDINE

1. Chemical and Physical Data

1.1 Synonyms and trade names

Chem. Abstr. Services Reg. No.: 930-55-2

Chem. Abstr. Name: 1-Nitrosopyrrolidine

N-Pyr; NO-Pyr; NPYR

1.2 Structural and molecular formulae and weight

O=N—N (pyrrolidine ring)

$C_4H_8N_2O$ Mol. wt: 100.2

1.3 Chemical and physical properties of the pure substance

(a) Description: Yellow liquid

(b) Boiling-point: 214°C (760 mm); 98°C (12 mm)

(c) Spectroscopy data: λ_{max} 230 and 333 nm (E^1_1 = 812.8 and 10.7) in water (Druckrey *et al.*, 1967); mass spectroscopy data are given by Pensabene *et al.* (1972) and Rainey *et al.* (1978).

(d) Solubility: Miscible with water in all proportions; soluble in organic solvents and lipids

(e) Volatility: Can be steam-distilled (Eisenbrand *et al.*, 1970)

(f) Stability: Stable at room temperature for more than 14 days in neutral or alkaline aqueous solutions in the dark (Druckrey *et al.*, 1967); slightly less stable in acidic solutions; light-sensitive, especially to ultra-violet light

(g) Reactivity: Strong oxidants (peracids) oxidize it to the corresponding nitramine; can be reduced to the corresponding hydrazine and/or amine; relatively resistant to hydrolysis, but can be split by hydrogen bromide in acetic acid (Eisenbrand & Preussmann, 1970).

1.4 Technical products and impurities

No data were available to the Working Group.

2. Production, Use, Occurrence and Analysis

2.1 Production and use

(a) Production

N-Nitrosopyrrolidine (NPYR) was first prepared by Petersen in 1888 by the reaction of pyrrolidine with potassium nitrite in a weak hydrochloric acid solution (Prager & Jacobson, 1935). No evidence was found that NPYR has been produced commercially.

(b) Use

No data were available to the Working Group.

2.2 Occurrence

NPYR is formed during the heating of *N*-nitrosoproline at 185-200°C (Eisenbrand *et al.*, 1977).

(a) Air

In the frying of bacon, 70-80% of the NPYR present normally is found in the vapour (Gough *et al.*, 1976); Sen *et al.* (1976) showed an average of 50% in the vapour during frying. These results are corroborated by those of Eisenbrand *et al.* (1977).

(b) Tobacco

McCormick *et al.* (1973) reported the presence of 1-110 ng/cigarette NPYR in tobacco smoke condensate; Klimsch *et al.* (1976) reported levels of 7-113 ng/cigarette.

From 5.1-34 ng/cigarette were found in 5 kinds of cigarettes (Brunnemann & Hoffmann, 1978). Levels of 115-1600 μg/kg have been found in the scrapings of pipes used for smoking tobacco in Transkei; these scrapings are believed to be consumed by the local inhabitants (IARC, 1977).

(c) Waste-water

Cohen & Bachman (1978) reported 0.09-0.20 μg/l[1] in water from 2/19 chemical factories.

(d) Food and feed

For details of the occurrence of NPYR in various foods, see Table 1.

Meat and fish products: Gray (1976) has reviewed the literature on the presence of NPYR and of its possible precursors in bacon. NPYR has been found in grilled or fried bacon; it is found mainly in residual fatty tissue and less in the lean and rind (Patterson *et al.*, 1976). Gough *et al.* (1976) found 25% NPYR in the rasher itself and 30% in cooked-out fat. In the US, the average content in bacon is decreasing: a study in 1971-1974 showed 67 μg/kg; in 1975-1976, the value was 17 μg/kg. This has been attributed to the use of ascorbate and to lower permissible levels of nitrite (Greenberg, 1977).

Spices: Dry premixed cures containing spices and sodium nitrite were found to contain up to 40 μg/kg NPYR when received; this could increase up to 520 μg/kg during 6-months' storage (Gough & Goodhead, 1975). Havery *et al.* (1976) found 730 μg/kg NPYR in a spice-cure mixture buffered with sodium carbonate.

Feed: NPYR was found in 50% of 46 samples of several types of animal feed at levels of 1-26 μg/kg (Kann *et al.*, 1978). Mirna *et al.* (1976) found levels of 2-8 μg/kg in 5/6 fishmeal samples.

(e) *In vivo*

Fine *et al.* (1977) were unable to detect NPYR in the blood of 6 students who ingested 170 g cooked bacon, although *N*-nitrosodimethylamine and *N*-nitrosodiethylamine were detected.

---

[1]This result was not confirmed by mass spectrometry (see also 'General Remarks on the Substances Considered', p. 40).

Table 1

Levels of *N*-nitrosopyrrolidine in various foods from several countries[1]

Product	Country	No. of samples	Number positive	Level (μg/kg)	References
Bacon (fried)	Canada	14	14	10-44	Greenberg (1977)
Spiced meat products	"	19	9	7-33	Sen *et al.* (1976b)
Sausage	"	66	14	10-105	Panalaks *et al.* (1974)
Bacon (fried)	"	12	3	3-8	" " "
Fried cured meat products	FRG	34	17	0.6-8	Eisenbrand *et al.* (1978)
Cheese	"	173	2	1.4-3.4	" " "
Bacon (raw)	"	5	1	17	" " (1977)
" (cooked)	"	5	5	10-40	" " "
Liver, meatloaf (raw)	"	4	0	NR	" " "
" " (cooked)	"	4	2	5-6	" " "
Pepper salami (raw)	"	5	1	2	" " "
" " (cooked)	"	5	5	7-12	" " "
Ham (raw)	"	6	3	8-15	" " "
" (cooked)	"	4	4	3-46	" " "
Fish products	Hong Kong	61	23	2-37	Fong & Chan (1977)
Fried bacon-like products	The Netherlands	NR[2]	NR	3.3-55	Stephany *et al.* (1976)
Nitrite-preserved meats	"	NR	NR	0-5.4	" " "
Assorted meats (raw and cooked)	"	48	0	<10	Groenen *et al.* (1977)

[1]No data were available to the Working Group from other countries.
[2]NR = not reported

Product	Country	No. of samples	Number positive	Level (µg/kg)	References
Bacon (fried)	UK	56	28	1-20	Gough *et al.* (1977)
Assorted cured and cooked meat products	"	107	0	<1	" " "
Fish	"	104	NR	0-3	Telling *et al.* (1974)
Bacon (fried)	USA	18	5	5-10	Havery *et al.* (1978)
			12	10-100	
" "	"	22	22	8-139	" " (1976)
Cured beef and pork	"	34	0	<1	" " (1978)
Souse and jellied cured meat products	"	10	1	19	Fiddler *et al.* (1975)
Fried ham	"	20	19	10-50	Greenberg (1975)
Bacon (fried) with added ascorbate	"	154	25	>5[3]	Birdsall (1977)
Bacon (fried)	"	12	12	8-47	Greenberg (1977)
Ham (fried)	"	20	3	19-50	" "

[3]Values only reported as less than or greater than 5 µg/kg

2.3 Analysis

An IARC Manual gives selected methods for the analysis of volatile *N*-nitrosamines, including NPYR (Preussmann *et al.*, 1978).

3. Biological Data Relevant to the Evaluation of Carcinogenic Risk to Man

3.1 Carcinogenicity studies in animals

(a) Oral administration

Mouse: Groups of 20 male and 20 female 5-7-week-old Swiss mice were given 5 ml of a solution containing 0.01% *N*-nitrosopyrrolidine (NPYR) 5 times/week in the drinking-water (total dose, 0.015 g/mouse). Many treated animals died early in the experiment (mean survival time, 12 weeks). Of animals that survived the subacute hepatic injury resulting from administration of the compound 4/34 animals examined had 51 lung adenomas. Only 8 adenomas were seen in 7/53 untreated controls examined (Greenblatt & Lijinsky, 1972a).

Rat: A group of 25 BD rats were given 5 or 10 mg/kg bw/day NPYR in the drinking-water; the doses were doubled 150 days after the start of treatment. After an average induction time of 470 or 290 days, respectively, 23/25 animals developed hepatocellular carcinomas (average total doses that caused tumours in 50% of animals, 3.9 or 4.2 g/kg bw) (Druckrey *et al.*, 1967).

This result was confirmed in MRC rats. In addition to hepatocellular carcinomas (25/25), 7/12 male rats developed 4 papillary mesotheliomas of the tunica vaginalis, 2 interstitial-cell tumours and 1 cavernous haemangioma of the testis (Greenblatt & Lijinsky, 1972b).

NPYR was administered to 14 male and 15 female 8-week-old Sprague-Dawley rats at a concentration of 0.02% in the drinking-water (20 ml/day) on 5 days/week for 50 weeks (total dose, 1 g/animal). Treated animals died after 45-105 weeks, and 26/29 animals developed hepatocellular carcinomas. In addition, 4 cholangiocarcinomas and 2 olfactory carcinomas were found (Lijinsky & Taylor, 1976).

Groups of 24-62 100-day-old Sprague-Dawley rats of both sexes were given NPYR in the drinking-water at doses of 0 (control), 0.3, 1, 3 or 10 mg/kg bw/day, respectively, for lifetime. At dose levels of 1, 3 and 10 mg/kg bw, 13/62, 30/38 and 9/24 animals, respectively, had hepatocellular carcinomas, which were not observed in animals given the lowest dose level (0.3 mg/kg bw) or in control animals. On the other hand, 3-20% of hepatocellular adenomas and a slight increase of the overall incidence of malignant tumours and leukaemias was found in all experimental groups but not in controls. The mean times of death of tumour-bearing animals were at 664 days (0.3 mg/kg bw), 685 days (1 mg/kg bw), 533 days (3 mg/kg bw) and 444 days (10 mg/kg bw). The authors indicated that the commercial diet fed to both control and treated rats contained trace quantities of volatile nitrosamines, as analysed by gas chromatography-thermal energy analysis (up to 60 μg/kg *N*-nitrosodimethylamine and up to 10 μg/kg NPYR) (Preussmann *et al.*, 1977).

(b) Subcutaneous and/or intramuscular administration

Hamster: The induction of lung tumours in Syrian golden hamsters by s.c. injection of NPYR was reported (Dontenwill, 1968) [Full details were not given].

(c) Carcinogenicity of derivatives

Administration of *N*-nitroso-2,5-dimethylpyrrolidine to Sprague-Dawley rats induced liver tumours in only 2/29 animals. Administration of *N*-nitroso-3,4-dichloropyrrolidine induced tumours of the oesophagus in 13/14 animals and tumours of the nasal turbinals in 4/14 (Lijinsky & Taylor, 1976).

3.2 Other relevant biological data

(a) Experimental systems

Toxic effects

In rats, the oral LD_{50} of NPYR was 900 mg/kg bw (Druckrey *et al.*, 1967), and the i.p. LD_{50}, 650 mg/kg bw (Lee & Lijinsky, 1966).

No data on the embryotoxicity or teratogenicity of this compound were available to the Working Group.

Metabolism

After i.p. administration of 6 mg/kg bw [2,5-^{14}C]- or [3,4-^{14}C]-NPYR to rats, these compounds were converted to $^{14}CO_2$ to the extent of 18-25% within 6 hours; 7% of the radioactivity was excreted in the urine and only 1-2% in the faeces (Krüger & Bertram, 1975). An oral dose of 4 mg/kg bw [2,5-^{14}C]-NPYR was converted to $^{14}CO_2$ to the extent of 77%, while only 14% of a dose of 650 mg/kg bw appeared as $^{14}CO_2$ in 24 hours (Snyder *et al.*, 1977).

Less than 1% of an i.p. dose of NPYR appeared as *N*-nitroso-3-hydroxy-pyrrolidine in the urine of rats. An alkylated base, which was not identified but was shown not to be 7-methylguanine, was isolated from hydrolysates of liver DNA (Krüger & Bertram, 1975). ^{3}H-NPYR administered to rats reacted with hepatic DNA and RNA; however, no products were characterized (Lijinsky *et al.*, 1973).

Mutagenicity and other short-term tests

NPYR produces reverse mutations in *Escherichia coli* and *Salmonella typhimurium* strains TA 1530, TA 1535, TA 1537 and TA 1538 in the presence of a liver microsomal fraction from phenobarbital- or Aroclor 1254-treated rats or from human biopsies (Bartsch *et al.*, 1976; Elespuru & Lijinsky, 1976; Gomez *et al.*, 1974; McCann *et al.*, 1975; Stoltz & Sen, 1977).

In the presence of a rat-liver microsomal system from phenobarbital-treated rats, NPYR induced 8-azaguanine-resistant mutants in Chinese hamster V79 cells (Kuroki *et al.*, 1977).

(b) Humans

No data were available to the Working Group.

3.3 Case reports and epidemiological studies

No data were available to the Working Group.

4. Summary of Data Reported and Evaluation

4.1 Experimental data

N-Nitrosopyrrolidine is carcinogenic in rats after its oral administration: it produces hepatocellular carcinomas. It also increases the incidence of lung adenomas in mice following its oral administration. A study in rats has been reported in which a dose-response relationship was established.

4.2 Human data

No case reports or epidemiological studies were available to the Working Group. Available information on occurrence suggests that the general population may be exposed to low levels of *N*-nitrosopyrrolidine; however, no exposed group suitable for an epidemiological investigation has yet been identified.

4.3 Evaluation

There is *sufficient evidence* of a carcinogenic effect of *N*-nitrosopyrrolidine in one experimental animal species. Although no epidemiological data were available, *N*-nitrosopyrrolidine should be regarded as if it were carcinogenic to humans.

5. References

Bartsch, H., Camus, A. & Malaveille, C. (1976) Comparative mutagenicity of *N*-nitrosamines in a semi-solid and in a liquid incubation system in the presence of rat or human tissue fractions. Mutation Res., 37, 149-162

Birdsall, J.J. (1977) *N*-Nitrosopyrrolidine in bacon obtained from 10 commercial bacon production plants. In: Tinbergen, B.J. & Krol, B., eds, Proceedings of the Second International Symposium on Nitrite in Meat Products, Zeist, 1976, Wageningen, Centre for Agricultural Publishing and Documentation, pp. 211-213

Brunnemann, K.D. & Hoffmann, D. (1978) Chemical studies on tobacco smoke. LIX. Analysis of volatile nitrosamines in tobacco smoke and polluted indoor environments. In: Walker, E.A., Castegnaro, M., Griciute, L. & Lyle, R.E., eds, Environmental Aspects of *N*-Nitroso Compounds, Lyon (IARC Scientific Publications No. 19) (in press)

Cohen, J.B. & Bachman, J.D. (1978) Measurement of environmental nitrosamines. In: Walker, E.A., Castegnaro, M., Griciute, L. & Lyle, R.E., eds, Environmental Aspects of *N*-Nitroso Compounds, Lyon (IARC Scientific Publications No. 19) (in press)

Dontenwill, W. (1968) Experimental studies on the organotropic effect of nitrosamines in the respiratory tract. Fd Cosmet. Toxicol., 6, 571

Druckrey, H., Preussmann, R., Ivankovic, S. & Schmähl, D. (1967) Organotrope carcinogene Wirkungen bei 65 verschiedenen *N*-Nitroso-Verbindungen an BD-Ratten. Z. Krebsforsch., 69, 103-201

Eisenbrand, G. & Preussmann, R. (1970) Eine neue Methode zur kolorimetrischen Bestimmung von Nitrosaminen nach Spaltung der *N*-Nitrosogruppe mit Bromwasserstoff in Eisessig. Arzneimittel-Forsch., 20, 1513-1517

Eisenbrand, G., Hodenberg, A. von & Preussmann, R. (1970) Trace analysis of *N*-nitroso compounds. II. Steam distillation at neutral, alkaline and acid pH under reduced and atmospheric pressure. Z. analyt. Chem., 251, 22-24

Eisenbrand, G., Janzowski, C. & Preussmann, R. (1977) Analysis, formation and occurrence of volatile and non-volatile *N*-nitroso compounds: recent results. In: Tinbergen, B.J. & Krol, B., eds, Proceedings of the Second International Symposium on Nitrite in Meat Products, Zeist, 1976, Wageningen, Centre for Agricultural Publishing and Documentation, pp. 155-169

Eisenbrand, G., Spiegelhalder, B., Janzowski, C., Kann, J. & Preussmann, R. (1978) Volatile and non-volatile *N*-nitroso compounds in foods and other environmental media. In: Walker, E.A., Castegnaro, M., Griciute, L. & Lyle, R.E., eds, Environmental Aspects of *N*-Nitroso Compounds, Lyon (IARC Scientific Publications No. 19) (in press)

Elespuru, R.K. & Lijinsky, W. (1976) Mutagenicity of cyclic nitrosamines in *Escherichia coli* following activation with rat liver microsomes. Cancer Res., 36, 4099-4101

Fiddler, W., Feinberg, J.I., Pensabene, J.W., Williams, A.C. & Dooley, C.J. (1975) Dimethylnitrosamine in souse and similar jellied cured-meat products. Fd Cosmet. Toxicol., 13, 653-654

Fine, D.H., Ross, R., Rounbehler, D.P., Silvergleid, A. & Song, L. (1977) Formation *in vivo* of volatile *N*-nitrosamines in man after ingestion of cooked bacon and spinach. Nature (Lond.), 265, 753-755

Fong, Y.Y. & Chan, W.C. (1977) Nitrate, nitrite, dimethylnitrosamine and *N*-nitrosopyrrolidine in some Chinese food products. Fd Cosmet. Toxicol., 15, 143-145

Gomez, R.F., Johnston, M. & Sinskey, A.J. (1974) Activation of nitrosomorpholine and nitrosopyrrolidine to bacterial mutagens. Mutation Res., 24, 5-7

Gough, T.A. & Goodhead, K. (1975) Occurrence of volatile nitrosamines in spice premixes. J. Sci. Fd Agric., 26, 1473-1478

Gough, T.A., Goodhead, K. & Walters, C.L. (1976) Distribution of some volatile nitrosamines in cooked bacon. J. Sci. Fd Agric., 27, 181-185

Gough, T.A., McPhail, M.F., Webb, K.S., Wood, B.J. & Coleman, R.F. (1977) An examination of some foodstuffs for the presence of volatile nitrosamines. J. Sci. Fd Agric., 28, 345-351

Gray, J.I. (1976) *N*-Nitrosamines and their precursors in bacon: a review. J. Milk Fd Technol., 39, 686-692

Greenberg, R.A. (1975) Update on nitrite, nitrate and nitrosamines. In: Proceedings of Meat Industry Research Conference, Chicago, American Meat Institute Foundation, pp. 71-76

Greenberg, R.A. (1977) Nitrosopyrrolidine in United States cured meat products. In: Tinbergen, B.J. & Krol, B., eds, Proceedings of the Second International Symposium on Nitrite in Meat Products, Zeist, 1976, Wageningen, Centre for Agricultural Publishing and Documentation, pp. 203-210

Greenblatt, M. & Lijinsky, W. (1972a) Failure to induce tumors in Swiss mice after concurrent administration of amino acids and sodium nitrite. J. nat. Cancer Inst., 48, 1389-1392

Greenblatt, M. & Lijinsky, W. (1972b) Nitrosamine studies: neoplasms of liver and genital mesothelium in nitrosopyrrolidine-treated MRC rats. J. nat. Cancer Inst., 48, 1687-1696

Groenen, P.J., de Cock-Bethbeder, M.W., Jonk, R.J.G. & van Ingen, C. (1977) Further studies on the occurrence of volatile *N*-nitrosamines in meat products by combined gas chromatography and mass spectrometry. In: Tinbergen, B.J. & Krol, B., eds, Proceedings of the Second International Symposium on Nitrite in Meat Products, Zeist, 1976, Wageningen, Centre for Agricultural Publishing and Documentation, pp. 227-237

Havery, D.C., Kline, D.A., Miletta, E.M., Joe, F.L., Jr & Fazio, T. (1976) Survey of food products for volatile *N*-nitrosamines. J. Ass. off. analyt. Chem., 59, 540-546

Havery, D.C., Fazio, T. & Howard, J.W. (1978) Survey of cured meat products for volatile *N*-nitrosamines: comparison of two analytical methods. In: Walker, E.A., Castegnaro, M., Griciute, L. & Lyle, R.E., eds, Environmental Aspects of *N*-Nitroso Compounds, Lyon (IARC Scientific Publications No. 19) (in press)

IARC (1977) Annual Report 1977, Lyon, International Agency for Research on Cancer, p. 64

Kann, J., Spiegelhalder, B., Eisenbrand, G. & Preussmann, R. (1978) Occurrence of volatile *N*-nitrosamines in animal diets. Z. Krebsforsch. (in press)

Klimsch, H.-J., Stadler, L. & Brahm, S. (1976) Quantitative Bestimmung flüchtiger Nitrosamine in Zigarettenrauchkondensat. Z. Lebensmittel-Untersuch., 162, 131-138

Krüger, F.W. & Bertram, B. (1975) Metabolism of nitrosamines *in vivo*. IV. Isolation of 3-hydroxy-1-nitrosopyrrolidine from rat urine after application of 1-nitrosopyrrolidine. Z. Krebsforsch., 83, 255-260

Kuroki, T., Drevon, C. & Montesano, R. (1977) Microsome-mediated mutagenesis in V79 Chinese hamster cells by various nitrosamines. Cancer Res., 37, 1044-1050

Lee, K.Y. & Lijinsky, W. (1966) Alkylation of rat liver RNA by cyclic *N*-nitrosamines *in vivo*. J. nat. Cancer Inst., 37, 401-407

Lijinsky, W. & Taylor, H.W. (1976) The effect of substituents on the carcinogenicity of *N*-nitrosopyrrolidine in Sprague-Dawley rats. Cancer Res., 36, 1988-1990

Lijinsky, W., Keefer, L., Loo, J. & Ross, A.E. (1973) Studies of alkylation of nucleic acids in rats by cyclic nitrosamines. Cancer Res., 33, 1634-1641

McCann, J., Choi, E., Yamasaki, E. & Ames, B.N. (1975) Detection of carcinogens as mutagens in the *Salmonella*/microsome test: assay of 300 chemicals. Proc. nat. Acad. Sci. (Wash.), 72, 5135-5139

McCormick, A., Nicholson, M.J., Baylis, M.A. & Underwood, J.G. (1973) Nitrosamines in cigarette smoke condensate. Nature (Lond.), 244, 237-238

Mirna, A., Harada, K., Rapp, U. & Kaufmann, H. (1976) *N*-Nitrosamine in Futtermitteln. Fleischwirtschaft, 56, 1014

Panalaks, T., Iyengar, J.R., Donaldson, B.A., Miles, W.F. & Sen, N.P. (1974) Further survey of cured meat products for volatile *N*-nitrosamines. J. Ass. off. analyt. Chem., 57, 806-812

Patterson, R.L.S., Taylor, A.A., Mottram, D.S. & Gough, T.A. (1976) Localised occurrence of *N*-nitrosopyrrolidine in fried bacon. J. Sci. Fd Agric., 27, 257-260

Pensabene, J.W., Fiddler, W., Dooley, C.J., Doerr, R.C. & Wasserman, A.E. (1972) Spectral and gas chromatographic characteristics of some *N*-nitrosamines. J. agric. Fd Chem., 20, 274-277

Prager, B. & Jacobson, P., eds (1935) Beilsteins Handbuch der Organischen Chemie, 4th ed., Vol. 20, Syst. No. 3037, Berlin, Springer, p. 6

Preussmann, R., Schmähl, D. & Eisenbrand, G. (1977) Carcinogenicity of *N*-nitrosopyrrolidine: dose-response study in rats. Z. Krebsforsch., 90, 161-166

Preussmann, R., Walker, E.A., Wasserman, A.E. & Castegnaro, M., eds (1978) Environmental Carcinogens - Selected Methods of Analysis, Vol. 1, Nitrosamines, Lyon (IARC Scientific Publications No. 18) (in press)

Rainey, W.T., Christie, W.H. & Lijinsky, W. (1978) Mass spectrometry of *N*-nitrosamines. Biomed. Mass Spectrom. (in press)

Sen, N.P., Donaldson, B., Iyengar, J.R. & Panalaks, T. (1973) Nitrosopyrrolidine and dimethylnitrosamine in bacon. Nature (Lond.), 241, 473-474

Sen, N.P., Seaman, S. & Miles, W.F. (1976a) Dimethylnitrosamine and nitrosopyrrolidine in fumes produced during the frying of bacon. Fd Cosmet. Toxicol., 14, 167-170

Sen, N.P., Iyengar, J.R., Miles, W.F. & Panalaks, T. (1976b) Nitrosamines in cured meat products. In: Walker, E.A., Bogovski, P. & Griciute, L., eds, Environmental *N*-Nitroso Compounds Analysis and Formation, Lyon (IARC Scientific Publications No. 14), pp. 333-342

Snyder, C.M., Farrelly, J.G. & Lijinsky, W. (1977) Metabolism of three cyclic nitrosamines in Sprague-Dawley rats. Cancer Res., 37, 3530-3532

Stephany, R.W., Freudenthal, J. & Schuller, P.L. (1976) Quantitative and qualitative determination of some volatile nitrosamines in various meat products. In: Walker, E.A., Bogovski, P. & Griciute, L., eds, Environmental *N*-Nitroso Compounds Analysis and Formation, Lyon (IARC Scientific Publications No. 14), pp. 343-354

Stoltz, D.R. & Sen, N.P. (1977) Mutagenicity of five cyclic *N*-nitrosamines: assay with *Salmonella typhimurium*. J. nat. Cancer Inst., 58, 393-394

Telling, G.M., Bryce, T.A., Hoar, D., Osborne, D. & Welti, D. (1974) Progress in the analysis of volatile *N*-nitroso compounds. In: Bogovski, P. & Walker, E.A., eds, *N*-Nitroso Compounds in the Environment, Lyon (IARC Scientific Publications No. 9), pp. 12-17

N-NITROSOSARCOSINE

1. Chemical and Physical Data

1.1 Synonyms and trade names

Chem. Abstr. Services Reg. No.: 13256-22-9

Chem. Abstr. Name: *N*-Methyl-*N*-nitroso-glycine

N-Nitrosomethylglycine; NSAR

1.2 Structural and molecular formulae and weight

$$O{=}N{-}N(CH_3){-}CH_2{-}C({=}O){-}OH$$

$C_3H_6N_2O_3$ Mol. wt: 118.1

1.3 Chemical and physical properties of the pure substance

From Lijinsky *et al.* (1970), unless otherwise specified

(a) Description: Pale-yellow crystals

(b) Melting-point: 66-67°C

(c) Spectroscopy data: λ_{max} 234 and 337 nm (E_1^1 = 499 and 6.5) in water (Druckrey *et al.*, 1967); mass spectroscopy data have been reported (Rainey *et al.*, 1978).

(d) Solubility: Miscible with water in all proportions; soluble in polar organic solvents

(e) Stability: The free acid is unstable in aqueous solution; a concentration decrease of more than 10% in 24 hours has been observed (Druckrey *et al.*, 1967); light-sensitive, especially to ultra-violet light (*f*) Reactivity: Partially decarboxylates on heating at 180-190°C to form *N*-nitrosodimethylamine; it is oxidized by strong oxidants (peracids) to the corresponding nitramine (Eisenbrand *et al.*, 1977).

1.4 Technical products and impurities

No data were available to the Working Group.

2. Production, Use, Occurrence and Analysis

2.1 Production and use

(*a*) Production

N-Nitrososarcosine (NSAR) has been prepared by passing nitrous acid fumes through a sarcosine solution (Brookes & Walker, 1957) and by the reaction of sarcosine with sodium nitrite in an acid solution (Bergel *et al.*, 1963; Hammick & Voaden, 1961; Lijinsky *et al.*, 1970). NSAR has also been formed by nitrosating *N*-methylsarcosine (dimethylglycine) hydrochloride (Friedman, 1975) and by treating *N*-amidinosarcosine (creatine) in an acid medium with an aqueous solution of sodium nitrite (Archer *et al.*, 1971; Velisek *et al.*, 1975).

No evidence was found that NSAR has been manufactured commercially.

(*b*) Use

No data were available to the Working Group.

2.2 Occurrence

NSAR was not found in bacon, but 1 smoked meat sample contained 10 μg/kg (Dhont & van Ingen, 1976). Eisenbrand *et al.* (1978) found NSAR in 5/8 meat samples: boiled ham, 2 μg/kg; bologna, 2 and 56 μg/kg; meatloaf, 2 and 15 μg/kg.

2.3 Analysis

Meat has been extracted with methanol:water, separated on an ion-exchange column, converted into the methyl ester and determined by gas chromatography-mass spectrometry (Dhont, 1977; Dhont & van Ingen, 1976).

Eisenbrand *et al.* (1978) extracted meat with acetone:water, purified the sample by column chromatography, converted it to the trimethylsilyl derivative and determined NSAR by gas chromatography-thermal energy analysis.

Chromatographic conditions suitable for use with high-pressure liquid chromatography-thermal energy analysis are described by Fan *et al.* (1978). Separation of *syn-anti* conformers by high-pressure liquid chromatography-ultra-violet is described by Iwaoka & Tannenbaum (1976). A thin-layer technique has been described by Rao & Bejnarowicz (1976).

A collaborative study on several analytical methods for 3 *N*-nitroso amino acids, including *N*-nitrososarcosine, showed good agreement between the methods (Castegnaro & Walker, 1978).

3. Biological Data Relevant to the Evaluation of Carcinogenic Risk to Man

3.1 Carcinogenicity and related studies in animals

(a) Oral administration

Mouse: In a study reported as an abstract, a group of 65 male and 65 female Swiss (IRC) mice were fed a diet containing 0.25% *N*-nitrososarcosine (NSAR) for 13 months. At that time, 21 male and 20 female survivors were killed, and 10 male and 11 female mice had squamous-cell carcinomas of the nasal region. Several other tumours were observed at necropsy, including 5 tumours of the lung, 2 of the small intestine, 2 of the vagina and 1 each of the testis, kidney, skin, thymus, bladder and pancreas. No tumours were observed in either male or female control mice which died or were sacrificed at 13 months (Sawyer & Friedman, 1974).

Rat: Twenty BD rats received 100 or 200 mg/kg bw/day NSAR in the drinking-water; treatment was terminated after 286 days when total doses of 28.6 and 57 g/kg bw, respectively, had been reached. Of animals given the lower dose (100 mg/kg bw), 5/14 died with oesophageal carcinomas 357-631 days after the start of treatment. Of those given the higher dose (200 mg/kg bw), 3/6 rats developed papillomas and 3/6, squamous-cell carcinomas of the oesophagus at 414-548 days (Druckrey *et al.*, 1967; Thomas & So, 1969).

(b) Intraperitoneal administration

Newborn mouse: Newborn (C57BL/6JxC3HeB/FeJ)F_1 mice received i.p. injections of 75 mg/kg bw NSAR suspended in trioctanoin on days 1, 4 and 7 after birth; all survivors were killed after 78 weeks. Of 12 male mice that survived for 50-78 weeks after dosing, 8 had liver-cell carcinomas, and 3 had lesions described as liver-cell hyperplasia. Three of 17 females that survived for the same period also showed liver-cell hyperplasia. In the control group, which received 3 x 5 mg/kg bw trioctanoin, 1/12 females that survived for 50-85 weeks had a liver-cell carcinoma and 2/14 males had liver-cell hyperplasia (Wogan *et al.*, 1975).

(c) Carcinogenicity of derivatives

N-Nitrososarcosine ethyl ester

(i) Oral administration

A group of 20 BD rats were given 50 or 100 mg/kg bw/day *N*-nitrososarcosine ethyl ester in the drinking-water. After average induction times of 200 or 160 days, respectively, all animals developed squamous-cell carcinomas of the oesophagus (average total dose that induced a 50% tumour incidence, 9.7 or 16 g/kg bw) (Druckrey *et al.*, 1967). Both carcinomas and various preneoplastic lesions were described in an abstract (Pozharisskii & Savost'yanov, 1972).

(ii) Intravenous administration

Twenty BD rats were injected intravenously with 100 mg/kg bw *N*-nitrososarcosine ethyl ester once weekly (14 animals) or twice weekly (6 animals). Nineteen of 20 treated rats developed squamous-cell carcinomas of the oesophagus after average induction times of 300 or 254 days, respectively (average total dose that induced a 50% tumour incidence, 3.9 or 5.7 g/kg bw) (Druckrey *et al.*, 1967).

3.2 Other relevant biological data

(a) Experimental systems

Toxic effects

The LD_{50} of NSAR in mice following a single i.p. injection 24 hours after birth was 184 mg/kg bw (Wogan *et al.*, 1975). The LD_{50} by an unspecified route in mice was reported to be 3.5 g/kg bw (Friedman & Couch, 1976). Single oral doses of 5 g/kg bw NSAR were non-toxic in rats (Druckrey *et al.*, 1967).

No data on the embryotoxicity or teratogenicity of this compound were available to the Working Group.

Metabolism

Administration of 1 g/kg bw NSAR to mice inhibits hepatic aminopyrine demethylase and aniline hydroxylase activities (Friedman, 1974); doses of 100-500 mg/kg bw inhibited hepatic *N*-nitrosodimethylamine *N*-demethylase activity (Friedman & Couch, 1976).

Mutagenicity and other short-term tests

NSAR (1 g/kg bw) administered to mice by gavage was not mutagenic in the host-mediated assay using *Salmonella typhimurium* strain G-46 (Couch & Friedman, 1976).

(b) Humans

No data were available to the Working Group.

3.3 Case reports and epidemiological studies

No data were available to the Working Group.

4. Summary of Data Reported and Evaluation

4.1 Experimental data

N-Nitrososarcosine is carcinogenic in mice and rats. It produces carcinomas of the nasal cavities in mice and oesophageal carcinomas in rats after its oral administration, and liver-cell carcinomas in newborn mice after its intraperitoneal injection.

4.2 Human data

No case reports or epidemiological studies were available to the Working Group. Available information on occurrence suggests that the general population may be exposed sporadically to low levels of this substance; however, no exposed group suitable for an epidemiological investigation has yet been identified.

4.3 Evaluation

There is *sufficient evidence* of a carcinogenic effect of *N*-nitrososarcosine in two experimental animal species. Although no epidemiological data were available, *N*-nitrososarcosine should be regarded for practical purposes as if it were carcinogenic to humans.

5. References

Archer, M.C., Clark, S.D., Thilly, J.E. & Tannenbaum, S.R. (1971) Environmental nitroso compounds: reaction of nitrite with creatine and creatinine. Science, 174, 1341-1343

Bergel, F., Brown, S.S., Leese, C.L., Timmis, G.M. & Wade, R. (1963) Some potentially cytotoxic methylnitrosamines. J. chem. Soc., 846-853

Brookes, P. & Walker, J. (1957) Formation and properties of sydnone imines, a new class of meso-ionic compound, and some sydnones related to natural α-amino-acids. J. chem. Soc., 4409-4416

Castegnaro, M. & Walker, E.A. (1978) New data on collaborative studies on analysis of nitrosamines. In: Walker, E.A. Castegnaro, M., Griciute, L. & Lyle, R.E., eds, Environmental Aspects of *N*-Nitroso Compounds, Lyon (IARC Scientific Publications No. 19) (in press)

Couch, D.B. & Friedman, M.A. (1976) Suppression of dimethylnitrosamine mutagenicity by nitrososarcosine and other nitrosamines. Mutation Res., 38, 89-96

Dhont, J.H. (1977) Development of a method of estimating *N*-nitrosamino acids and its use on some meat products. In: Tinbergen, B.J. & Krol, B., eds, Proceedings of the Second International Symposium on Nitrite in Meat Products, Zeist, 1976, Wageningen, Centre for Agricultural Publishing and Documentation, pp. 221-225

Dhont, J.H. & van Ingen, C. (1976) Identification and quantitative determination of nitrosoproline and nitrososarcosine and preliminary investigations on nitrosohydroxyproline in cured meat products. In: Walker, E.A., Bogovski, P. & Griciute, L., eds, Environmental *N*-Nitroso Compounds Analysis and Formation, Lyon (IARC Scientific Publications No. 14), pp. 355-360

Druckrey, H., Preussmann, R., Ivankovic, S. & Schmähl, D. (1967) Organotrope carcinogene Wirkungen bei 65 verschiedenen *N*-Nitroso-Verbindungen an BD-Ratten. Z. Krebsforsch., 69, 103-201

Eisenbrand, G., Janzowski, C. & Preussmann, R. (1977) Analysis, formation and occurrence of volatile and non-volatile *N*-nitroso compounds: recent results. In: Tinbergen, B.J. & Krol, B., eds, Proceedings of the Second International Symposium on Nitrite in Meat Products, Zeist, 1976, Wageningen, Centre for Agricultural Publishing and Documentation, pp. 155-169

Eisenbrand, G., Spiegelhalder, B., Janzowski, C., Kann, J. & Preussmann, R. (1978) Volatile and non-volatile *N*-nitroso compounds in foods and other environmental media. In: Walker, E.A., Castegnaro, M., Griciute, L. & Lyle, R.E., eds, Environmental Aspects of *N*-Nitroso Compounds, Lyon (IARC Scientific Publications No. 19) (in press)

Fan, S.T., Krull, I.S., Ross, R.D., Wolff, M.H. & Fine, D.H. (1978) Comprehensive analytical procedures for the determination of volatile and nonvolatile, polar and nonpolar *N*-nitroso compounds. In: Walker, E.A., Castegnaro, M., Griciute, L. & Lyle, R.E., eds, Environmental Aspects of *N*-Nitroso Compounds, Lyon (IARC Scientific Publications No. 19) (in press)

Friedman, M.A. (1974) Inhibitory effects of nitrososarcosine on mouse liver mixed function oxidase activity. Experientia, 30, 857-859

Friedman, M.A. (1975) Reaction of sodium nitrite with dimethylglycine produces nitrososarcosine. Bull. environm. Contam. Toxicol., 13, 226-232

Friedman, M.A. & Couch, D.B. (1976) Suppression of hepatic DMN demethylase activity by nitrososarcosine and other nitrosamines. Biochem. Pharmacol., 25, 2709-2712

Hammick, D.L. & Voaden, D.J. (1961) Chemical and physical properties of some sydnones. J. chem. Soc., 3303-3308

Iwaoka, W. & Tannenbaum, S.R. (1976) Liquid chromatography of *N*-nitroso-amino acids and their *syn* and *anti* conformers. J. Chromat., 124, 105-110

Lijinsky, W., Keefer, L. & Loo, J. (1970) The preparation and properties of some nitrosamino acids. Tetrahedron, 26, 5137-5153

Pozharisskii, K.M. & Savost'yanov, G.A. (1972) Pathomorphological and electron-microscope study of experimental oesophagus tumors. In: Kavetskii, R.E., ed., Proceedings of a Symposium on Mechanisms of Carcinogenesis, 1972, Kiev, Institute of Problems on Oncology, pp. 84-85 [Chem. Abstr., 82, 94017d]

Rainey, W.T., Christie, W.H. & Lijinsky, W. (1978) Mass spectrometry of *N*-nitrosamines. Biomed. Mass Spectrom. (in press)

Rao, G.S. & Bejnarowicz, E.A. (1976) Thin-layer chromatography of sarcosine and its *N*-lauroyl and *N*-nitroso derivatives. J. Chromat., 123, 486-489

Sawyer, D.R. & Friedman, M.A. (1974) Effects of dietary nitrososarcosine on body weight, mortality and carcinogenicity in mice (Abstract No. 2176). Fed. Proc., 33, 596

Thomas, C. & So, B.T. (1969) Zur Morphologie der durch *N*-Nitroso-Verbindungen erzeugten Tumoren im oberen Verdauungstrakt der Ratte. Arzneimittel-Forsch., 19, 1077-1081

Velisek, J., Davidek, J., Klein, S., Karaskova, M. & Vykoukova, I. (1975) The nitrosation products of creatine and creatinine in model systems. Z. Lebensmittel-Untersuch., 159, 97-102

Wogan, G.N., Paglialunga, S., Archer, M.C. & Tannenbaum, S.R. (1975) Carcinogenicity of nitrosation products of ephedrine, sarcosine, folic acid, and creatinine. Cancer Res., 35, 1981-1984

STREPTOZOTOCIN

This substance was considered previously by an IARC Working Group, in June 1973 (IARC, 1974). Since that time new data have become available, and these have been incorporated into the monograph and taken into account in the present evaluation.

1. Chemical and Physical Data

1.1 Synonyms and trade names

Chem. Abstr. Services Reg. No.: 18883-66-4

Chem. Abstr. Name: 2-Deoxy-2{[(methyl-nitrosoamino)carbonyl]amino}-D-glucopyranose

2-Deoxy-2-(3-methyl-3-nitrosoureido)-D-glucopyranose; *N*-D-glucosyl-(2)-*N*'-nitroso-*N*'-methylurea; NSC 85998; STR; streptozocin; streptozoticin

1.2 Structural and molecular formulae and weight

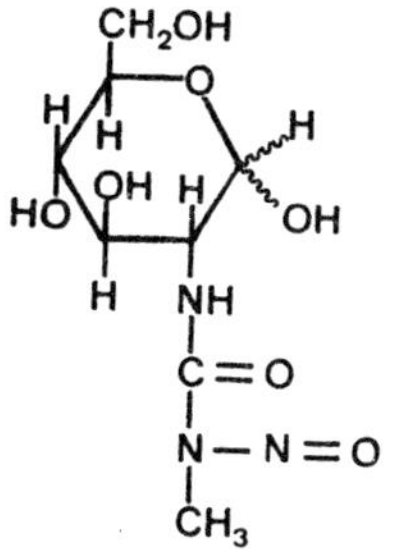

CH2OH, H, H, H, OH, H, HO, OH, H, NH, C=O, N—N=O, CH3

$C_8H_{15}N_3O_7$ Mol. wt: 265

1.3 Chemical and physical properties of the pure substance

(a) Description: Pale-yellow crystals

(b) Melting-point: Approximately 115°C (decomposition) (White, 1963)

(c) Optical rotation: Streptozotocin is a mixture of α and β stereoisomers; $[\alpha]_D^{25}$ varies widely between +15 and +68°; aqueous solutions rapidly undergo mutarotation to an equilibrium value of $[\alpha]_D^{25}$ = +39° (Herr *et al.*, 1967; Rudas, 1972).

(d) Spectroscopy data: λ_{max} 228 nm (E^1_1 = 240) (Herr *et al.*, 1967), 380, 394 and 412 nm (Rudas, 1972) in ethanol

(e) Solubility: Very soluble in water; only slightly soluble in polar organic solvents; insoluble in non-polar organic solvents

(f) Stability: Decomposes to diazomethane in alkaline solutions at 0^oC (Herr *et al.*, 1967)

(g) Reactivity: Can be acetylated to form a tetraacetate (Herr *et al.*, 1967)

1.4 Technical products and impurities

The specifications of a product offered for research purposes only by one company are as follows: off-white to tan crystalline solid, 7% max. moisture, 0.5% max. residue on ignition, and 7% max. loss on drying.

2. Production, Use, Occurrence and Analysis

2.1 Production and use

For background information on this section, see preamble, p. 22.

(a) Production

Streptozotocin was first isolated as an antibiotic (Lewis & Barbiers, 1960; Vavra *et al.*, 1960). It can be obtained from *Streptomyces achromogenes* fermentation broth; it also has been synthesized by three different procedures: (i) from tetra-*O*-acetylglucosamine hydrochloride (Herr *et al.*, 1967), (ii) from D-glucosamine and *N*-nitrosomethylcarbamylazide (Hardegger *et al.*, 1969) and (iii) from D-glucosamine and *N*-methylisocyanate (Hessler & Jahnke, 1970). The method of synthesis used commercially is not known.

Streptozotocin is produced commercially in the US by two manufacturers of research biochemicals in undisclosed amounts (see preamble, p. 23) (US International Trade Commission, 1977). It is not believed to be produced commercially in Japan or Europe.

(b) Use

Streptozotocin has been investigated as a potential antibacterial agent (Lewis & Barbiers, 1960) but has never been used as such commercially.

It has also been investigated for use in diabetes, since it has a specific toxic action on pancreatic β-cells, inducing hyperglycaemia (Rakieten *et al.*, 1963).

It has been shown to have a cytotoxic effect against several experimental tumours in animals (Evans *et al.*, 1965; Rudas, 1972; Schein *et al.*, 1967; White, 1963) and has been used clinically in the treatment of tumours of the pancreatic β-cells (Broder & Carter, 1973; Rudas, 1972). It is also active in the treatment of malignant carcinoid tumours; it is administered as weekly i.v. or i.a. doses of 1 g/m^2 of body surface for 4 weeks (Calabresi & Parks, 1975).

2.2 Occurrence

Streptozotocin is produced by the soil microorganism, *Streptomyces achromogenes* var. 128, first isolated from soil samples collected near Blue Rapids, Kansas, US (Vavra *et al.*, 1960). No information on the occurrence of streptozotocin in soil was available to the Working Group.

2.3 Analysis

A colorimetric procedure first described by Forist (1964) has been improved upon by Preussmann & Schaper-Druckrey (1972).

3. Biological Data Relevant to the Evaluation of Carcinogenic Risk to Man

3.1 Carcinogenicity and related studies in animals

(a) Intraperitoneal administration

Mouse: Two groups of 25 male and 25 female 6-week-old Swiss Webster mice received thrice-weekly i.p. injections of streptozotocin (6 or 12 mg/kg bw/dose) for 6 months and were observed for a further 12 months. Lung tumours developed in 18/30 males and 33/39 females, and kidney tumours occurred in 18/30 males and 7/39 females. The incidences were significantly greater than in untreated mice (P<0.001-<0.01). Uterine tumours occurred in 6/39 females (P=0.001) (Weisburger *et al.*, 1975) [The tumour types were not specified].

Rat: Two groups of 25 male and 25 female 6-week-old Sprague-Dawley-derived Charles River CD rats received thrice-weekly i.p. injections of streptozotocin (6 or 12 mg/kg bw/dose) for 6 months and were observed for a further 12 months. Kidney tumours occurred in 19/42 males and 16/46 females; pancreatic tumours were observed in 3/42 males and in 4/46 females; 19/46 females developed liver tumours; and 4/42 males developed peritoneal sarcomas. These tumour incidences were statistically significant in comparison with controls (P<0.001-P=0.006) (Weisburger *et al.*, 1975) [The tumour types were not specified].

Hamster: A group of 84 young adult Chinese hamsters (*Cricetulus griseus*) received single i.p. injections of 100 mg/kg bw streptozotocin (in some cases the dose was given as 4 divided doses at monthly intervals) and were observed for 14-18 months. Cholangiomas (13%) and hepatomas (13%) and non-hepatic benign or malignant tumours (24%) were observed in the treated animals (Berman *et al.*, 1973).

(b) Intravenous administration

Rat: Following a single i.v. injection of 50 mg/kg bw streptozotocin in saline and citric acid to adult male Holtzman rats, 10/19 animals killed between 8-16 months after the injection had tumours; 9 rats developed adenomas of the renal cortex, and 1 rat, a tumour of the pancreas (Arison & Feudale, 1967). Of 37 Holtzman rats treated in the same way, 6 males and 6 females survived for more than 8 months, and 5 males and 1 female had kidney tumours, which appeared between 304 and 485 days after the start of the experiment. Experiments designed to show that streptozotocin itself was carcinogenic and that an accompanying substance, also derived from *Streptomyces achromogenes*, zedalan, was not responsible for the observed tumorigenicity, gave similar results in Sherman and Holtzman rats; an 85:15 mixture of streptozotocin:zedalan was used. Kidney tumours were not seen in rats treated with zedalan alone (10 mg/kg bw i.p.) or in controls that received saline and citric acid only (Rakieten *et al.*, 1968). Some of the kidney tumours observed were adenocarcinomas and sarcomas, and these were shown to metastasize (Rakieten & Gordon, 1975). Administration of a single i.v. dose of 50 mg/kg bw streptozotocin to 28 male Holtzman rats induced a pancreatic tumour in 1/21 animals surviving for 8 months or longer.

No kidney tumours were observed. Controls given saline and citric acid developed no tumours within 550 days, by which time all experimental animals were dead (Rakieten *et al.*, 1971).

Sixty Sprague-Dawley and 100 Lewis rats were treated with single i.v. injections of 65 mg/kg bw streptozotocin. Of the 130 animals that survived the accompanying diabetes for more than 2 months, 27 developed renal tumours of the epithelial type, 40% of which were bilateral; 3/56 were found in animals killed before 8 months and 24/74 in animals killed after 8 months (Mauer *et al.*, 1974a).

After a single i.v. dose of 50 mg/kg bw streptozotocin, 20/21 male Holtzman rats (77%) developed adenomas of the kidney (Rakieten *et al.*, 1976a).

Hamster: Of 35 Chinese hamsters injected with streptozotocin, 13 developed tumours of the liver. The tumours affected mainly the parenchyma (hepatomas) and the biliary epithelium, but 3 sarcomas, possibly of extra-hepatic origin, were also seen in the liver (Sibay & Hayes, 1969) [The dose and period of observation were not recorded].

(c) Other experimental systems

Transplantation

Lewis rats injected intravenously with 65 mg/kg bw streptozotocin demonstrated chronic diabetes, but none had evidence of renal tumours. When the kidneys from these rats were transplanted 6 months after treatment into unilaterally nephrectomized recipients, 4 of the 11 transplanted kidneys developed tumours within the next 4 months (Mauer *et al.*, 1974b).

(d) Factors that modify carcinogenicity in animals

In two groups of 25 male and 25 female 6-week-old Swiss Webster mice that received thrice-weekly i.p. injections of 6 or 12 mg/kg bw streptozotocin plus 250 mg/kg bw nicotinamide at the same for 6 months, the incidence of kidney tumours was lower than in animals that received streptozotocin alone (2/46 *versus* 18/30 in males; 1/45 *versus* 7/39 in females), and a low incidence (P=0.2-0.3) of pancreatic tumours was observed (1/46 and 1/45) (Weisburger *et al.*, 1975) [The tumour types were not specified].

Administration of 250 mg/kg bw nicotinamide with 6 or 12 mg/kg bw streptozotocin intraperitoneally thrice weekly for 6 months to two groups of 25 male and 25 female 6-week-old Sprague-Dawley Charles River CD rats did not alter the tumour incidences produced by streptozotocin alone (Weisburger *et al.*, 1975) [The tumour types were not specified].

Co-administration intraperitoneally of 2 doses of 350 mg/kg bw nicotinamide after a single i.v. dose of 50 mg/kg bw streptozotocin to 28 male Holtzman rats induced pancreatic islet-cell tumours (nesidioblastomas) in 18/26 rats that lived longer than 8 months, whereas streptozotocin alone produced a single pancreatic tumour in 1/21 animals (Rakieten *et al.*, 1971).

When male Holtzman rats were given 2 i.p. injections of 350 mg/kg bw nicotinamide 10 minutes before and 180 minutes after an i.v. injection of 50 mg/kg bw streptozotocin, 5/26 (18%) of animals developed kidney tumours *versus* 20/21 rats given streptozotocin alone (Rakieten *et al.*, 1976a).

Twenty-two hypoglycaemic Holtzman rats bearing insulin-screening islet-cell adenomas induced by one i.v. injection of 50 mg/kg bw streptozotocin plus 2 i.p. injections of 350 mg/kg bw nicotinamide were injected intravenously 18 months after the initial treatment with 50 mg/kg bw streptozotocin weekly for 1-8 weeks. An antitumour response was observed, consisting of an increased blood glucose level and a reduction in plasma and tumour immuno-reactive insulin; there was also a reduction in histopathological changes in the β-cell neoplasm, which included cellular necrosis, degeneration and haemorrhages (Rakieten *et al.*, 1976b).

3.2 Other relevant biological data

(a) Experimental systems

Toxic effects

The oral LD_{50} in mice is 260 mg/kg bw (Evans *et al.*, 1965).

I.v. injection of 50-200 mg/kg bw streptozotocin causes destruction of the pancreatic β-cells and subsequent diabetes in a range of animal species, including dogs, rodents and monkeys (Rakieten *et al.*, 1963; Schein *et al.*, 1973). It has been postulated that the glucose residue in the streptozotocin molecule potentiates its β-cytotoxic effect (Gunnarsson *et al.*, 1974). Prior or simultaneous injection of nicotinamide protects against β-cell destruction (Schein *et al.*, 1973). Increased urinary excretion of β-glucoronidase, indicating renal damage, was found in rats treated with 50 or 100 mg/kg bw streptozotocin (Conzelman & Gribble, 1973).

I.p. injection of 100 mg/kg bw resulted in a transient diabetic state and in hepatic lesions, including parenchymal necrosis, cirrhosis, biliary and nodular hepatic hyperplasia, in Chinese hamsters (Berman *et al.*, 1973).

No data on the embryotoxicity or teratogenicity of this compound were available to the Working Group.

Absorption, distribution and excretion

Streptozotocin is well absorbed from the gastrointestinal tract in mice, but absorption was poor in monkeys and negligible in dogs (White, 1963). ^{14}C-Labelled streptozotocin given by i.v. injection was rapidly cleared from the blood of rats, so that less than 1% remained after 10 minutes (Karunanayake *et al.*, 1976).

Metabolism

Radioactive products derived from streptozotocin remained bound to liver, kidney and pancreas for at least 6 hours (Karunanayake *et al.*, 1976) [The data suggest that streptozotocin decomposes rapidly *in vivo*, but no products have yet been characterized, and it is not clear whether enzymatic reactions are required for this decomposition].

Mutagenicity and other short-term tests

Streptozotocin does not appear to require enzymatic conversion into mutagenic metabolites, since it was shown to be mutagenic for *Salmonella typhimurium* in the absence of a liver microsomal activation system (Kolbye & Legator, 1968). It causes X-linked recessive lethal mutations in *Drosophila melanogaster* (Browning, 1973).

Its mutagenic activity was also demonstrated in host-mediated assays, using *S. typhimurium* G46, in rats (1 or 10 mg/kg bw) and in mice (400 μg/mouse) (Ficsor *et al.*, 1971; Gabridge *et al.*, 1969).

(b) Humans

Data on the toxic effects of clinical exposure to streptozotocin used for the treatment of pancreatic islet-cell carcinomas has been reviewed (Rudas, 1972; Schein *et al.*, 1974). Nausea and vomiting were seen in almost all of 52 patients treated for islet-cell carcinoma (Broder & Carter, 1973). Renal or hepatic toxicity was seen in 2/3 patients, and bone-marrow damage was observed in about 10%; renal toxicity was responsible for 5 deaths. Anaemia, leucopenia or thrombocytopenia was observed in 20% of patients and was responsible for 1 death (Broder & Carter, 1973; Calabresi & Parks, 1975).

Nephrosis and cytoproliferative changes in the kidneys were observed at autopsy in a patient given a total dose of 15 g streptozotocin for the treatment of a pancreatic islet-cell carcinoma (Myerowitz *et al.*, 1976).

After its i.v. injection in patients with advanced cancer, streptozotocin was rapidly cleared from the plasma so that none was detectable within 3 hours. Up to 15% of the unchanged streptozotocin was excreted in the urine within 2 hours (Adolphe *et al.*, 1975).

3.3 Case reports and epidemiological studies

No data were available to the Working Group.

4. Summary of Data Reported and Evaluation

4.1 Experimental data

Streptozotocin is carcinogenic in mice, rats and Syrian golden and Chinese hamsters following its intravenous or intraperitoneal administration. It produces benign and malignant tumours of the liver and kidney and islet-cell tumours of the pancreas. It is carcinogenic after its administration in single doses.

4.2 Human data

No adequate data on humans were available to the Working Group, but the chemotherapeutic use of streptozotocin indicates the existence of an exposed group.

4.3 Evaluation

There is *sufficient evidence* of a carcinogenic effect of streptozotocin in several experimental animal species. Although no epidemiological data were available (and efforts should be directed toward this end), streptozotocin should be regarded for practical purposes as it it were carcinogenic to humans.

5. References

Adolphe, A.B., Glasofer, E.D., Troetel, W.M., Ziegenfuss, J., Stambaugh, J.E., Weiss, A.J. & Manthei, R.W. (1975) Fate of streptozotocin (NSC-85998) in patients with advanced cancer. Cancer Chemother. Rep., Part 1, 59, 547-556

Arison, R.N. & Feudale, E.L. (1967) Induction of renal tumour by streptozotocin in rats. Nature (Lond.), 214, 1254-1255

Berman, L.D., Hayes, J.A. & Sibay, T.M. (1973) Effect of streptozotocin in the Chinese hamster (*Cricetulus griseus*). J. nat. Cancer Inst., 51, 1287-1294

Broder, L.E. & Carter, S.K. (1973) Pancreatic islet cell carcinoma. II. Results of therapy with streptozotocin in 52 patients. Ann. intern. Med., 79, 108-118

Browning, L.S. (1973) Mutagenicity of various chemicals and their metabolites in *Drosophila* (Abstract). Genetics, 74, s33

Calabresi, P. & Parks, R.E., Jr (1975) Alkylating agents, antimetabolites, hormones, and other antiproliferative agents. In: Goodman, L.S. & Gilman, A., eds, The Pharmacological Basis of Therapeutics, 5th ed., New York, Macmillan, p. 1268

Conzelman, G.M., Jr & Gribble, D.H. (1973) Urinary excretion of β-glucuronidase after administration of streptozotocin (NSC-85998) to Fischer rats. Cancer Chemother. Rep., Part 1, 57, 235-236

Evans, J.S., Gerritsen, G.C., Mann, K.M. & Owen, S.P. (1965) Antitumor and hyperglycemic activity of streptozotocin (NSC-37917) and its cofactor, U-15,774. Cancer Chemother. Rep., 48, 1-6

Ficsor, G., Beyer, R.D., Janca, F.C. & Zimmer, D.M. (1971) An organ-specific host-mediated microbial assay for detecting chemical mutagens *in vivo*: demonstration of mutagenic action in rat testes following streptozotocin treatment. Mutation Res., 13, 283-287

Forist, A.A. (1964) Spectrophotometric determination of streptozotocin. Analyt. Chem., 36, 1338-1339

Gabridge, M.G., Denunzio, A. & Legator, M.S. (1969) Microbial mutagenicity of streptozotocin in animal-mediated assays. Nature (Lond.), 221, 68-70

Gunnarsson, R., Berne, C. & Hellerström, C. (1974) Cytotoxic effects of streptozotocin and *N*-nitrosomethylurea on the pancreatic B cells with special regard to the role of nicotinamide-adenine dinucleotide. Biochem. J., 140, 487-494

Hardegger, E., Meier, A. & Stoos, A. (1969) Eine präparative Synthese von Streptozotocin. Helv. chim. acta, 52, 2555-2560

Herr, R.R., Jahnke, H.K. & Argoudelis, A.D. (1967) The structure of streptozotocin. J. Amer. chem. Soc., 89, 4808-4809

Hessler, E.J. & Jahnke, H.K. (1970) Improved synthesis of streptozotocin. J. org. Chem., 35, 245-246

IARC (1974) IARC Monographs on the Evaluation of Carcinogenic Risk of Chemicals to Man, 4, Some Aromatic Amines, Hydrazine and Related Substances, *N*-Nitroso Compounds and Miscellaneous Alkylating Agents, Lyon, pp. 221-227

Karunanayake, E.H., Baker, J.R.J., Christian, R.A., Hearse, D.J. & Mellows, G. (1976) Autoradiographic study of the distribution and cellular uptake of [^{14}C]streptozotocin in the rat. Diabetologia, 12, 123-128

Kolbye, S.M. & Legator, M.S. (1968) Mutagenic activity of streptozotocin. Mutation Res., 6, 387-389

Lewis, C. & Barbiers, A.R. (1960) Streptozotocin, a new antibiotic. *In vitro* and *in vivo* evaluation. In: Marti-Ibañez, F., ed., Antibiotics Annual 1959-1960, Vol. 7, New York, Antibiotica Inc., pp. 247-254

Mauer, S.M., Lee, C.S., Najarian, J.S. & Brown, D.M. (1974a) Induction of malignant kidney tumors in rats with streptozotocin. Cancer Res., 34, 158-160

Mauer, S.M., Sutherland, D.E.R., Steffes, M.W., Lee, C.S., Najarian, J.S. & Brown, D.M. (1974b) Effects of kidney and pancreas transplantation on streptozotocin-induced malignant kidney tumors in rats. Cancer Res., 34, 1643-1645

Myerowitz, R.L., Sartiano, G.P. & Cavallo, T. (1976) Nephrotoxic and cytoproliferative effects of streptozotocin. Report of a patient with multiple hormone-secreting islet cell carcinoma. Cancer, 38, 1550-1555

Preussmann, R. & Schaper-Druckrey, F. (1972) Investigation of a colorimetric procedure for determination of nitrosamides and comparison with other methods. In: Bogovski, P., Preussmann, R. & Walker, E.A., eds, *N*-Nitroso Compounds Analysis and Formation, Lyon (IARC Scientific Publications No. 3), pp. 81-86

Rakieten, N. & Gordon, B.S. (1975) Metastatic renal adenocarcinoma produced by streptozotocin (NSC-85998). Cancer Chemother. Rep., Part 1, 59, 891-892

Rakieten, N., Rakieten, M.L. & Nadkarni, M.V. (1963) Studies on the diabetogenic action of streptozotocin (NSC-37917). Cancer Chemother. Rep., 29, 91-98

Rakieten, N., Gordon, B.S., Cooney, D.A., Davis, R.D. & Schein, P.S. (1968) Renal tumorigenic action of streptozotocin (NSC-85998) in rats. Cancer Chemother. Rep., 52, 563-567

Rakieten, N., Gordon, B.S., Beaty, A., Cooney, D.A., Davis, R.D. & Schein, P.S. (1971) Pancreatic islet cell tumors produced by the combined action of streptozotocin and nicotinamide. Proc. Soc. exp. Biol. (N.Y.), 137, 280-283

Rakieten, N., Gordon, B.S., Beaty, A., Cooney, D.A. & Schein, P.S. (1976a) Modification of renal tumorigenic effect of streptozotocin by nicotinamide: spontaneous reversibility of streptozotocin diabetes. Proc. Soc. exp. Biol. (N.Y.), 151, 356-361

Rakieten, N., Gordon, B.S., Beaty, A., Bates, R.W. & Schein, P.S. (1976b) Streptozotocin treatment of streptozotocin-induced islet cell adenomas in rats. Proc. Soc. exp. Biol. (N.Y.), 151, 632-635

Rudas, B. (1972) Streptozotocin. Arzneimittel-Forsch., 22, 830-861

Schein, P.S., Cooney, D.A. & Vernon, M.L. (1967) The use of nicotinamide to modify the toxicity of streptozotocin diabetes without loss of antitumor activity. Cancer Res., 27, 2324-2332

Schein, P.S., Rakieten, N., Cooney, D.A., Davis, R. & Vernon, M.L. (1973) Streptozotocin diabetes in monkeys and dogs, and its prevention by nicotinamide. Proc. Soc. exp. Biol. (N.Y.), 143, 514-518

Schein, P.S., O'Connell, M.J., Blom, J., Hubbard, S., Magrath, I.T., Bergevin, P., Wiernik, P.H., Ziegler, J.L. & DeVita, V.T. (1974) Clinical antitumor activity and toxicity of streptozotocin (NSC-85998). Cancer, 34, 993-1000

Sibay, T.M. & Hayes, J.A. (1969) Potential carcinogenic effect of streptozotocin. Lancet, ii, 912

US International Trade Commission (1977) Synthetic Organic Chemicals, US Production and Sales, 1975, USITC Publication 804, Washington DC, US Government Printing Office, p. 105

Vavra, J.J., DeBoer, C., Dietz, A., Hanka, L.J. & Sokolski, W.T. (1960) Streptozotocin, a new antibacterial antibiotic. In: Marti-Ibañez, F., ed., Antiobiotics Annual 1969-1960, Vol. 7, New York, Antiobiotica Inc., pp. 230-235

Weisburger, J.H., Griswold, D.P., Prejean, J.D., Casey, A.E., Wood, H.B. & Weisburger, E.K. (1975) The carcinogenic properties of some of the principal drugs used in clinical cancer chemotherapy. Recent Results Cancer Res., 52, 1-17

White, F.R. (1963) Streptozotocin. Cancer Chemother. Rep., 30, 49-53

SUPPLEMENTARY CORRIGENDA TO VOLUMES 1 - 16

Corrigenda covering Volumes 1 - 6 appeared in Volume 7, others appeared in Volumes 8, 10, 11, 12, 13, 15 and 16.

Volume 14	Asbestos	
p. 33	(a) Air 1st para.	*replace* "some factories using asbestos" *by* "asbestos mills"
	last line	*delete* "Rickards, 1973"
p. 44	Table 14 2nd line	*add* "1 papillary carcinoma of the lung" *to* "Amosite"
	2nd para.	*delete*
p. 45	Other species	*delete* "however ..." *to* "reported"
p. 55	Table 21	*delete* "Reeves (1976)" *all data*
p. 67	Amosite: 1st para.	*replace* "Selikoff (1976a)" *by* "Selikoff (1976b)"
p. 72	3.4 2nd para.	*replace* "Timbrell (1972) has shown" *by* "Timbrell (1972) reported"
		add "Timbrell *et al.*, 1971" *after* "Langer *et al.*, 1974"
p. 78	Table 22	*replace* "Selikoff, 1976a" *by* "Selikoff, 1976b"
p. 100	References	*delete* "Rickards *et al.* (1973) ..."
p. 104	References	*add* "Timbrell, V., Griffiths, D.M. & Pooley, F.D. (1971) Possible biological importance of fibre diameters in South African amphiboles. Nature (Lond.), 232, 55-56"

CUMULATIVE INDEX TO IARC MONOGRAPHS ON THE EVALUATION OF THE CARCINOGENIC RISK OF CHEMICALS TO HUMANS

Numbers underlined indicate volume, and numbers in italics indicate page. References to corrigenda are given in parentheses.